THE IRON DISORDERS INSTITUTE PRESENTS . . .

EXPOSING THE
HIDDEN
DANGERS
OF IRON

THE IRON DISORDERS INSTITUTE PRESENTS . . .

EXPOSING THE
HIDDEN
DANGERS
OF IRON

*What Every Medical Professional Should Know About
the Impact of Iron on the Disease Process*

E. D. Weinberg, Ph.D.

Edited by Cheryl Garrison
Foreword by Lois K. Lambrecht, M.D.
Introduction by Randy S. Alexander

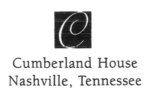

Cumberland House
Nashville, Tennessee

Published by
Cumberland House Publishing, Inc.
431 Harding Industrial Drive
Nashville, TN 37211

Exposing the Hidden Dangers of Iron is for educational and informational
purposes only and is not intended to replace the advice given by a patient's
physician. Reviewers, contributors, and advisors who contributed text,
images, or remarks for portions of this book are not responsible for errors,
omissions, or overall content.

Cover design: Gore Studio, Inc.
Text design: Lisa Taylor

Library of Congress Cataloging-in-Publication Data

Weinberg, Eugene D.
  Exposing the hidden dangers of iron : what every medical professional
should know about the impact of iron on the disease process / E. D.
Weinberg ; edited by Cheryl Garrison.
      p. ; cm.
  Includes bibliographical references and index.
  ISBN 1-58182-336-3 (pbk.)
  1. Iron—Metabolism—Disorders. 2. Iron—Metabolism—Disorders—
Complications.
  [DNLM: 1. Iron Overload—diagnosis. 2. Iron Overload—therapy.
3. Anemia, Iron-Deficiency—diagnosis. 4. Anemia, Iron-Deficiency—
etiology. 5. Anemia, Iron-Deficiency—therapy. 6. Iron Overload—
etiology. WD 200.5.I7 W423e 2004] I. Garrison, Cheryl D., 1945–
II. Title.
  RC632.I7W45 2004
  616.3'99—dc22

                                                          2004010114

1 2 3 4 5 6 7 8 — 08 07 06 05 04 03

To the hundreds of scientists and clinicians
whose work on raising awareness of the
hazards of iron loading is resulting in marked
improvements in human and animal health.

Contents

CONTENTS

Part III: Practical Guide to Diagnosis, Treatment, and Prevention

Foreword

I recall my first meeting several years ago with Dr. Weinberg and his ever so slightly anemic yet lovely wife, Fran. I was the appropriately cautious and investigative internist.

The new client was anemic and my mind went clicking to unexplained iron-deficiency anemia in the over-forty age group. I recommended additional iron studies and, if warranted, a colonoscopy. Dr. Weinberg's eyes seemed to twinkle a bit as he smiled understandingly. He explained that his wife's iron stores were deliberately low due to regularly scheduled phlebotomies in order to avoid undue iron overload in the post-menopausal state. I made a mental note to review the topic of iron storage disorders and quickly moved on to their next health concern. A week or so after the visit I received a neatly addressed envelope from Dr. Weinberg with several articles on iron metabolism and hemochromatosis. I placed these in the large stack of "To Do's" and kept working. Then came another meeting with the Weinbergs and a second packet of information on the iron topic. Somewhere in this process I discovered that Dr. Weinberg was one of the world's leading scientific authorities on iron. I realized that I had best get busy and read that material. I started in on the growing pile of papers.

Although I was familiar with the clinical features of iron storage disease, its common occurrence, presenting signs and symptoms, ease of diagnosis and treatment, I realized that my practical knowledge in this area was relatively blunted and my prevention acumen poor. As I completed one packet, the next would be delivered, accompanied by lively discussions with Gene on subjects ranging from the deleterious effects of iron overloading through supplements to the use of phlebotomy products to feed my rosebushes. I made certain that the multivitamin carried in my clinic was "sans iron." As fate would have it, the laboratory I used in my office practice included serum ferritin as part of a routine comprehensive metabolic panel. This simple test coupled with my heightened awareness allowed me to diagnose three new cases of hemochromatosis in one year! The preventive aspect of medicine has always been a thrill to me.

I have been exceedingly fortunate in having Dr. Weinberg's tutelage. Now it is available for other professionals in his book *Exposing the Hidden Dangers of Iron*, a compilation of all those packets of carefully prepared information and much more. It is clearly written and quite informative . . . certainly "what every medical professional should know about the impact of iron on the disease process." Having read Dr. Weinberg's book, I have a much greater understanding for iron-related diseases, as well as a new appreciation for Mrs. Weinberg's ever-so-slight anemia.

From firsthand experience I know that the family practice physician can be the first line of defense for early detection of iron overload, and with cooperation by the patient there is a high probability for prevention of chronic disease.

Lois Lambrecht, M.D.
Internal Medicine
Bloomington, Indiana

Preface

A question often asked is why have I been occupied exclusively with iron for the past half century—why not zinc or copper or manganese or several other important elements? In 1952, my wife Fran was prescribed tetracycline for a mild infection. I wondered if any item in her food might be neutralizing or interfering with the antibiotic (in those olden times, no instructions were provided by the pharmaceutical companies).

I asked my lab assistant to mix each of a large number of organic and elemental nutrients with tetracycline to see if any specific ingredient(s) could affect activity with the drug. A few days later she said, "I think I've made a mistake. Look at the Petri plate. It's loaded with bacteria; I must have forgotten to put in the tetracycline." But when she repeated the experiment, the results were the same. The neutralizing substance was iron!

Fran's physician did not think much of my advice to either halt her iron supplement or the tetracycline. However, within a few years, we were able to persuade the several companies that produce tetracyclines to include an iron warning label on the packages of these drugs.

It was a logical step then to envision that what we saw on the bacteria-loaded Petri plate might also be occurring within our bodies. That is, what if we are sending our defense cells and chemicals into an infected wound but there is an excess of iron in the tissue? Who would win—the person or the bacterial invader? No other element—not zinc, nor copper, nor manganese—has the enormous broad-spectrum ability to favor microbial or cancer cells over the defending animal or human. That is why I have been fascinated with iron for more than five decades.

If iron is so critical in the outcome of encounters between invaders and hosts, perhaps our bodies could actually attempt to withhold the metal from the microbial or cancer cell invaders. But if iron is so helpful to invaders, why have iron-loading disorders survived in populations for many centuries?

Hundreds of clinicians and scientists have provided information on these and other matters compiled in this book. I have also been greatly helped by provocative questions from my microbiology and medical students and, not least, from iron-loaded patients and members of their families.

Fran has continued to provide encouragement in my exploration of the many aspects of the impact of excessive iron on disease. In turn, I was reassured that she actually believed in my work with iron because, following menopause, she decided to prevent post-menopausal iron loading by donating blood every two months to our blood bank.

The stimulus to write this book was supplied by Cheryl Garrison of the Iron Disorders Institute. Having taught medical students, I saw a real need for a book about iron that would give physicians an edge in their practice. So, I agreed to do the book providing that Cheryl would edit and invigorate my pedantic prose. My thanks also to Chris Kieffer, Randy Alexander, Laura Main, Cheryl Mellan, David Garrison, and other members of the Iron Disorders Institute for their encouragement and contributions. I am grateful to all of the scientists whose excellent work helped to shape this book and to those who made a direct contribution: Drs. Clara Camaschella, Leah Harris, James Connor, and Lewis Wesselius. I especially want to thank Dr. Lois Lambrecht for reading the entire manuscript and for writing the foreword. And, last but not least, my thanks to Lisa Taylor, Ron Pitkin, and all of Cumberland House for the finished product.

Introduction

As a patient who has hereditary hemochromatosis, I am very pleased about the book *Exposing the Hidden Dangers of Iron*. A decade ago medical students were taught a great deal about "too little iron," but they had only a few pages that addressed the issue of "too much iron." With incomplete knowledge about iron's dangerous potential, these physicians unknowingly missed opportunity upon opportunity to prevent chronic disease. Not because they lacked caring or compassion for the patient but because of what they learned in medical school, they likely treated their patients' various diseases of diabetes, heart trouble, joint pain, liver disease, impotence, depression, or infertility without ever giving thought to the idea that there might be one common underlying cause: excess iron.

The former US Surgeon General, Dr. David Satcher, publicly stated that "early detection of iron overload disease represents a major chronic disease prevention opportunity." When we prevent disease we are reducing mortality, morbidity, and the overall cost of health care.

The problem is that physicians can only completely diagnose excess body iron with very specific tests. Once part of a routine blood panel, abnormal levels of serum iron prompted physicians to investigate and properly diagnose thousands of patients. I am one of those patients. Sadly, as of 1999 due to changes to the Medicare Reimbursement Policy, serum iron is no longer part of any routine panel. Doctors must suspect iron overload and know which tests to order before the complete diagnosis can be reached.

One could argue that a person becomes a doctor so that he or she can diagnose and treat patients. However, today's medicine is more intricate than ever before, and doctors no longer have the time they once had to spend delving into and researching possible causes. Even seasoned physicians miss the opportunity to test a patient's iron levels. Complaints of chronic fatigue, joint pain, impotence, depression, and heart fluttering are many times attributed to psychiatric problems. The patient's various complaints are addressed with pain medication, antidepressants, beta-blockers, and a plethora of other medications, none of which addresses the underlying cause: iron overload.

Prior to seeing Dr. Mark Princell in Greenville, SC, I was miserable. I wanted an explanation for my severe depression, headaches, abdominal pain, impotence, and chronic fatigue. I had been summarily dismissed by several doctors as a "nut case" and, quite frankly, I was beginning to believe that they were correct. Discouraged at the thought that I might have to live the rest of my life with the pain and paralyzing depression, I contemplated taking my own life.

If it had not been for an abnormally high serum iron on a routine panel and the perseverance of Dr. Princell, I would not be here today. After a year of tests, including a liver biopsy, Dr. Princell finally settled on the diagnosis of hemochromatosis for me.

I remember being surprised—I had never heard the word before that day. My head was spinning with questions. Was I going to die? Dr. Princell looked grim when he told me that hemochromatosis was a "rare, older man's disease—and often fatal." Could someone catch this disease from me? I did not understand at the time that this was an inherited condition of iron metabolism. And then I was told of the treatment: phlebotomy! Being terrified of needles, I nearly passed out with fear. In fact, I hid from treatment for a while, but eventually I had the life-saving phlebotomies once a week for 18 months. Back then, I had no insurance and had to pay out of pocket at one hundred dollars per treatment. I can recall times that I literally had to choose between treatment and paying my bills. Often, I went without the phlebotomy.

It was during this time that I decided that no other person should suffer as I did. I knew that physicians needed to know about this easy-to-diagnose and simple-to-treat condition. Other grass roots organizations were trying to raise awareness, but I knew that we must have the support of our government health agencies—US Centers for Disease Control and Prevention and the National Institutes of Health—to be credible to the medical community.

I formed an organization that focused on hemochromatosis. With the help of co-founders Chris Kieffer, whose husband Harry has hemochromatosis, and Cheryl Garrison, whose son David has some yet to be identified iron loading disorder, eventually the organization became the Iron Disorders Institute with a broader emphasis on iron out of balance.

Our vision was to create a national voluntary health agency that was not centered on an individual or just a web address, but as bricks and mortar for all the patients diagnosed and undiagnosed. Our mission remains to reduce pain, suffering, and unnecessary death due to disorders of iron through awareness, education, and research. We set high standards, creating professional-looking, evidence-based educational products. We are also committed to annual events where patients can meet one-another and experts can share their knowledge. We sought the support of alliances such as the Arthritis Foundation, American Diabetes Association, and The American Liver Foundation. These three organizations now acknowledge elevated iron as a risk factor for arthritis, diabetes, and liver disease. We also sought strategic partnerships with the US Centers for Disease Control and Prevention, The National Institutes of Health, The American Academy of Family Physicians, The American Society of Hematology (ASH), and The American Association for the Study of Liver Diseases (AASLD). And finally, we were invited by Penn State University and the University of Connecticut to establish Centers of Excellence, where physicians could attend seminars about iron and where patients could participate in focused research.

Our first books, *Iron Disorders Institute Guide to Hemochromatosis* and *Guide to Anemia*, were written for the patient and families of patients. *Exposing the Hidden Dangers of Iron* is the first in a series of books for the medical student and the family practice physician. Our hope is that this book and others about specific body systems become required reading for medical students. If we can sensitize one physician, he or she will diagnose hundreds!

In closing, I invite you to visit our web site: *www.irondisorders.org* and enter the portal for medical professionals. Here you can link to the CDC physician online hemochromatosis study course, receive CME credits, learn about seminars and conferences, patient services, our products, our timeline of achievements, our supporters, alliances, and strategic partners, as well as submit details about your practice for our national physician's registry.

As you read *Exposing the Hidden Dangers of Iron*, I hope that you are enlightened about the importance of iron out of balance and that you begin to see every patient through new eyes.

Best Wishes,

Randy S. Alexander
Founder & Chairman, Iron Disorders Institute
C282Y/C282Y hemochromatosis patient

THE IRON DISORDERS INSTITUTE PRESENTS . . .

EXPOSING THE
HIDDEN
DANGERS
OF *IRON*

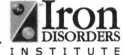

PART ONE

Iron Loading in the Body Systems

1

Basics of Iron Loading

"... as humans have no means to control iron excretion; excess iron, regardless of the route of entry, accumulates in parenchymal organs and threatens cell viability. In fact, a number of disease states (that is, iron overload diseases) attributable to genetic or acquired factors are pathogenetically linked to excess body iron stores, and iron removal therapy is an effective lifesaving strategy."

—A. Pietrangelo

Iron enters the body in various ways. Iron can be inhaled, ingested, injected, or accumulate as a result of decompartmentalization due to chronic hemolysis or liver cell destruction. Age, gender, behavior, nutrition, and genetics all influence the mechanisms that regulate the metal once it enters the body.

Millions of humans worldwide have inherited one of the several iron-loading disorders or have acquired physiologic deficits that contribute to iron loading. Examples of some of the more common conditions that lead to iron mismanagement are hereditary hemochromatosis (HHC), African siderosis, beta-thalassemia, sickle cell anemia, alcohol abuse, and viral hepatitis. Some of the more rare and less known but still devastating conditions that result in iron overload are aceruloplasminemia, atransferrinemia, sideroblastic anemia, non-alcoholic steatohepatitis (NASH), dysmetabolic iron overload syndrome (DIOS), GRACILE, neonatal hemochromatosis, juvenile hemochromatosis, and enzymopathies,

iron enters the body in various ways

●INHALATION●

Mining iron
Grinding and cutting steel
Crocidolite, amosite, tremolite asbestos
Tobacco smoke
Urban air particulates

●INGESTION●

High amount of red meat
High amount of alcohol
Iron supplements
Additive iron (fortified foods)

●INJECTION●

Intramuscular
Barefoot walking on iron oxide
Multiple units of blood transfused

●DECOMPARTMENTALIZATION●

Hemolysis (red blood cell destruction)
Hepatitis (liver cell destruction)

such as glucose-6-phosphate dehydrogenase (G6PD), pyruvate kinase deficiency, or congenital dyserythropoietic anemia type II (CDAII). Other acquired means of iron overload include portacaval shunting, repeated parenteral iron injections or infusions, chronic blood transfusions, and excessive, long-term consumption of oral iron supplements.

Iron is life-sustaining, but when in excess in the tissues of the body, iron can be fatal. Since there is no physiological means of excreting excessive iron from the body, except for blood loss, over time the excess iron accumulates at toxic levels in the heart, liver, endocrine glands, and joints. Overwhelmed with iron, these systems can no longer function optimally and the disease process takes over. Arthritis, diabetes, hyperpigmentation, hepatic cirrhosis; hormone imbalances leading to hypothyroidism, impotence, infertility, and premature cessation of menstruation; cancer, infection, and early death by heart attack are among the consequences of untreated iron loading.

Hereditary hemochromatosis is a leading known cause of iron overload disease in humans. Hemochromatosis was first described in 1865 by a French physician named Armand Trousseau who noted a relationship between skin color and diabetes. Due to the bronze coloring of skin, which was noted among many of his diabetic patients, he called this condition "bronze diabetes." In 1889 a German scientist named H. von Recklinghausen noted a relationship between tissue injury, as in cirrhosis, and increased tissue iron. He termed this phenomenon "haemochromatosis." "Haem" for blood, "chroma" for bronze-colored skin, and "osis" for the condition. In 1927, a British physician named J. H. Sheldon suggested that iron deposition is caused by an inherited metabolic disorder. He conducted an exhaustive review of opinion, compiling all information he could obtain on the subject of hemochromatosis. In 1935 Sheldon published his consolidated effort in an Oxford University Press book entitled *Haemochromatosis*. In this monograph Sheldon wrote, "The most reasonable explanation of haemochromatosis is that it should be classed as an inborn error of metabolism, which has an overwhelming incidence in males, and which at times actually has a familial incidence."

In the 1970s Marcel Simon and his team of investigators determined that hemochromatosis was inherited in an autosomal recessive pattern due to mutation(s) on chromosome 6. In 1996, a team of geneticists identified *HFE*, the gene for hemochromatosis and two major mutations: C282Y and H63D. Since this important discovery, other scientific advances have made significance contributions to a better understanding of how the body regulates iron. As these new iron regulatory proteins and other gene discoveries have emerged, hemochromatosis has been more definitively classified.

There are both primary (inherited) and secondary forms of hemochromatosis. *HFE*-related hemochromatosis is the most common type known, occurring in about 1:200–400 Caucasians. About 85 percent of patients with hemochromatosis are homozygous for

7

the C282Y mutations of *HFE*, which results in abnormal dietary iron absorption.

Normally the body employs various sophisticated maneuvers to regulate the amount of iron absorbed. The total amount of body iron in healthy adults is maintained at a level of about 4 grams, which are distributed in proteins and serum. The daily 1–2 mg of iron absorbed from diet is prudently balanced by daily excretion in perspiration, urine, and feces of 1–2 mg.

IRON DISTRIBUTION	males 4 grams females 3.5 grams children 3 grams
Hemoglobin	70%
Myoglobin and Enzymes	15%
Ferritin	14%
In transit in serum	1%

In hemochromatosis patients, however, the daily amount of iron absorbed is 2–4 mg, but the daily excretion remains unchanged. Accordingly, were the imbalance to begin in a 20-year-old person, about 1 gram/year would be accumulated and would need to be hidden away in innocuous packages throughout the various organs. By the time that 10–15 grams have accumulated, clinical symptoms in one or more organs might have begun to appear. Untreated, some HHC patients have been reported to collect as much as 50 grams during their lifetime. The enormous challenge of where in the body to sequester high quantities of this hazardous metal is daunting, especially since the disorder suppresses macrophage iron deposition. However, for whatever reason some persons are able to hide the metal without harm to their organs, while others suffer symptoms in their twenties or thirties. This difference in expression is highly suggestive of other influences, such as gene modifiers and environmental factors.

Regardless of the cause of iron loading, early detection and prompt treatment of iron overload offers a physician an opportunity to lower the risk of heart trouble, arthritis, liver disease, diabetes, impotence, infertility, hormone imbalances, and depression in his or her patients. Hemochromatosis, once thought to be a rare, older male's disease, is now known to be common, to affect both males and females, and to have the potential to be fatal if not detected and treated.

In 1996, the US Centers for Disease Control and Prevention (CDC) in Atlanta sent surveys to nearly 3000 individuals diagnosed with hemochromatosis; 80 percent (2851 individuals) responded. Of the 2851 respondents, 67 percent of those with symptoms had been given multiple, various diagnoses prior to receiving the proper diagnosis of hemochromatosis. Among the misdiagnoses were arthritis, gallbladder and liver disease, stomach disorders, hormonal deficiencies, psychiatric disorders, and diabetes. These patients indeed had these conditions, but the true underlying cause of iron overload was missed. Respondents reported that they saw an average of three different physicians and that it took more than 9 years before they received the complete diagnosis of hemochromatosis and the primary cause for their illness: iron overload.

Prevalence of Selected Signs or Symptoms and Response to Treatment in 2,851 Patients with Hemochromatosis Treated with Phlebotomy			
Symptom	Reported Sign or Symptom, Number (%)	Improved with Therapy, Number (%)	Worse Despite Therapy, Number (%)
Extreme fatigue	1,296 (45-5)	705 (54.4)	223 (17.2)
Joint pain	1,241 (43.5)	115 (9.2)	422 (34.0)
Impotence (or loss of libido)	735 (25.8)	93 (12.7)	204 (27.8)
Skin bronzing	733 (25.7)	431 (58.8)	30 (4.1)
Heart fluttering	679 (23.8)	42 (6.2)	69 (10.1)
Depression	592 (20.8)	242 (40.8)	61 (10.3)
Abdominal pain	578 (20.3)	129 (22.3)	69 (11.9)

Source S M McDonnell et al

9

Frequency of Conditions Reported in the General US Population and US Participants in the Hemochomatosis (HHC) Survey, by Age*

Condition	WOMEN NUMBER (%)		MEN NUMBER (%)	
	General Population	HHC Survey	General Population	HHC Survey
Arthritis				
17-39 years	1,921 (5.9)	10 (10.3)	1,680 (5.2)	15 (8.9)
40-59 years	5,070 (23.4)	147 (34.9)	3,120 (14.7)	194 (22.2)
60-84 years	9,154 (51.1)	212 (42.8)	4,725 (33.8)	203 (31.5)
Diabetes mellitus				
17-39 years	538 (1.6)	3 (3.1)	457 (1.4)	2 (1.2)
40-59 years	950 (4.4)	31 (7.4)	1,087 (1.5)	65 (7.5)
60-84 years	2,437 (13.6)	31 (6.3)	1,991 (12.1)	62 (9.6)
Liver disease or gallbladder disease				
17-39 years	1,887 (7.2)	5 (5.2)	700 (2.7)	16 (9.5)
40-59 years	2,674 (16.9)	84 (20.0)	1,106 (7.3)	154 (17.7)
60-84 years	2,135 (25.6)	115 (23.2)	932 (12.2)	113 (17.5)
Extreme fatigue				
17-39 years	14,235(43.4)	48 (49.5)	9,647 (29.9)	61 (36.0)

Source: S. M. McDonnell et al.

* General population data for liver disease or gallbladder disease from NHANES 11 (1976-1980, reference 19); other general population data from NHANES 111 (1988-1994, reference 20). Arthritis, diabetes, and liver or gallbladder disease based on response to the question: "Have you ever been diagnosed with fatigue by a physician?" Based on self-reported severe fatigue. Data include only white subjects, ages 17 to 84. These data not available in NHANES for older subjects.

Social Implications
Expressed in Percent Reporting (%)

Type of Change	Severe HHC* (n=1,255)	Without Severe HHC* (n=1,596)
Divorce or breakup with significant other	6.5	2.0
Troubles with spouse or significant other	7.7	14
Marriage or relationship stronger	13.4	4.8
Family members in denial of my disease	12.3	3.8
Family members in denial of own risk	25.2	12.7
Family members supportive	44.5	38.1
Job loss	19.6	2.8
Reduced ability to do daily tasks	33.4	7.3
Loss of health insurance	8.7	5.8
Loss of life insurance	7.7	6.4
Other	5.6	3.3
No real change	28.7	60.0

Source S M McDonnell et al   * HHC = Hemochromatosis

The average age of the patients surveyed was 41. Of those who reported symptoms, 75 percent experienced chronic fatigue, 75 percent had joint pain, 58 percent reported a loss of libido or loss of interest in sex, 44 percent had skin color changes, 41 percent experienced heart irregularities, and 35 percent reported abdominal pain. Thirty percent had no symptoms. Seventeen percent had been found anemic and prescribed iron supplements, having been misdiagnosed with iron deficiency. It is still not widely recognized that iron overload can cause anemia, just as iron deficiency can; the mechanisms are quite different, however! Another 18 percent reported they had taken iron supplements for their health.

Even though the CDC survey included a relatively small sample of the US population, the survey results documented many similarities among patients with hemochromatosis. Patients who participated in focus groups felt that the results of the survey allowed a closer look and a better understanding of a hemochromatosis patient profile. Symptoms such as depression, which had not previously been attributed to iron overload, emerged as a major problem for hemochromatotics.

HFE-related hemochromatosis is seen mostly in Caucasians, but other ethnicities also exhibit iron loading. The genetic makeup, however, is different.

African siderosis

In sub-Saharan African countries, dietary iron overload is a common, although often unrecognized, health problem. In some rural populations, more than 10 percent of persons are affected. The disorder has been reported most often in South Africa but also has been recorded in Ghana, Kenya, Malawi, Mozambique, Nigeria, Swaziland, Tanzania, Uganda, Zambia, and Zimbabwe.

In rural areas, intestinal absorption of excessive iron often is associated with ingestion of acid-fermented grains such as sour porridge and sorghum beer that are processed in non-galvanized iron containers at pH 3–3.5. The daily intake of iron can exceed the amount from a US diet by sevenfold. However, persons in urban areas of Africa also are at risk of becoming iron loaded.

11

Because the condition has familial aspects, an underlying genetic disorder has been postulated. The putative homozygotes might become iron loaded regardless of diet, whereas the heterozygote carriers would develop the condition only were they to consume excessive amounts of the metal. In a study of 808 African Americans for transferrin iron saturation values, approximately 86 percent had normal levels, 13 percent had moderately elevated values, and 1 percent had strongly elevated values. The authors observed that these results are consistent with percentages for normal persons, heterozygote carriers, and homozygotes, respectively, of an as yet undiscovered gene mutation.

Unlike HHC, persons with African siderosis load iron in macrophages throughout the course of the disorder. Therefore, as iron is accumulated, their risk of tuberculosis (primarily an infection of iron-rich alveolar macrophages) is increased. As with HHC, iron loading in hepatocytes (liver parenchymal cells) markedly enhances risk of cirrhosis and hepatocellular carcinoma. Also elevated in African siderosis are risks for diabetes and osteoporosis.

In African, but not Caucasian, populations, a Q284H mutation in the ferroportin 1 gene has been detected. This mutation in the export protein, ferroportin 1, is associated with a mild anemia and a tendency for macrophage iron loading.

Ferroportin disease

A new inherited disorder of iron metabolism, ferroportin disease is increasingly recognized worldwide. The disorder is due to pathogenic mutations in the SLC40A1 gene encoding for a main iron export protein in mammals, ferroportin1/IREG1/MTP1, and it was originally identified as an autosomal-dominant form of iron overload not linked to the hemochromatosis (*HFE*) gene. It has distinctive clinical features such as early increase in serum ferritin in spite of low-normal transferrin saturation; progressive iron accumulation in organs, predominantly in reticuloendothelial macrophages; and marginal anemia with low tolerance to phlebotomy. Ferroportin mutations have been reported in many countries, regardless of ethnicity. They may lead to a loss of protein function responsible for reduced iron export from cells, particularly reticu-loendothelial cells. Now, the disorder appears to be the most common cause of hereditary iron overload beyond *HFE* hemochromatosis.

Beta-thalassemia

In ß-thalassemia, an inherited disorder in which hemoglobin is produced incorrectly, patients absorb as much as 2–5 grams/year of excess iron in a futile attempt to produce useful hemoglobin. Hemolysis occurs as the body senses abnormal red cells; iron is released from the lysed cells and released back into the reticuloendothelial system (RES). Compounding the iron burden of the RES are the necessary chronic blood transfusions, as each pint of transfused blood delivers one-fourth gram of iron.

The ß-thalassemias are widespread throughout the Mediterranean region, Africa, the Middle East, the Indian sub-continent and Burma, Southeast Asia including the Malay peninsula, Indonesia, and southern China. In some areas, the altered ß-globin gene frequencies have been estimated to range from 3–10 percent of the population. The more severe forms generally result from homozygosity or compound het-erozygosity.

When the ß-globin gene is altered by mutation, the synthesis of hemoglobin becomes inefficient and the patient constantly attempts to increase red blood cell production to compensate for the defect. The increased red cell synthesis leads to enhanced iron absorption with progressive accumulation of iron in the tissues. Most affected is the heart, leading to death by heart failure by the second or third decade of life. Even in patients who are not receiving blood transfusions (to provide efficient red blood cells), the iron burden can increase from 2–5 grams per year.

After approximately 50 units of blood have been transfused (loading the body with 10 grams of unexcretable iron), the iron holding limits of macrophages are well exceeded and iron over-flow into parenchymal cells occurs. The organs damaged by iron in ß-thalassemia are essentially the same as in HHC and African siderosis. However, in ß-thalassemia, iron loading and the consequent organ deterioration begins much earlier in the life of the patient as compared with the other two disorders.

In sicklemia, another inherited disease in which hemoglobin synthesis has been altered by mutation, transfusional iron overload also has been reported. As with other causes of iron loading, elevated ferritin levels in sicklemic patients predict organ failure and enhanced mortality. However, persons with either sicklemic or thalassemic gene mutations tend to have increased resistance to malaria, a life-threatening disease caused by a protozoan. This pathogen obtains growth-essential iron from normal hemoglobin but cannot acquire the metal from altered hemoglobin molecules or from iron bound to transferrin.

In both ß-thalassemia and sicklemia, the spleen can become excessively swollen due to accumulation of red blood cells with nonfunctional hemoglobin. Thus the spleen often is surgically removed. Unfortunately, after splenectomy, iron loading becomes intensified. Both transferrin iron saturation and serum ferritin rise markedly. In one survey of ß-thalassemia, for instance, the mean ferritin value in 50 nonsplenectomized patients was 400 ng/mL and in 41 splenectomized patients 2400 ng/mL. Possibly the spleen produces an as yet undiscovered factor that participates in the blocking of dietary iron from intestinal absorption.

Predictably, splenectomized persons are at much increased risk for specific bacterial and protozoan infections. Especially important is Streptococcus pneumoniae, which can cause severe septicemia, even in normal persons who have lost their spleens because of accidents. This prominent pneumonia-causing pathogen likewise is very troublesome in patients who have been splenectomized because of sicklemia or ß-thalassemia.

Sideroblastic anemias (SA)

Sideroblastic anemias (SA) can be inherited or acquired. Some forms are reversible, such as pyridoxine responsive SA which can be due to chronic alcohol abuse or exposure to certain medications such as hormone replacement or birth control pills. The acquired form is often seen in the elderly because of nutritional deficiencies due to irregular dietary habits or possibly hemodialysis. In a study of 452 patients (approximately 60

14

percent males and 40 percent females) with primary acquired sideroblastic anemia, the median age of occurrence was determined to be 74.4 years. Sideroblastic anemias are characterized by two findings: (1) the body is impaired in its ability to use iron to synthesize heme to form hemoglobin; (2) this results in iron that collects around the nuclei of immature red blood cells (called ringed sideroblasts). Persons who have SA are likely to experience anemia ranging from mild to severe, and are also likely to have iron overload. Some forms of SA are pyridoxine responsive. Therapeutic doses of oral pyridoxine (vitamin B₆) can completely eliminate ringed sideroblasts in these patients. In other SA cases where there is concomitant anemia and iron overload, the patients are not able to tolerate therapeutic phlebotomy and may require iron chelation therapy with deferoxamine (DF) (Desferal).

Atransferrinemia

Atransferrinemia is a condition in which transferrin, the plasma protein that binds with and transports iron, is absent or deficient (hypotransferrinemia). Severe microcytic, hypochromic (small, pale) red blood cells are detected at birth. Dietary iron is readily absorbed and circulates as unbound iron in plasma. Almost none of this iron can be used to make red blood cells and is instead deposited in the liver, pancreas, kidneys, heart, and thyroid. Little iron is found in the spleen and none in bone marrow. These individuals usually receive transferrin by whole red blood transfusions, which can lead to acquired iron overload. However, purified human transferrin is becoming available; read more about this in chapter 17 on treatment.

Aceruloplasminemia

A recently recognized uncommon disorder of iron metabolism is aceruloplasminemia. A mutation in a gene that controls formation of a copper-containing molecule, ceruloplasmin (CP), causes a deficiency in quantity of this plasma protein. Ceruloplasmin, a multi-copper oxidase (enzyme), is required for regulating the efficiency of cellular iron efflux, although the exact mechanism of this is not completely known. In iron metabolism, CP is essential because it oxidizes ferrous to ferric ions, a process needed in normal iron cycling. Individuals who are deficient in serum ceruloplasmin develop both systemic and central nervous system iron overload. In these patients, iron accumulates mainly in liver, pancreas, and brain and presents with insulin-dependent diabetes mellitus, retinal degeneration, and progressive neuro-degeneration, resulting in a Parkinson-like disease. Iron metabolism in specific brain cells called astrocytes is especially impaired in these patients.

Often these individuals are misdiagnosed with hemochromatosis and are phlebotomized. In the sera of these individuals, there is absent circulating serum ceruloplasmin (carriers for the disease have half the normal levels of ceruloplasmin), mildly lowered serum iron, elevated serum ferritin, and a mild anemia.

Alcoholism

It was formerly held that hemochromatosis was caused by alcohol abuse. Many hemochromatotics were falsely accused of excess alcohol consumption and inappropriately diagnosed. Investigators have found that there is increased iron absorption in chronic alcoholics, though the exact mechanism is not completely understood. Iron and alcohol have been shown to result in increased oxidative stress, resulting in lipid peroxidation and tissue injury. Together, the two toxins accentuate disease expression and increase the risk of cirrhosis and cancer.

Hepatitis

Chronic viral hepatitis can contribute to iron overload because iron is decompartmentalized during the destruction of liver cells. The iron load is worsened when patients are homozygous for the gene mutation for hereditary hemochromatosis, *HFE*. These patients have higher hepatic iron concentrations and develop fibrosis at an earlier age.

Non-alcoholic steatohepatitis (NASH)

Non-alcoholic steatohepatitis, also called non-alcoholic fatty liver disease (NAFLD), was first described in the 1980s and today is gaining recognition as a serious liver disease. NASH patients are not consumers of alcohol and exhibit type II diabetes, obesity, and fatty livers, possibly with cirrhosis. About

16

half of the NASH patients have increased liver iron. In these patients, iron's role may be to increase oxidative stress, enhancing the progression of steatosis to fibrosing steatohepatitis.

Dysmetabolic iron overload syndrome (DIOS)

Dysmetabolic-associated liver iron overload syndrome, also called dysmetabolic hepatosiderosis, is characterized by normal serum iron, low or normal transferrin saturation levels, elevated ferritin (hyperferritinemia) and hepatic iron overload. Patients with these characteristics have been described in France and Italy, and it is hypothesized that these individuals represent a subgroup of hemochromatosis. Liver biopsy is very useful in the diagnostic approach to iron overload disorders, by defining the amount and the distribution of iron within the organ.

Congenital dyserythropoietic anemia type II (CDAII)

CDAs comprise a group of hereditary disorders of red blood cell production. They are considered to be rare diseases, with fewer than 300 cases identified worldwide. The classical types are CDAI, II, and III. Each of these types have in common a distinct abnormality of structure and form (morphology) of the majority of erythroblasts in the bone marrow. The types differ in inheritance patterns, consequences, such as iron overload, hemolysis, gallstones, vacuoles (a clear space in the center of a red blood cell that is filled with fluid or air), and the type of morphology observed such as binuclearity or multinuclearity (more than one nucleus) or fragmentation of the chromatin, which is the colored genetic material within the nucleus that normally remains intact. The hepatic iron overload in these patients is due to the ongoing hemolysis with continued increased iron absorption in response to the need for new red blood cells.

Glucose-6-phosphate dehydrogenase (G6PD) deficiency

G6PD deficiency is an inheritable x-linked recessive disorder, which means that the gene defect occurs on the x chromosome and must be passed by both parents. This condition is estimated to affect about 400 million people worldwide. The highest prevalence rates are found in tropical Africa, the Middle East,

17

tropical and subtropical Asia, Papua New Guinea, and some parts of the Mediterranean, such as Italy and Greece.

In the United States, the incidence of G6PD is much higher among the African American population with a heterozygote frequency (carrier state with one normal gene and one abnormal gene) of 24 percent. Approximately 10–14 percent of the African American male population is affected. The disorder may occasionally affect a few black females to a mild degree (depending on their genetic inheritance). Persons with the disorder are not normally anemic and display no evidence of the disease until the red cells are exposed to an oxidant, chemical or stress.

Neonatal hemochromatosis

This pediatric liver disease is characterized by massive iron accumulation in hepatocytes, leading to death within a few days to weeks of birth. The livers of these infants are massively iron-loaded and fibrotic, while lesser amounts of iron are found in parenchymal cells of the heart, pancreas, kidneys, adrenals, thyroid, and pituitary gland. Also, very little iron is present in cells of the reticuloendothelial system.

GRACILE

GRACILE is the acronym for growth retardation, aminoaciduria, cholestasis, iron overload, lactacidosis, and early death. This syndrome is a rare inherited metabolic disorder seen primarily in the Finnish population. Inheritance is in an autosomal recessive pattern. Infants with this disease are severely growth retarded; the average birth weight is less than 4 pounds (1700 grams). Immediately at birth, these newborns develop fulminant lactic acidosis with an average arterial blood pH of 7.0. Other findings include nonspecific aminoaciduria, cholestasis, and iron overload, including hemosiderosis of the liver. Findings include increased serum ferritin, low transferrin, increased free plasma iron, and increased transferrin iron saturation. Survival is poor; half of the infants die during the first days of life and the remainder within 4 months.

Juvenile hemochromatosis (JH)

Juvenile hemochromatosis is an iron-loading condition seen in youths, but it is not associated with *HFE* mutations. Onset of symptoms of iron overload is prior to age 30. Clara Cameschella and her team of investigators have made significant contributions to a better understanding of the cause of JH, especially in Northern Italian families with iron overload, noting that the gene for JH was located somewhere on chromosome #1 with possible modulating genes on chromosome #19.

In late 2003 a team of scientists at the University of Athens, and other associated research facilities, were successful in the cloning of the gene for JH, which they named "hemojuvelin," and reported their findings in *Nature Genetics*, November 2003. One particular mutation of the hemojuvelin gene, G320V, is among the first to be identified.

The inheritance pattern of hemojuvelin is autosomal-recessive, the same as type I hemochromatosis (*HFE* related). Individuals most at risk are those of Greek or French ancestry.

As with *HFE*-related hemochromatosis, juvenile onset hemochromatosis also involves excessive iron absorption from the diet. As described by James Barton et al. following a study of eight South Carolinian patients within one family: Six of the seven patients had hypogonadotrophic hypogonadism, two had severe cardiomyopathy, seven had hepatomegaly, two had hepatic cirrhosis, and five had hyperpigmentation. Two of four siblings with JH also had Hashimoto thyroiditis. One patient with severe cardiomyopathy improved with therapeutic phlebotomy, medical therapy for congestive heart failure, and a permanent pacemaker; the other died before phlebotomy was initiated. The authors concluded that juvenile hemochromatosis may be unusually prevalent in the Southeastern region of the United States.

Though the mechanisms differ, all of these conditions have in common excessive accumulation of iron and increased risk of disease.

References:

Anuwatanakulchai, M., P. Pootrakul, P. Thuvasethakul, and P. Wasi. "Nontransferrin Iron in ß-thalassemia/Hb E and Hemoglobin H Diseases." *Scandinavian Journal of Haematology* 32 (1984): 153–58.

Ballas, S. K. "Iron Overload Is a Determinant of Morbidity and Mortality in Adult Patients with Sickle Cell Disease." *Seminars in Hematology* 38 (2001): 30–36.

Barton, J. C., and C. Q. Edwards, eds. *Genetics, Pathophysiology, Diagnosis and Treatment.* Cambridge: Cambridge University Press, 2000.

Barton, J. C., S. V. Rao, N. M. Pereira, T. Gelbart, E. Beutler, C. A. Rivers, and R. T. Acton. "Juvenile Hemochromatosis in the Southeastern United States: A Report of Seven Cases in Two Kinships." *Blood Cells, Molecules, and Diseases* 29 (2002): 104–15.

Beutler, E., T. Gelbart, and W. Miller. "Severe Jaundice in a Patient with a Previously Undescribed Glucose-6-Phosphate Dehydrogenase (G6PD) Mutation and Gilbert Syndrome." *Blood Cells, Molecules, and Diseases* 28 (2002): 104–7.

Bonkovsky, H. L. "Iron and the Liver." *American Journal of Medical Science* 301 (1991): 32–43.

Bonkovsky, H. L., N. Troy, K. McNeal, B. F. Banner, A. Sharma, J. Obando, S. Mehta, R. S. Koff, Q. Liu, and C. C. Hsieh. "Iron and *HFE* or TfR1 Mutations as Comorbid Factors for Development and Progression of Chronic Hepatitis C." *Journal of Hepatology* 37 (2002): 848–54.

Bottomley, S. S. "Secondary Iron Overload Disorders." *Seminars in Hematology* 35 (1999): 77–86.

Brandhagen, D. J., V. F. Fairbanks, and W. Baldus. "Recognition and Management of Hereditary Hemochromatosis." *American Family Physician* 65 (2002): 853–60.

Camaschella, C., A. Roetto, and M. De Gobbi. "Juvenile Hemochromatosis." *Seminars in Hematology* 39 (2002): 242–48.

Chitturi, S., and J. George. "Interaction of Iron, Insulin Resistance, and Non-alcoholic Steatohepatitis." *Current Gastroenterology Reports* 5 (2003): 18–25.

Duane, P., K. A. Raja, R. J. Simpson, and T. J. Peters. "Intestinal Iron Absorption in Chronic Alcoholics." *Alcohol and Alcoholism* 27 (1992): 539–44.

Ellervik, C., T. Mandrup-Poulsen, B. G. Nordestgaard, L. E. Larsen,

M. Appleyard, M. Frandsen, P. Petersen, P. Schlichting, T. Saermark, A. Tybjaerg-Hansen, and H. Birgens. "Prevalence of Hereditary Haemochromatosis in Late-Onset Type I Diabetes Mellitus: A Retrospective Study." *The Lancet* 358 (2001): 1405–9.

Fargion, S., M. Mattioli, A. L. Fracanzani, M. Sampietro, D. Tavazzi, P. Fociani, E. Taioli, L. Valenti , and G. Fiorelli. "Hyperferritinemia, Iron Overload, and Multiple Metabolic Alterations Identify Patients at Risk for Non-alcoholic Steatohepatitis." *American Journal of Gastroenterology* 96 (2001): 2448–55.

Fleming, D. J., K. L. Tucker, P. F. Jacques, G. E. Dallal, P. W. Wilson, and R. J. Wood. "Dietary Factors Associated with the Risk of High Iron Stores in the Elderly Framingham Heart Study Cohort." *American Journal of Clinical Nutrition* 76 (2002): 1375–84.

Fleming, R. E., and W. S. Sly. "Mechanisms of Iron Accumulation in Hereditary Hemochromatosis." *Annual Reviews in Physiology* 64 (2002): 663–80.

Fletcher, L. M., K. R. Bridle, and D. H. Crawford. "Effect of Alcohol on Iron Storage Diseases of the Liver." *Best Practices in Clinical Gastroenterology* 17 (2003): 663–77.

Gordeuk, V. R., A. Caleffi, E. Corradini, F. Ferrara, R. A. Jones , O. Castro, O. Onyekwere, R. Kittles, E. Pignatti, G. Montosi, C. Garuti, I. T. Gangaidzo, Z. A. Gomo, V. M. Moyo, T. A. Rouault, P. MacPhail, and A. Pietrangelo. "Iron Overload in Africans and African Americans and a Common Mutation in the SCL40A1 (ferroportin 1) Gene." *Blood Cells, Molecules, and Diseases* 31 (2003): 299–304.

Gordeuk, V. R., C. P. McLaren, A. C. Looker, V. Hasselblad, and G. M. Brittenham. "Distribution of Transferrin Saturation in the African American Population." *Blood* 91 (1998): 2175–79.

Harrison, S. A, and B. R. Bacon. "Hereditary Hemochromatosis: Update for 2003." *Journal of Hepatology* 38 (2003): S14–S23.

Iolascon, A., V. J. Delaunay, S. N. Wickramasinghe, S. Perrotta, M. Gigante, and C. Camaschella. "Natural History of Congenital Dyserythropoietic Anemia Type II." *Blood* 98 (2001): 1258–60.

McDonnell, S. M., B. L. Preston, S. A. Jewell, J. C. Barton, C. Q. Edwards , P. Adams, and R. Yip. "A Survey of 2,851 Patients with Hemochromatosis: Symptoms and Response to Treatment." *American Journal of Medicine* 106 (1999): 619–24.

Murray, K. F., and K. V. Kowdley. "Neonatal Hemochromatosis." *Pediatrics* 108 (2001): 960–64.

21

Niederau, C., R. Fischer, A. Sonnenberg, W. Stremmel, H. J. Trampisch, and G. Strohmeyer. "Survival and Causes of Death in Cirrhotic and in Noncirrhotic Patients with Primary Hemochromatosis." *New England Journal of Medicine* 313 (1985): 1256–62.

Nittis, T., and J. D. Gitlin. "The Copper-Iron Connection: Hereditary Aceruloplasminemia." *Seminars in Hematology* 39 (2002): 282–89.

Olivieri, N. F. "The Beta-thalassemias." *New England Journal of Medicine* 341 (1999): 99–109.

Papanikolaou, G., M. E. Samuels, E. H. Ludwig, M. L. MacDonald, P. L. Franchini, M. P. Dube, L. Andres, J. MacFarlane, N. Sakellaropoulos, M. Politou, E. Nemeth, J. Thompson, J. K. Risler, C. Zaborowska, R. Babakaiff, C. C. Radomski, T. D. Pape, O. Davidas, J. Christakis, P. Brissot, G. Lockitch, T. Ganz, M. R. Hayden, and Y. P. Goldberg. "Mutations in HFE2 Cause Iron Overload in Chromosome 1 Linked Juvenile Hemochromatosis." *Nature Genetics* 34 (2004): 77–82.

Pietrangelo, A. "EASL International Consensus, Conference on Haemochromatosis." *Journal of Hepatology* 33 (2000): 485–504.

———. "Haemachromatosis." *Gut* 52, suppl. 2 (2003): 23–30.

———. "The Ferroportin Disease." *Blood Cells, Molecules, and Disease.* 32 (2004): 131–38.

Piperno, A. "Classification and Diagnosis of Iron Overload." *Haematologica* 83 (1998): 447–55.

Roetto, A., F. Daraio, F. Alberti, P. Porporato, A. Cali, M. De Gobbi, C. Camaschella. "Hemochromatosis Due to Mutations in Transferrin Receptor 2." *Blood Cells Molecule Discovery* 29 (2002): 465–70.

Scotet, V., M. C. Merour, A. Y. Mercier, B. Chanu, T. Le Faou, O. Raguenes, G. Le Gac, C. Mura, J. B. Nousbaum, and C. Ferec. "Hereditary Hemochromatosis: Effect of Excessive Alcohol Consumption on Disease Expression in Patients Homozygous for the C282Y Mutation." *American Journal of Epidemiology* 158 (2003): 129–34.

Sheth, S., and G. M. Brittenham. "Genetic Disorders Affecting Proteins of Iron Metabolism: Clinical Implications." *Annual Review of Medicine* 51 (2000): 443–64.

Strachan, A. S. "Haemosiderosis and Haemochromatosis in South Africanes with a Comment on Etiology of Haemocromatosis." Thesis, University of Glasgow, 1929.

Visapää, I., V. Fellman, J. Vesa, A. Dasvarma, J. L. Hutton, V. Kumar, G. S. Payne, M. Makarow, R. Van Coster, R. W. Taylor, D. M. Turnbull, A. Suomalainen, and L. Peltonen. "GRACILE Syndrome, a Lethal Metabolic Disorder with Iron Overload, Is Caused by a Point Mutation in *BCS1L*." *American Journal of Human Genetics* 71 (2002): 863–76.

Weinberg, E. D. "The Role of Iron in Cancer." *European Journal of Cancer Prevention* 5 (1996): 19–36.

Witte, D. L., W. H. Crosby, C. Q. Edwards, V. F. Fairbanks, and F. A. Mitros. "Hereditary Hemochromatosis." *Clinica Chimica Acta* 245 (1996): 139–200.

Worwood, M. "Inborn Errors of Metabolism: Iron." *British Medical Bulletin* 55 (1999): 556–67.

2

Genetics of Iron Loading

"Remarkable progress is being made in understanding the molecular basis of disorders of human iron metabolism. . . . work has uncovered unanticipated relationships with the immune and nervous systems, intricate interconnections with copper metabolism, and striking homologies between yeast and human genes involved in the transport of transition metals."

—S. Sheth and G. Brittenham

Beta-thalassemia, congenital dyserythropoietic anemia type II (CDAII), enzymopathies such as G6PD or pyruvate kinase deficiencies, juvenile hemochromatosis, and classical (type I) hemochromatosis are inherited conditions where iron loading is directly influenced by specific gene mutations. Modifier genes for iron regulatory, binding, and transport proteins, such as transferrin receptor mutations, heavy and light ferritin chains, hepcidin, ferroportin 1, frataxin, haptoglobin, and ceruloplasmin also contribute to iron loading. Type I or classical hemochromatosis (HHC), however, remains the leading inherited condition to influence abnormal accumulation of iron. When seen in combination with other disorders, HHC increases the mortality and morbidity of the patient.

Prior to the availability of molecular analysis, scientists relied on HLA (human leukocyte antigen) typing to determine paternity and inherited conditions such as hemochromatosis within families. The HLA test detects genetic markers (antigens) on white blood cells (leukocytes). The HLA antigens are grouped in four sets: HLA-A, HLA-B, HLA-C, and HLA-D. Today the HLA test continues to be used to determine tissue compatibility for blood donors and transfusion recipients. Antigen markers associated with hereditary hemochromatosis include HLA-A3, B7, and B14. HLA-A3 is present in approximately 70 percent of patients who have hemochromatosis. However, since the discovery in 1996 of the *HFE* gene, HLA typing no longer is used to determine susceptibility to hereditary hemochromatosis. Physicians can use molecular analysis to confirm the diagnosis of iron overload, yet with the potential of genetic testing comes the legal and ethical implications for the patient. Physicians will want to inform patients prior to ordering a DNA sample, so that the patient is clear on the possible consequences.

Known Mutations or Inherited Conditions that Result in Iron Loading

* Mutations of *HFE* Chromosome #6: C282Y, H63D, S65C, C282S, V53M, Q127H, P160delC, E168X, Q283P, R6S

* Mutations of the Transferrin Receptor II E60X, M172K, Y250X, Q690P, AVAQ594-597del

* Mutations of Ferroportin I Chromosome #19 N144H, V162del, A77D, Y64N, D157G, Q182H, G323V

* Mutations of hepcidin gene R56X, 93delG, G71D

* CDA II

* X-linked sideroblastic anemia

* Enzymopathies: pyruvate kinase or G6PD deficiencies

* Cystic fibrosis

* GRACILE

* aceruloplasmin
* atransferrinemia
* African siderosis
* neonatal hemochromatosis
* juvenile hemochromatosis (a & b)
* beta thalassemia

Source: C. Camaschella et al.

HFE encodes a major histocompatibility complex (MHC) class I–like protein that is mutated in nearly 90 percent of all individuals known to have hemochromatotic iron overload.

Mutations explained

Type I or classical hemochromatosis is an autosomal recessive disorder because both copies of the *HFE* gene, residing on the two homologs of the autosomal chromosome 6, need to have a particular mutation in order for the disorder to present itself. To date, several different mutations in the *HFE* gene have been described, but two in particular, when present in the appropriate arrangement, can lead to the development of HHC.

The major disease-causing mutation is a replacement of the amino acid cysteine with a different amino acid called tyrosine. This mutation is referred to as C282Y. The second disease-causing mutation is a replacement of the amino acid histidine with another amino acid called aspartic acid. This mutation is referred to as H63D. There are additional mutations within the *HFE* gene, such as S65C, C282S, E168Q, Q283P, etc. It is not yet known how significantly these new mutations will contribute to abnormal metabolism of iron. C282Y presently is the most significant for causing iron loading. Whether a person is homozygous, heterozygous, or compound heterozygous contributes variably to the increased risk of increased iron absorption.

Approximately 0.2–0.5 percent of the Caucasian population are C282Y homozygotes and approximately 5 to 15 percent are carriers (heterozygotes) of the C282Y mutation. Homozygotes are the most at risk for iron loading and consequent disease.

Homozygosity for the H63D mutation is not presently considered as much of a risk for iron loading as is homozygosity for C282Y. The C282Y mutation is believed to cause a change in structural shape in the *HFE* protein, which would cause a disruption in how the protein connects with its receptor. The H63D variation may cause the *HFE* protein to be unstable, causing it to have a shortened existence.

Compound heterozygotes, or those who have one C282Y mutation and one H63D mutation, can develop serious iron overload. Studies of how iron overload manifests in heterozygotes will contribute greatly to how iron loading occurs in the general population.

To understand what the terms "homozygote," "heterozygote," and "compound heterozygote" mean with respect to hereditary hemochromatosis, it is useful to keep in mind a few basic facts about human genetics. (The following material is used with permission by Iron Disorders Institute, publications 1998–2004.)

The genetic material (DNA) comprising a human being is arranged into 46 chromosomes. One half or 23 chromosomes are inherited from each of the parents. Twenty-two of the 23 chromosomes are called the autosomes and the remaining chromosome, the X or Y chromosomes, are called the sex chromosomes, because the arrangement of these two chromosomes determines if an individual is a male (XY) or female (XX). Therefore, every human being, with rare exceptions, carries two copies, called homologs, of each of the 22 autosomal chromosomes and either an X and Y or two X chromosomes, depending on their sex.

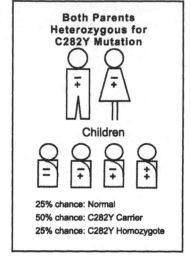

Heterozygote: If an individual has only one chromosome mutated, with any of the *HFE* mutations, C282Y, H63D, S65C, C282S, etc., the person is referred to as a heterozygote. The remaining nonmutated copy of the *HFE* gene is sufficient in most carriers to prevent the onset of symptoms.

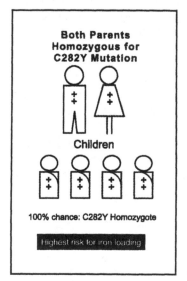

Homozygote: If an individual has the C282Y mutation on both chromosomes, that person is referred to as being a homozygote for the C282Y mutation. These individuals have a very

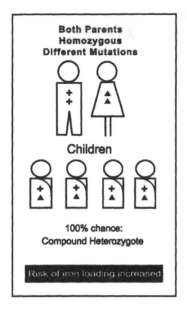

Both Parents Homozygous Different Mutations

Children

100% chance: Compound Heterozygote

Risk of iron loading increased

good chance of developing HHC. An individual can also have the H63D mutation on both chromosomes, and this person would also be called homozygous for this mutation.

Compound heterozygote: Patients with the C282Y mutation on one of their chromosomes and the H63D mutation on the other chromosome are compound heterozygotes. These individuals can sometimes develop HHC. In fact, of the HHC patients who have the C282Y mutation on only one copy of chromosome 6, approximately 77 percent have H63D on the other chromosome 6. This arrangement is referred to as a compound heterozygote because two different mutations are found together in the same individual.

As of mid-2003, more than 19 mutations of *HFE* have been identified and 4 types of hemochromatosis have been established. Some of these types are inherited in an autosomal-recessive pattern; some are inherited in an autosomal-dominant pattern.

Autosomal: located on chromosome 1–22
Sex linked: located on chromosome 23
Recessive: disease requires two mutated copies of the gene
Dominant: disease requires only one mutated copy of the gene

Type I is *HFE*-related; Type II is juvenile onset; Type III involves a receptor mutation; Type IV is autosomal dominant due to mutations in ferroportin 1. African siderosis and neonatal hemochromatosis represent other serious forms of iron loading, which are believed to be inherited, but the genes for these conditions are not yet identified.

Genetic
TYPES OF HEMOCHROMATOSIS

	Genetic Description	Most at Risk	Characterization
TYPE ONE Classical Hemochromatosis	HFE-gene autosomal recessive Chromosome: 6q21 Key mutations: C282Y, H63D	Caucasian: Northern European heritage Males age 30+ Females who no longer menstruate	Adult onset, iron loading in parenchymal cells of major organs. Iron loading not seen in macrophages (until very late in the disease). Associated with chronic fatigue and arthropathy and later diabetes, cirrhosis, heart failure, hypothyroidism, and hypogonadism.
TYPE TWO Juvenile Hemochromatosis	Type 2a:Hemojuvelin autosomal recessive (G320V) chromosome 1q Type 2b autosomal recessive hepcidin mutation chromosome #19	Caucasian: Greek, French, Northern Italian ancestry	Onset prior to age 30; affects both genders and is associated with severe cardiomyopathy and hypogonadism.
TYPE THREE Mutations of the transferrin receptor 2 gene (TfR2)	autosomal recessive chromosome 7q22	Any ethnicity	The consequences of type 3 are similar to those of type 1.
TYPE FOUR Mutations of the ferroportin 1 gene	autosomal dominant chromosome 2q32	African, African Americans	Iron deposition is predominantly in the macrophages.
OTHER TYPES African siderosis (African iron overload)	mutation Q248H of ferroportin-1	African	Hepatic portal fibrosis and micronodular cirrhosis prominent in both macrophages and hepatic parenchymal cells.
Neonatal hemochromatosis	unknown	Any ethnicity	Unknown origin characterized by congenital cirrhosis or fulminant hepatitis with hepatic and extra-hepatic iron deposits. Survival beyond a few weeks is rare.

Source: C. Camaschella et al.

The extent to which iron loading and consequent clinical problems develop is called expressivity or penetrance. The amount of penetrance in C282Y homozygotes has been reported to be a low as 1 percent and as great as 78 percent. The discrepancy in penetrance of *HFE* lies in ascertainment bias and in the definition of penetrance.

When applied to hemochromatosis (HHC), penetrance refers to the development of one or more iron-loading disease manifestations: cirrhosis, diabetes, hyperpigmentation, heart failure, arthritis, impotence, infertility, hypogonadism, hypothyroidism, or depression. The persons examined usually have either double C282Y mutations (homozygotes) or have one C282Y and one H63D mutation (compound heterozygote). However, it is recognized that HHC can underlie iron-loading tissue destruction even in the absence of known gene mutations.

In most genetically based disorders, penetrance is less than 100 percent. That is, some persons have the mutation(s) but still display normal longevity and remain free of development of specific diseases. In regard to HHC, there is uncertainty as to the percentage of persons with various gene mutations who will eventually proceed to develop iron-loading disease manifestations.

Clinicians and scientists who study large numbers of hemochromatotic patients are currently debating the extent of "penetrance" of this disorder. Beutler et al. at Scripps Research Institute, La Jolla, California, reported findings in a 2002 article in *The Lancet* that *HFE* is not highly penetrant; that only about 1 percent of individuals with genetic hemochromatosis develop disease. In contrast, others report penetrance significantly higher.

The discrepancies in *HFE* penetrance reported by Beutler or Ryan occur primarily because of the definition of penetrance used, as well as participant selection (ascertainment bias). Central to Beutler's definition of penetrance is whether or not the patient will develop severe organ damage, such as cirrhosis, whereas Ryan's definition of penetrance is based on whether the patient has elevated iron indices with symptoms. In another study, Asberg et al. provide support for either Beutler's or Ryan's definition of penetrance. Among 65,238 Norwegians, those with elevated serum ferritin and transferrin iron saturation percentages were studied. Asberg found that 34 percent of the females and 68 percent of males had elevated iron indices, but only 4 men had cirrhosis.

In an extensive review in a 2003 issue of *Blood*, hematologists R. S. Ajioka and J. P. Kushner noted that use of a single clinical criterion (biopsy-proven hepatic fibrosis or cirrhosis) has been observed in various studies in 4 to 25 percent of C282Y homozygotes. If diseases in addition to liver fibrosis or cirrhosis are considered, penetrance may be higher. For instance, when elevated liver enzymes and HHC arthropathy of metacarpal-phalangeal joints were included, 52 percent of males over age 40 and 38 percent of females over the age of 50 had at least one of the three medical problems related to C282Y homozygosity.

To illustrate the considerable variety of disease problems that can develop in C282Y homozygotes, a study by Olynyk et al. might be cited. Three hundred and sixty-six C282Y homozygotes who were first- or second-degree relatives of persons initially identified as C282Y homozygotes were studied. Relatives often, but not always, are younger than the first member of the family identified to have HHC. At the time of the sampling, symptoms had already emerged in 64 relatives (17 percent): arthralgia in 54 (15 percent), diabetes in 32 (8.7 percent), enlarged liver in 27 (7.4 percent), gonadal atrophy in 6 males (3 percent), and cardiomyopathy in 2 (0.5 percent). Of course it would be unethical to withhold treatment (i.e., phlebotomies) for the relatives so as to observe subsequent decay of their tissues and organs due to long-term, continuous iron loading.

In Dublin, Ireland, Ryan and colleagues studied 79 C282Y homozygotes who reported the nonspecific symptoms of fatigue, arthropathy, and impotence. Transferrin iron saturation percentage, serum ferritin, and hepatic iron levels of these patients were analyzed. Seventy-eight percent of the men (mean age 42 years) and 36 percent of women (mean age 39 years) who were identified as C282Y homozygotes had iron overload, as defined by a transferrin saturation equal to or greater than 52 percent combined with a serum ferritin greater than or equal to 300 ng/mL for the men and greater than or equal to 200 ng/mL for the women. The frequency of nonspecific symptoms reported by the individuals with iron overload was not significantly different from those who did not have iron overload. These investigators concluded that underdiagnosis of hemochromatosis "may be due to the nonspecific nature of early symptoms and less frequently to the incomplete penetrance of the C282Y mutation."

A comparison of two major studies where penetrance of *HFE* differ are illustrated in the following image.

Other investigators have noted that in studies of large numbers of persons from the United States, Europe, and Australia, 50–100 percent of C282Y homozygotes have abnormal iron metabolism as determine by increased transferrin iron saturation and/or elevated serum ferritin.

Investigators:	Definition of penetrance	Participants	Liver Assessment	Blood Donation	Lifestyle	Findings
Beutler, E., Felitti, V., Koziol, J., Ho, N., Gelbart, T. Scripps Research Institute, La Jolla, California	Severe organ damage	41,038 screened 152 homozygotes Insured as members of Kaiser Permanente Health Appraisal or MediCare age >26 73 males; 79 females	Surrogate collagen IV*	Blood donors were identified as treated (therapeutic phlebotomy as prescribed by a physician) or untreated (those who had donated more than 20 units of blood ever; also called frequent blood donors)	Not considered	Less than 1% had severe organ damage: (cirrhosis) TS% was elevated above 50% in 76% of males and 41% of females; ferritin> 250 in 77% of males and 66% of females (After disqualifying "frequent" blood donors)
Olynyk, J., Cullen, D., Aquilia, S., Rossi, E., Summerville, L., Powell, L. Department of Medicine, University of Western Australia, Fremantle Australia	Clinical signs with elevated iron indices	5,000 screened 3,011 randomly chosen,16 homozygotes Randomly selected cross section of an urban Australian population, unrelated age 20-79; 7 males, 9 females	Liver biopsy in subjects with serum ferritin >300ng/mL	Anyone who had donated blood was disqualified	Alcoholism investigated and noted in one male homozygote.	25% had cirrhosis 100% had elevated iron indices; 50% had symptoms of hyperpigmentation, arthritis, or hepatomegaly

*Type IV collagen, Biomedicals, Aurora, OH (Use limited to research; not presently available to US clinicians)

Source: E. Beutler et al. and J. Olynyk et al.

These clinicians observed that in such other inherited metabolic disorders as hyperchlolesteremia we do not require patients to wait for evidence of atherosclerosis before recommending the use of cholesterol-lowering drugs. Thus they suggest that penetrance in HHC be based on evidence of iron loading and that de-ironing therapy be considered prior to appearance of disease manifestations.

Carriers

Several studies have monitored the incidence of iron loading in carriers. In each of the groups of carriers examined for iron loading, a minority of the population had elevated iron values. In those examined for specific diseases known to be increased in people with hereditary hemochromatosis, the risk to carriers was often significantly higher than the controls.

In one study, risk of premature death was observed to be increased in C282Y heterozygotes but not in H63D heterozygotes as compared with controls. In contrast, another study found no increased risk among C282Y homozygotes or C282Y/H63D compound heterozygotes.

Contributing factors such as diet remain in question. One study found that the serum ferritin values of C282Y/H63D compound heterozygotes were elevated by 36 percent in women and 42 percent in men who ate red meat daily as compared with those who ate meat only 1 to 2 days per week. Ferritin values were 17 percent higher in women and 46 percent higher in men who drank more than 50 grams (about 1.76 ounces) of alcohol per day.

Risk of Disease in *HFE* heterozygotes

Clinical Condition	*HFE* Mutation C282Y H63D WT ND	Contributing Factors	Clinical Observation
Iron loading	CY/wt	Not Determined	In men and women, respectively, mean elevation of 15 and 18% in Tf sat % and of 3 and 8% in serum ferritin Beutler, *et al.* 2002
Iron loading	CY/HD	Not Determined	In men and women, respectively, mean elevation of 48 and 41% in Tf sat % and of 62 and 35% in serum ferritin Beutler, *et al.* 2002
Iron loading	CY/HD	Alcohol	In some patients, elevated Tf sat % serum ferritin and hepatic iron Jeffrey, *et al.* 2001
Iron loading	CY/wt & CY/HD	Alcohol & Red meat	In some CY/wt males, elevated Tf sat % in some CY/wt males & females, elevated Tf% and serum ferritin Rossi, *et al.* 2001
Infection	CY/wt	Alcohol; Raw shellfish	In an hepatic iron loaded patient, death due to Vibrio vulnificus septicemia Gerhard *et al.* 2001
Arthritis	Not Determined	Not Determined	Increased risk (2.1X) for arthritis Nelson *et al.* 2001
Vascular Disease	CY/wt	Smoking	Increased risk (3.5X) for cardiovascular disease Roest *et al.* 2001
Vascular Disease	CY/wt	Not Determined	Increased risk (2.3X) for myocardial infarction Tuomainen *et al.* 1999
Vascular Disease	CY/wt	Not Determined	Increased risk (6.6X) for ischemic cardiomyopathy Pereira *et al.* 2001
Vascular Disease	CY/HD	Not Determined	Increased risk (4.1X) for ischemic heart disease George *et al.* 2001
Cancer	CY/wt	Ser/Ser mutation in TfR gene	Increased risk 2.2X multiple myeloma 2.2X breast cancer 1.6X colorectal cancer Beckman *et al.* 1999
Cancer	CY/HD	Ser/Ser mutation in TfR gene	Increased risk 6.5X multiple myeloma 7.3X breast cancer 8.7X colorectal cancer Beckman *et al.* 1999
Cancer	HD/wt	Not Determined	Increased risk for malignant glioma Montemuros *et al.* 2001
Shortened Life Expectancy	CY/wt	Not Determined	Increased mortality prior to age 65 Bathum *et al.* 2001

Source: E. D. Weinberg

Chart Source: Weinberg, E.D., "Do Some Carriers of Hemochromatosis Gene Mutations Have a Higher Than Normal Rates of Disease and Death?" *BioMetals* 15: (2002) 347-50.

Indeed both CY and HD carriers are recommended to have their serum iron values tested periodically and, if values begin to rise, consider phlebotomy therapy to prevent development of clinical disease.

Concomitant disorders

When a person has more than one iron disorder, molecular analysis might explain the potential consequences. Investigators find that patients who have beta-thalassemia and who are homozygous for H63D, the lesser mutation of *HFE*, have significantly elevated ferritin. In a study of 152 healthy males heterozygous for beta-thalassemia, 45 subjects were H63D heterozygotes and 4 were H63D homozygotes. Both groups (H63D heterozygotes and homozygotes) exhibited elevated serum ferritin levels significantly higher than in controls, suggesting that this mutation of *HFE* might have an enhancing effect on iron absorption when accompanied by the genetic mutations for beta-thalassemia.

Gene mutations revealed as a result of liver transplantation

At the Department of Gastroenterology and Hepatology, Flinders Medical Centre, Adelaide, South Australia, investigators Wigg, Harley, and Casey observed an unusual case. They transplanted a liver into a 54-year-old Caucasian male with cirrhosis, who did not possess the C282Y or H63D mutations of *HFE*.

As part of the pre-transplantation work-up, a liver biopsy was performed on the recipient's existing liver. He had cirrhosis with minor grade 1 siderosis, which means that less than 25 percent of the hepatocytes were affected. The patient had abstained from alcohol use for the previous 6 months and there was no family history of iron overload or liver disease.

The first 4 years following the transplantation were uneventful until a hernia operation was required. During surgery to repair the hernia, the surgeon obtained a liver biopsy specimen. It came as a surprise that the biopsy revealed significant iron deposition. The man had grade 4 siderosis, which means that 75 percent of his hepatocytes were affected. A second liver biopsy was performed to confirm the iron content; the findings were identical. HIC (hepatic iron content) was 252 µmol/g dry weight; normal is 80. His HII (hepatic iron index) was 5.0; normal is 1.9 or less.

Somewhat baffled, Wigg and his colleagues began to rule out possible causes one by one. Review of postoperative blood work showed no evidence that the patient had resumed alcohol consumption. They ruled out acquired means of iron overload such as ingestion of iron supplements or blood transfusions. Next they ruled out viral hepatitis C, non-alcoholic steatohepatitis (NASH), and portal systemic shunting. Chronic hemolytic anemia was ruled out with a variety of tests.

The investigators noted that the iron deposition was in the parenchymal hepatocytes, which is highly suggestive of an inherited cause rather than an acquired cause of iron loading. So they decided to take a closer look at the genetic makeup of both the donor and recipient. The donor, a 44-year-old Caucasian female, was a C282Y heterozygote.

The recipient had a novel, not yet identified mutation of *HFE*, which the investigators named R6S. The mutation, they think, interacts with the C282Y mutation and leads to significant iron overload.

In 1999 Adams, Jeffrey, Alanen, Preshaw, Howson, and Grant, Department of Medicine, University of Western Ontario, reported a case of iron loading in a liver-intestine transplantation recipient. The donor of the liver-intestine transplant was discovered posthumously to be a C282Y homozygote. The recipient was normal (wild type) for the gene. Within 21 months after the transplantation, his transferrin saturation had risen to 94 percent. This case supports the hypothesis that a fundamental defect in hemochromatosis is at the level of the intestine rather than a systemic abnormality.

These two events are significant because they prompt a strong case that both the liver and intestine must have defects before greater than normal iron loading will take place. Recent discoveries such as hepcidin, an iron-regulating protein produced by the liver, strengthens this premise. Apparently the donor liver was incapable of forming hepcidin.

In addition to the known mutations of *HFE*, investigators have discovered several other gene abnormalities that modify iron homeostasis. Among these are mutations in the protein transferrin, transferrin receptor 1, transferrin receptor 2, ferritin-L, ferritin-H, IRP1, IRP2, beta(2) microglobulin, mobilferrin/cal-reticulin, ceruloplasmin, ferroportin, NRAMP1, NRAMP2 (DMT1), haptoglobin, heme oxygenase-1, heme oxygenase-2, USF2, ZIRTL, duodenal cytochrome b ferric reductase (DCYTB), TNF alpha, keratin 8, and keratin 18. The most significant modifier is the recently discovered hepcidin, a small peptide, a chain of 25 amino acids produced by the liver. Hepcidin production is increased when iron stores are adequate, suggesting that this protein regulates iron absorption based on body needs. Read more about hepcidin in chapter 4.

References:

Adams, P. C., G. Jeffrey, K. Alanen, S. Chakrabarti, R. Preshaw, W. Howson, and D. Grant. "Transplantation of Haemochromatosis Liver and Intestine into a Normal Recipient." *Gut* 45 (1999): 783.

Aguilar-Martinez, P. A., C. Biron, F. Banc, C. Masmejean, P. Jeanjean, H. Michel, and J. F. Schved. "Compound Heterozygotes for Hemochromatosis Gene Mutations: May They Help to Understand the Pathophysiology of the Disease?" *Blood Cells, Molecules, and Diseases* 23 (1997): 269–76.

Ajioka, R. S., and J. P. Kushner. "Clinical Consequences of Iron Overload in Hemochromatosis Homozygotes." *Blood* 101 (2003): 3351–53.

Asberg, A., K. Hveem, K. Thorstensen, E. Ellekjter, K. Kannelonning, U. Fjosne, T. B. Halvorsen, H. B. Smethurst, E. Sagen, and K. S. Bjerve. "Screening for Hemochromatosis: High Prevalence and Low Morbidity in an Unselected Population of 65,238 Persons." *Scandinavian Journal of Gastroenterology* 36 (2001): 1108–15.

Barton, J. C., R. T. Acton, C. A. Rivers, L. F. Bertoli, T. Gelbart, C. West, and E. Beutler. "Genotypic and Phenotypic Heterogeneity of African Americans with Primary Iron Overload." *Blood Cells, Molecules, and Diseases* 31 (2003): 310–19.

Bassett, M. L., S. R. Wilson, and J. A. Cavanaugh. "Penetrance of *HFE* Related Hemochromatosis in Perspective." *Hepatology* 36 (2002): 500–503.

Beutler, E., J. C. Barton, V. J. Felitti, T. Gelbart, C. West, P. L. Lee, J. Waalen, and C. Vulpe. "Ferroportin 1 (SCL40A1) Variant

Associated with Iron Overload in African-Americans." *Blood Cells, Molecules, and Diseases* 31 (2003): 305–9.

Beutler, E., V. Felitti, J. Koziol, N. J. Ho, and T. Gelbart. "Penetrance of 845G A (C282Y) *HFE* Hereditary Hemochromatosis Mutation in the USA." *The Lancet* 359 (2002): 211–18.

Burke, W., G. Imperatore, S. M. McDonnell, R. C. Baron, and M. J. Khoury. "Contribution of Different *HFE* Genotypes to Iron Overload Disease: A Pooled Analysis." *Genetic Medicine* 2 (2000): 271–77.

Camaschella, C., A. Roetto, A. Cali, M. De Gobbi, G. Garozzo, M. Carella, N. Majorano, A. Totaro, and P. Gasparini. "The Gene TFR2 Is Mutated in a New Type of Haemochromatosis Mapping to 7q22." *Nature Genetics* 25 (2000): 14–15.

Camaschella, C., A. Roetto, and M. De Gobbi. "Genetic Haemochromato-sis: Genes and Mutations Associated with Iron Loading." *Best Practices in Research Clinical Haematology* 15 (2002): 261–76.

Cazzola, M., L. Cremonesi, M. Papaioannou, N. Soriani, A. Kioumi, A. Charalambidou, R. Paroni, K. Romtsou, S. Levi, M. Ferrari, P. Arosio, and J. Christakis. "Genetic Hyperferritinaemia and Reticuloendothelial Iron Overload Associated with a Three Base Pair Deletion in the Coding Region of the Ferroportin Gene (SLC11A3)." *British Journal of Haematology* 119 (2002): 539–46.

Cox, T. M., and D. J. Halsall. "Hemochromatosis-Neonatal and Young Subjects." *Blood Cells, Molecules, and Diseases* 29 (2002): 411–17.

De Gobbi, M., A. Roetto, A. Piperno, R. Mariani, F. Alberti, G. Papanikolaou, M. Politou, G. Lockitch, D. Girelli, S. Fargion, T. M. Cox, P. Gasparini, M. Cazzola, and C. Camaschella. "Natural History of Juvenile Haemochromatosis." *British Journal of Haematology* 117 (2002): 973–79.

De Gobbi, M., F. Daraio, C. Oberkanins, A. Moritz, F. Kury, G. Fiorelli, and C. Camaschella. "Analysis of *HFE* and TFR2 Mutations in Selected Blood Donors with Biochemical Parameters of Iron Overload." *Haematologica* 4 (2003): 396–401.

Devalia, V., K. Carter, A. P. Walker, S. J. Perkins, M. Worwood, A. May, and J. S. Dooley. "Autosomal Dominant Reticuloendothelial Iron Overload Associated with a 3-Base Pair Deletion in the Ferroportin 1 Gene (SLC11A3)." *Blood* 100 (2002): 695–97.

Feder, J. N., A. Gnirke, W. Thomas, Z. Tsuchihashi, D. A. Ruddy, A. Basava, F. Dormishian, R. Domingo Jr, M. C. Ellis, A. Fullan,

L. M. Hinton, N. L. Jones, B. E. Kimmel, et al. "A Novel MHC Class I-Like Gene Is Mutated in Patients with Hereditary Haemochromatosis." *Nature Genetics* 13 (1996): 399–408.

Fellman, V. "The GRACILE Syndrome, a Neonatal Lethal Metabolic Disorder with Iron Overload." *Blood Cells, Molecules, and Diseases* 29 (2002): 444–50.

Gordeuk, V. R., A. Caleffi, E. Corradini, F. Ferrara, R. A. Jones, O. Castro, O. Onyekwere, R. Kittles, E. Pignatti, G. Montosi, C. Garuti, I. T. Gangaidzo, Z. A. Gomo, V. M. Moyo, T. A. Rouault, P. MacPhail, and A. Pietrangelo. "Iron Overload in Africans and African Americans and a Common Mutation in the SCL40A1 (ferroportin 1) Gene." *Blood Cells, Molecules, and Diseases* 31 (2003): 299–304.

Gordeuk, V. R., C. E. McLaren, A. C. Locker, V. Hasselblad, and G. M. Brittenham. "Distribution of Transferrin Saturation in the African American Population." *Blood* 91 (1998): 2175–79.

Gordeuk, V. R., R. Boyd, and D. Brittenham. "Dietary Iron Overload Persists in Rural Sub-Saharan Africa." *The Lancet* 1 (1986): 1310–13.

Hetet, G., I. Devaux, N. Soufir, B. Grandchamp, and C. Beaumont. "Molecular Analyses of Patients with Hyperferritinemia and Normal Serum Iron Values Reveal Both L Ferritin IRE and 3 New Ferroportin (Slc11a3) Mutations." *Blood* 102 (2003): 1904–10.

Imperatore, G., L. E. Pinsky, A. Motulsky, M. Reyes, L. A. Bradley, and W. Burke. "Hereditary Hemochromatosis: Perspectives of Public Health, Medical Genetics, and Primary Care." *Genetic Medicine* 5 (2003): 1–8.

Knutson, M. D., M. R. Vafa, D. J. Haile, and M. Wessling-Resnick. "Iron Loading and Erythrophagocytosis Increase Ferroportin1 (FPN1) Expression in J774 Macrophages." *Blood* 102 (2003): 4191–97.

Laine, F., M. Ropert, C. L. Lan, O. Loreal, E. Bellissant, C. Jard, M. Pouchard, A. Le Treut, and P. Brissot. "Serum Ceruloplasmin and Ferroxidase Activity are Decreased in *HFE* C282Y Homozygote Male Iron-Overloaded Patients." *Hepatology* 36 (2002): 60–65.

Lee, P., T. Gelbart, C. West, C. Halloran, and E. Beutler. "Seeking Candidate Mutations That Affect Iron Homeostasis." *Blood Cells, Molecules, and Diseases* 29 (2002): 471–87.

Lee, P. L., T. Gelbart, C. West, C. Halloran, V. Felitti, and E. Beutler. "A Study of Genes That May Modulate the Expression of Hereditary

Hemochromatosis: Transferrin Receptor-1, Ferroportin, Ceruloplasmin, Ferritin Light and Heavy Chains, Iron Regulatory Proteins (IRP)-1 and -2, and Hepcidin." *Blood Cells, Molecules, and Diseases* 27 (2001): 783–802.

Mattman, A., D. Huntsman, G. Lockitch, S. Langlois, N. Buskard, D. Ralston, Y. Butterfield, P. Rodrigues, S. Jones, G. Porto, M. Marra, M. De Sousa, and G. Vatcher. "Transferrin Receptor 2 (Tfr2) and *HFE* Mutational Analysis In Non-C282Y Iron Overload: Identification of a Novel Tfr2 Mutation." *Blood* 100 (2002): 1075–77.

Melis, M. A., M. Cau, F. Deidda, S. Barella, A. Cao, and R. Galanello. "H63D Mutation in the *HFE* Gene Increases Iron Overload in Beta-thalassemia Carriers." *Haematologica* 87 (2002): 242–45.

Merryweather-Clarke, A. T., E. Cadet, A. Bomford, D. Capron, V. Viprakasit, A. Miller, P. J. McHugh, R. W. Chapman, J. J. Pointon, V. L. Wimhurst, K. J. Livesey, V. Tanphaichitr, J. Rochette, and K. J. Robson. "Digenic Inheritance of Mutations in HAMP and *HFE* Results in Different Types of Haemochromatosis." *Human Molecular Genetics* 12 (2003): 2241–47.

Meyers, D. G., D. Strickland, P. A. Maloley, J. K. Seburg, J. E. Wilson, and B. F. McManus. "Possible Association of a Reduction in Cardiovascular Event with Blood Donation." *Heart* 78 (1997): 188–93.

Montosi, G., A. Donovan, A. Totaro, C. Garuti, E. Pignatti, S. Cassanelli, C. C. Trenor, P. Gasparini, N. C. Andrews, and A. Pietrangelo. "Autosomal-Dominant Hemochromatosis Is Associated with a Mutation in the Ferroportin (SLC11A3) Gene." *Journal of Clinical Investigation* 108 (2001): 619–23.

Moyo, V. M., I. T. Gangaidzo, Z. A. Gomo, H. Khumalo, T. Saungweme, C. F. Kiire, T. Rouault, and V. R. Gordeuk. "Traditional Beer Consumption and the Iron Status of Spouse Pairs from a Rural Community in Zimbabwe." *Blood* 89 (1997): 2159–66.

Niederau, C. "Hereditary Hemochromatosis." Internist (Berl), 2003. 191–205; quiz 206–7.

Olynyk, J., D. Cullen, S. Aquilia, E. Rossi, L. Summerville, and L. Powell. "A Population-Based Study of the Clinical Expression of the Hemochromatosis Gene." *New England Journal of Medicine* 341 (1999): 718–24.

Papanikolaou, G., M. E. Samuels, E. H. Ludwig, M. L. MacDonald, P. L. Franchini, M. P. Dube, L. Andres, J. MacFarlane,

N. Sakellaropoulos, M. Politou, E. Nemeth, J. Thompson, J. K. Risler, C. Zaborowska, R. Babakaiff, C. C. Radomski, T. D. Pape, O. Davidas, J. Christakis, P. Brissot, G. Lockitch, T. Ganz, M. R. Hayden, and Y. P. Goldberg. "Mutations In *HFE2* Cause Iron Overload in Chromosome 1q-Linked Juvenile Hemochromatosis." *Nature Genetics* 34 (2004): 77–82.

Phatak, P. D., D. H. Ryan, J. Cappuccio, D. Oakes, C. Braggins, K. Provenzano, S. Eberly, and R. L. Sham. "Prevalence and Penetrance of *HFE* Mutations in 4865 Unselected Primary Care Patients." *Blood Cells, Molecules, and Diseases* 29 (2002): 41–47.

Philpott, C. C. "Molecular Aspects of Iron Absorption: Insights into the Role of *HFE* in Hemochromatosis." *Hepatology* 35 (2002): 993–1001.

Roetto, A., A. T. Merryweather-Clarke, F. Daraio, K. Livesey, J. J. Pointon, G. Barbabietola, A. Piga, P. H. Mackie, K. J. Robson, and C. Camaschella. "A Valine Deletion of Ferroportin 1: A Common Mutation in Hemochromastosis Type 4." *Blood* 100 (2002): 733–34.

Roetto, A., G. Papanikolaou, M. Politou, F. Alberti, D. Girelli, J. Christakis, D. Loukopoulos, and C. Camaschella. "Mutant Antimicrobial Peptide Hepcidin Is Associated with Severe Juvenile Hemochromatosis." *Nature Genetics* 33 (2003): 21–22.

Rolfs, A., H. L. Bonkovsky, J. G. Kohlroser, K. McNeal, A. Sharma, U. V. Berger, and M. A. Hediger. "Intestinal Expression of Genes Involved in Iron Absorption in Humans." *American Journal of Physiology & Gastrointestinal Liver Physiology* 282 (2002): G598–607.

Rossi, E., M. K. Bulsara, J. K. Olynk, D. J. Cullen, L. Summerville, and L. W. Powell. "Effect of Hemochromatosis Genotype and Lifestyle Factors on Iron and Red Cell Indices in a Community Population." *Clinical Chemistry* 47 (2001): 202–8.

Roy, C. N., and C. A. Enns. "Iron Homeostasis: New Tales from the Crypt." *Blood* 96 (2000): 4020–27.

Ryan E., V. Byrnes, B. Coughlan, A. M. Flanagan, S. Barrett, J. C. O'Keane, and J. Crowe. "Underdiagnosis of Hereditary Haemochromatosis: Lack of Presentation or Penetration?" *Gut* 51 (2002): 108–12.

Sheth, S., and G. Brittenham. "Genetic Disorders Affecting Proteins of Iron Metabolism: Clinical Implications." *Annual Review of Medicine* 51 (2000): 443–64.

Weinberg, E. D. "Do Some Carriers of Hemochromatosis Gene Mutations Have Higher Than Normal Rates of Disease and Death?" *BioMetals* 15 (2002): 347–50.

Wigg, A. J., H. Harley, and G. Casey. "Heterozygous Recipient and Donor *HFE* Mutations Associated with a Hereditary Haemochromatosis Phenotype after Liver Transplantation." *Gut* 52 (2003): 433–35.

3

Absorption and Transport of Iron

"Iron is absorbed primarily by villus enterocytes of the duodenum."
—*S. A. Harrison and B. R. Bacon*

Our cells and tissues require a moderate amount of iron for such vital functions as DNA synthesis, oxygen transport, and numerous enzymatic processes. However, because the metal is quite dangerous, it must be handled and stored as safely as possible. Futhermore, the amount of iron absorbed from our diet must be carefully regulated. Should an excessive quantity be absorbed, it can be excreted only by bleeding. Thus our bodies have evolved an elaborate system of controls for absorption of necessary, but not excessive, quantities of iron. When iron enters the duodenum, its status greatly influences the degree of absorption. Ferric (Fe3+) is reduced to the soluble ferrous iron (Fe2+) form in the highly acidic environment of the stomach. When stomach acid is low, this change does not take place and absorption is poor.

Our knowledge of the details of the iron regulatory system continues to unfold. Just as adequate stomach acid and ascorbic acid enhance the absorption of iron, certain substances, especially tannin, fiber, and calcium, can impair absorption, as can defects in newly discovered proteins.

A critical site of control of absorption is contained in the epithelial cell lining of the duodenum. In this region, specialized enterocytes have developed that are capable of responding to

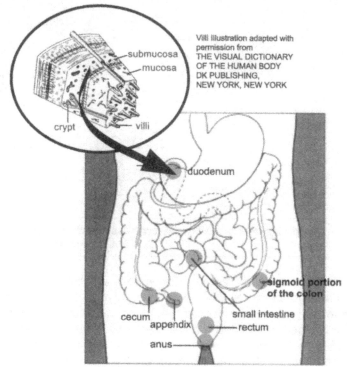

Villi Illustration adapted with permission from THE VISUAL DICTIONARY OF THE HUMAN BODY DK PUBLISHING, NEW YORK, NEW YORK

Image adapted from National Cancer Institutes.
http://www.cancer.gov

the body's needs for iron as well as to the danger of acquiring too much metal. The enterocytes absorb iron from the diet by several mechanisms.

Besides transferrin, two newly discovered proteins, divalent metal transporter 1 (DMT1) and ferroportin (FPN), are important to the transport of nonheme iron. DMT1 is located on the surface of the intestine that comes in contact with food. DMT1 is responsible for nearly all dietary iron uptake. DMT1 carries iron into the cell, while ferroportin carries iron out of the cell and into the bloodstream. Ferroportin also appears to have a role in iron recycling because of the rapid and strong induction of FPN1 expression noted after erythro-phagocytosis. Some patients with iron overload have a defective ferroportin gene.

As their macrophages fail to release iron properly, more dietary iron is absorbed to compensate. In addition to its functions ferroportin may modulate the activity of DMT1.

DMT1 is expressed in both the brush border and duodenal enterocytes and is activated only in an acidic environment. DMT1 has the ability to transport ferrous iron as well as other metals such as lead from the surface of the intestinal mucosa into cells via the villus and the crypt cells. Enterocyte expression of DMT1 differs in iron-deficiency anemia (IDA) and iron overload. In IDA, DMT1 is localized to both the microvillus membrane and cytoplasm; whereas in the iron-loaded state, DMT1 is expressed only in the cytoplasm.

A second method involves the absorption of heme iron, which is a different mechanism from nonheme iron. This system is much more efficient. Heme iron is in a form readily absorbed. Another possible method is that of a mobilferrin-integrin complex that would facilitate uptake of ferric iron. (Note that dietary iron consists of heme and ferric iron, but some of the latter is reduced to ferrous iron in the low pH of the stomach acid.)

The enterocytes are destined to detach from the intestine and to be excreted in the feces. But before they detach, they must decide how much of their absorbed iron should be passed into the bloodstream. In healthy adults on a well-balanced diet, only 10 percent of the iron is sent into the blood. An exception is made in the second trimester of pregnancy where the amount is increased sixfold and in the third trimester ninefold.

HFE—modifier of iron absorption

The export of iron from the enterocyte into the bloodstream involves several pathways. These include mechanisms catalyzed by the proteins located on the basolateral surface of the enterocyte: ferroportin, hephaestin, ceruloplasmin, and the transferrin receptor-*HFE* complex. Of these, the latter has been the most clearly characterized. The transferrin receptor is located at the enterocyte surface and strongly binds the transferrin protein that is circulating in the blood serum. The binding enables transferrin to acquire iron from the enterocyte. However, in normal individuals, the *HFE* protein in the serum competes with

45

transferrin for binding to the receptor, and thus it blocks excessive conveyance of the iron from the enterocyte to the serum. Unfortunately, in hemochromatosis, the C282Y gene mutation results in an altered structure of *HFE* and the H63D gene mutation may decrease its stability so that *HFE* is less efficient in binding to the receptors. Accordingly, in many persons with these mutations, absorption of dietary iron can be increased two- to threefold. Still to be determined is the role of hepcidin and the transferrin receptor 2 in the regulation of iron absorption. Additionally, the role of the multicopper oxidases, ceruloplasmin and hephaestin, as primary ferroxidases converting $Fe2+$ to $Fe3+$ has yet to be fully delineated as they play a role in iron trafficking and homeostasis. Exciting future directions will involve the characterization of iron-related proteins' expression in the brain and on the macrophage cell surface.

Transferrin—transporter and withholder of iron

The transferrin molecule can bind two atoms of iron. The protein has two functions—it transports iron through the body fluids, such as serum, lymph, and cerebrospinal fluid, and it also withholds iron from invading microorganisms. Normally, its iron-carrying capacity (saturation) is between 25 percent and 30 percent. During infections, its saturation can decrease to as little as 5 to 10 percent, which increases its ability to suppress microbial growth. In iron-loading conditions, saturation can increase to as much as 100 percent. Persons with saturation values above 40 percent are much more susceptible to many kinds of infection.

Transferrin accomplishes its transport function by combining with transferrin receptors on those body cells that need iron. The receptors can distinguish between transferrin molecules that contain iron and those that lack it and will bind only those molecules with iron. The complex then enters the cell and diffuses to an organelle called an endosome that has an acidic pH value. At the low pH, iron dissociates from transferrin. The receptor conveys the iron-free transferrin molecule to the cell surface to enable it to enter the serum and repeat its iron transport function. It has been calculated that a single transferrin molecule can repeat delivery of iron over 100 times during its existence.

Ferritin—packager of hazardous iron

The iron atoms that have been deposited in the endosome will then be diverted either into metabolic functions or into storage in ferritin within the cell. Ferritin is a very large spherical structure with a spacious cavity that can accommodate as many as 4500 atoms of iron. As ferritin molecules become satiated with iron, they are transformed into hemosiderin. The latter is an insoluble amalgam of degraded protein and ferric hydroxide. Although hemosiderin is highly effective in packaging dangerous amounts of iron, accumulation of excessive quantities of the amalgam can interfere with normal cell functions, and ultimately result in cell death.

The production of ferritin is increased during inflammatory conditions such as infection or cancer in order to withhold as much iron as possible from invading cells. Ferritin production is also increased in persons with iron loading. In some patients, serum iron and transferrin saturation may remain low but ferritin becomes highly elevated. An example is hyperferritinemia-cataract syndrome (HHCS), in which cataracts develop in both eyes of young adults. Another example is hemochromatosis type 4 (SLC11A3), in which patients have a mutation in the ferroportin gene.

Hepcidin—a coordinator of enterocytes and macrophages

Clearly there needs to be communication and coordination among numerous cells and proteins that are responsible for adjusting optimal levels of iron as we progress through various stages of growth, illness, good and poor nutrition, pregnancy, aging, etc. The chemicals assigned to these tasks generally are molecules much smaller than proteins and are termed cytokines or hormones.

During the 1970s and 1980s, several of these messenger molecules that regulate shifts in iron levels were discovered. These chemicals include various interleukins and interferons. However, the compounds have a variety of actions not only on iron but on many other body processes. Quite recently, a hormone has been discovered that has a very specific action on iron traffic. It is a small peptide (a chain of 25 amino acids) called hepcidin. A lack of hepcidin expression has been associated with

47

iron overload and overexpression of hepcidin results in iron-deficiency anemia in mice.

At the start of a microbial invasion, a cytokine called interleukin-6 signals the patient's hepatocytes to elevate production of hepcidin and secrete it into the bloodstream. The peptide then acts at two sites; it (1) suppresses enterocyte secretion of dietary iron into the blood and (2) stimulates macrophages to retain iron that these white blood cells have extracted from hemoglobin of aged red blood cells. These two actions lower the level of transferrin saturation and result in increased ferritin synthesis within macrophages. When the infection danger has passed, hepcidin synthesis is decreased.

Moreover, hepcidin synthesis is increased not only in response to microbial invasion but also to nutritional iron loading. Also, production of the hormone is lowered in iron deficiency. Unfortunately, however, in hemochromatosis (HHC) hepcidin synthesis is severely depressed. Thus in HHC not only is excessive iron absorbed from the enterocytes, but also macrophages fail to retain the surplus metal. Futhermore, persons who are heterozygous carriers of mutations of both the *HFE* gene and the hepcidin gene can have an increase in clinical problems. There is considerable hope that the hepcidin hormone might be developed into a useful drug to assist persons who have these mutations to adjust their iron traffic to normal ranges.

Lactoferrin is found in human secretions such as tears, perspiration, vaginal fluid, seminal

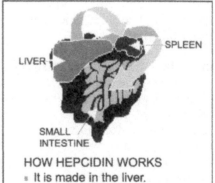

HOW HEPCIDIN WORKS
- It is made in the liver.
- It is increased by inflammation, or when iron stores are sufficient.
- It inhibits iron uptake by the small intestine.
- It inhibits recycled iron released from macrophages, many in the spleen.

Source: T. Ganz

fluids, and breast milk. Lactoferrin binds with iron, but it is not considered a transporter of iron; instead lactoferrin's role is entirely defense related. Lactoferrin can withhold iron from invading microorganisms. However, *H. pylori*, a cause of gastric ulcer, actually seeks out lactoferrin-bound iron contained in the lining of the stomach. Lactoferrin-bound iron gives *H. pylori* its initial nourishment, enabling the microorganism to bore through the stomach wall, where it will then obtain iron directly from heme.

Free or unbound iron, hemosiderin and free-radical activity

Normally, transferrin is about 25–35 percent saturated with the metal, but when too much iron is present for transferrin to carry, trouble can develop. Transferrin molecules that are heavily saturated lose the ability to tightly bind iron. Unbound or free iron is highly destructive and dangerous. Unbound iron can trigger free-radical activity, which can cause cell death and destroy DNA. Free iron can also provide nourishment for pathogens such as Yersinia, Listeria, and Vibrio bacteria. Many strains of these bacteria are harmless for people with normal iron levels, but when transferrin is highly saturated with iron the invaders can readily multiply to cause disease and death.

Like transferrin, iron-loaded ferritin can also become ineffective. Think of ferritin like a big sink; when this sink gets full, ferritin and its iron can be changed into an insoluble substance called hemosiderin.

Hemosiderin is like rust and can accumulate in cells of the heart, liver, lungs, pancreas, and other organs, restricting their ability to function. For example, when beta cells (insulin-producing cells of the pancreas) are loaded with hemosiderin, these cells become unable to produce or store adequate amounts of the hormone insulin, which results in diabetes.

"Indeed the management of iron in our body has been compared to the handling of fire in our homes. Confinement of fire to the furnace, the fireplace, and the stove provides essential services. Allowing fire to invade the walls of our homes ensures destruction."
—*Eugene Weinberg, 1962*

Unfortunately, excess iron that is not trapped by ferritin or bound to other proteins can catalyze production of free radicals. The latter can depolymerize polysaccharides, cause DNA strand breaks, inactivate enzymes, and initiate lipid peroxidation. Consequences include disease, premature aging, and death.

Iron that is not absorbed

For those with normal iron metabolism, unabsorbed iron (about 90 percent of iron ingested) is managed by enterocytes. These cells become engorged with iron, die, drop off, and are excreted in feces.

References:

Aisen, P., C. Enns, and M. Wessling-Resnick. "Chemistry and Biology of Eukaryotic Iron Metabolism." *International Journal of Biochemistry and Cell Biology* 33 (2001): 940–59.

Ajoika, R. S., J. E. Levy, N. C. Andrews, and J. P. Kushner. "Regulation of Iron Absorption in *HFE* Mutant Mice." *Blood* 100 (2002): 1465–69.

Anderson, G. J., D. M. Frazer, A. T. McKie, and C. D. Vulpe. "The Ceruloplasmin Homolog Hephaestin and the Control of Intestinal Iron Absorption." *Blood Cells, Molecules, and Diseases* 29 (2002): 367–75.

Barrett, J. F. R., P. G. Whittaker, J. G. Williams, and T. Lind. "Absorption of Non-Heme Iron from Food During Normal Pregnancy." *British Medical Journal* 309 (1994): 79–82.

Bendich, A. "Calcium Supplementation and Iron Status of Females." *Nutrition* 17 (2001): 46–51.

Conrad, M. E., J. N. Umbreit, E. G. Moore, L. N. Hainsworth, M. Porubcin, M. J. Simovich, M. T. Nakada, K. Dolan, and M. D. Garrick. "Separate Pathways for Cellular Uptake of Ferric and Ferrous Iron." *American Journal of Physiology & Gastrointestinal Liver Physiology* 279 (2000): G767–74.

Cook, J. D., and M. B. Reddy. "Ascorbic Acid Has a Pronounced Enhancing Effect on the Absorption of Dietary Nonheme Iron When Assessed by Feeding Single Meals to Fasting Subjects." *American Journal of Clinical Nutrition* 73 (2001): 93–98.

Fleming, D. J., K. L. Tucker, P. F. Jacques, G. E. Dallal, P. W. Wilson, and R. J. Wood. "Dietary Factors Associated with the Risk of High Iron Stores in the Elderly Framingham Heart Study Cohort." *American Journal of Clinical Nutrition* 76 (2002): 1375–84.

Ganz, T. "Hepcidin, a Key Regulator of Iron Metabolism and Mediator of Anemia of Inflammation." *Blood* 102 (2003): 783–88.

Garrison, Cheryl, ed. *The Iron Disorders Institute Guide to Anemia.* Nashville, TN: Cumberland House, 2003.

Hallberg, L., and L. Hulthen. "Prediction of Dietary Iron Absorption: An Algorithm for Calculating Absorption and Bioavailability of Dietary Iron." *American Journal of Clinical Nutrition* 71 (2000): 1147–60.

Harrison, S. A, and B. R. Bacon. "Hereditary Hemochromatosis: Update for 2003." *Journal of Hepatology* 38 (2003): S14–S23.

Hellman, N. E., and J. D. Gitlin. "Ceruloplasmin Metabolism and Function." *Annual Review Nutrition* 22 (2002): 439–58.

Hetet, G., I. Devaux, N. Soufir, B. Grandchamp, and C. Beaumont. "Molecular Analyses of Patients with Hyperferritinemia and Normal Serum Iron Values Reveal Both L Ferritin IRE and 3 New Ferroportin (SLC11A3) Mutations." *Blood* 102 (2003): 1904–10.

Knutson, M. D., M. R. Vafa, D. J. Haile, and M. Wessling-Resnick. "Iron Loading and Erythrophagocytosis Increase Ferroportin1 (FPN1) Expression in J774 Macrophages." *Blood* 102 (2003): 4191–97.

Leong, W. I., and B. Lonnerdal. "Hepcidin, the Recently Identified Peptide that Appears to Regulate Iron Absorption." *Journal of Nutrition* 134 (2004): 1–4.

Leong, W. I., C. L. Bowlus, J. Tallkvist, B. Lonnerdal. "DMT1 and FPN1 Expression During Infancy: Developmental Regulation of Iron Absorption." *American Journal of Physiology and Gastrointestinal Liver Physiology* 285 (2003): G1153–61.

Ludwiczek, S., E. Aigner, L. Theurl, and G. Weiss. "Cytokine-Medicated Regulation F Iron Transport in Human Monocytic Cells." *Blood* 101 (2003): 4148–54.

Merryweather-Clarke, A. T., et al. 2003. "Heterozygosity for Novel Hepcidin Mutations May Modify the C282Y Heterozygotes." Poster #80 presented at the Bioiron World Congress, Bethesda, MD.

Roy, C. N., and C. A. Enns. "Iron Homeostasis: New Tales from the Crypt." *Blood* 96 (2000): 4020–27.

Roy, C. N., E. J. Carlson, E. L. Anderson, A. Basava, S. M. Starnes, J. N. Feder, and C. A. Enns. "Interactions of the Ectodomain of

51

HFE with the Transferrin Receptor Are Critical for the Iron Homeostasis in Cells." *Federation of European Biological Society Letters* 484 (2000): 271–74.

Simovich, M., L. N. Hainsworth, P. A. Fields, J. N. Umbreit, and M. E. Conrad. "Localization of the Iron Transport Proteins Mobilferrin and DMT-1 in the Duodenum: The Surprising Role of Mucin." *American Journal of Hematology* 74 (2003): 32–45.

Stuart, K. A., G. J. Anderson, D. M. Frazer, L. W. Powell, M. McCullen, L. M. Fletcher, and D. H. Crawford. "Duodenal Expression of Iron Transport Molecules in Untreated Haemochromatosis Subjects." *Gut* 52 (2003): 953–59.

Thomas, C., and P. S. Oates. "Ferroportin/IREG-1/MTP-1/SLC40A1 Modulates the Uptake of Iron at the Apical Membrane of Enterocytes." *Gut* 53 (2004): 44–49.

Umbreit, J. N., M. E. Conrad, E. G. Moore, and L. F. Latour. "Iron Absorption and Cellular Transport: The Mobilferrin/Paraferritin Paradigm." *Seminars in Hematology* 35 (1998): 13–26.

Weinberg, E. D. "Iron and Susceptibility to Infectious Disease." *Science* 184 (1974): 952–56.

———. "The Therapeutic Potential of Human Lactoferrin." *Expert Opinion on Investigational Drugs* 12 (2003): 841–51.

4

Liver, Spleen, Gallbladder, Pancreas

"Of all the organs, the liver serves as the most important 'landfill' for the disposal of excessive iron. In untreated HHC, for example, the liver iron concentration reaches 50–100 times that of normal figures. A similar proportional increase occurs in the pancreas. . . . The iron deposits are mainly in the form of hemosiderin."

—*T. H. Bothwell et al.*

The liver serves as a principal depository for dangerous quantities of iron. Hepatic iron overload can be seen in conditions such as Type I hemochromatosis (*HFE* related), juvenile hemochromatosis (types a and b), African siderosis, neonatal hemochromatosis, beta-thalassemia, enzymopathies G6PD and pyruvate kinase, sickle cell disease, CDAII, GRACILE, PCT, cystic fibrosis, viral hepatitis B or C, NASH, and alcoholism. Depending upon the disorder, liver iron distribution can include the Kupffer cells, hepatocytes, and hepatic stellate cells, and involve multiple subcellular organelles such as the mitochondria, lysosomes, and smooth endoplasmic reticulum.

In conditions of chronic hemolysis or repeated transfusion, for example, hepatic hemosiderin in Kupffer cells is seen. With hereditary hemochromatosis, a progressive accumulation of the metal in hepatocytes causes these cells to lose their ability to function and to survive. The affected areas are invaded by connective tissue cells and become fibrotic. As damage continues,

Iron-loading conditions that lead to liver damage
Hereditary hemochromatosis
Thalassemia, sickle cell anemia, splenectomy or chronic blood transfusion
African siderosis
Porphyria cutanea tarda, cystic fibrosis
Decompartmentalization of iron due to hemolytic conditions or hepatitis
Deficiency in quantity of transferrin or ceruloplasmin
Defective functioning of haptoglobin Hp2-2

the normal architecture of the liver and its blood flow are disrupted, leading to cirrhosis. Patients with hemochromatosis are at twentyfold risk of liver cancer. When cirrhosis is present at the time of diagnosis of hemochromatosis the risk of liver cancer can be as high as two-hundred-fold.

Cirrhotic tissue provides a fertile ground for the initiation and promotion of cancer cell growth. Iron is a well-recognized mutagen and can cause development of liver cancer even in nonfibrotic tissue. Therefore, prompt treatment of any liver iron excess, even when mild, is prudent and integral to the patient's continued good health.

"The liver is a principal target for iron toxicity because it is chiefly responsible for taking up and storing excessive amounts of iron."
—*H. L. Bonkovsky and R. W. Lambrecht*

Persons with untreated iron overload have elevated values for transferrin iron saturation percentage (Tsat%) and serum ferritin, and they often have increased levels of serum transaminases. It is important to recognize, however, that desaturation of transferrin occurs in patients during inflammatory episodes.

In hemochromatosis, iron consistently accumulates in hepatocytes. In long-standing cases of HHC, probably as a result of hepatocyte death, iron begins to also appear in the Kupffer cells. Greater aggregation of iron occurs at the outer areas of the liver lobules than in their center. In the other iron-loading conditions, both hepatocytes and macrophages (Kupffer cells) throughout the course of the disease process become iron loaded. In patients with undiagnosed HHC, the enzymes that leak from hepatocytes into serum usually are only moderately elevated (less than 2.5 times normal). Detection of this modest elevation might suggest to the clinician that there exists only a mild chronic hepatitis. Unfortunately, unless transferrin iron saturation percentage and serum ferritin values are obtained, the diagnosis of HHC will be missed and the livers of the patients will continue to deteriorate.

The high incidence of cancer in patients who have cirrhosis due to iron is greater than in persons who have other causes of cirrhosis. For example, although copper (like iron) catalyzes formation of reactive radicals, patients with copper-induced cirrhosis rarely develop liver cancer. Unlike iron, copper is unable to function as an essential nutrient for the growth of cancer cells.

Additional research projects which investigate other dangerous aspects of liver iron loading are needed. As an example, in a group of 161 iron-loaded patients who were not homozygous for the C282Y HHC gene mutation, 52 percent developed fatty liver and resistance to insulin.

Many of the early studies of tissue iron excess centered around the reticuloendothelial system (RES) and intestinal absorption. Initial findings strengthen the suggestion that hemochromatosis is due to a faulty regulation system caused by mutations of *HFE* whereby inappropriate signals are sent to the villi of the intestinal mucosa from crypt cells. With the discovery of unique transporters DMT1 and ferroportin, iron absorption and transport are better understood. Ferroportin is increased in patients with hepatic iron overload and hepcidin is depressed in iron overload. Hepcidin is produced in the liver, which brings new emphasis to the role of the liver in iron regulation.

Hepcidin

Hepcidin is a small peptide (a chain of 25 amino acids so named because the compound is produced mainly by liver cells (hep) and can weakly inhibit growth of bacteria and yeasts in laboratory culture (cidin)). At the start of an invasion, a cytokine called interleukin-6 signals the patient's hepatocytes to produce hepcidin. The peptide circulates in the bloodstream and acts at two sites: it suppresses (1) duodenal cell absorption of dietary iron, and (2) macrophage release of iron (from recycled red blood cells). The second action then causes an increase in ferritin synthesis within the macrophages. Because hepcidin is a small peptide molecule, it is excreted into urine by the kidneys. Nevertheless, as long as the invasion emergency persists, the patient's hepatocytes continue to form more hepcidin under the influence of interleukin-6.

Remarkably, hepcidin synthesis is increased not only in response to invasion but also to iron overload, and production of the hormone is decreased in iron deficiency. Hepcidin levels decrease in mice fed a low-iron diet and increase in mice fed a high-iron diet; these findings support the role of hepcidin as a signal that limits intestinal iron absorption. In humans and in mice with hemochromatosis, hepcidin synthesis is severely depressed. Thus in hemochromatosis, not only is excessive iron absorbed in the duodenum but also macrophages fail to retain the surplus metal.

Hepcidin is decreased in *HFE* knockout mice, which demonstrates characteristics of iron overload as in hemochromatosis patients. Hence, *HFE* is suggested to act as a regulator of hepcidin expression. Furthermore, persons who are heterozygote carriers of both an HHC gene mutation and a hepcidin gene mutation may have an increase in clinical problems.

It is also possible for hepcidin to be overproduced. An example is seen in patients with adenomatous tumors of the liver. The tumor can form an excessive amount of hepcidin, leading to decreased absorption of dietary iron and increased retention of macrophage iron. Surgical removal of the tumor restores normal iron management.

Iron overload with concurrent disease

Age, male sex, chronic alcohol abuse, and concurrent disease such as viral hepatitis, AIDS, porphyria cutanea tarda, diabetes, cirrhosis, cystic fibrosis, cancer, or non-alcoholic steatohepatitis (NASH) dramatically increase liver morbidity and mortality. For example, except in hemochromatosis, iron-loaded livers are very susceptible to infection by tuberculosis pathogens (which require iron-loaded macrophages in order to grow in the body). In 1929, in 601 autopsies from a population that contained persons with African siderosis, a strong association between hepatic iron loading and tubercular liver infections was observed. Much more recently, it has become known that patients with AIDS develop iron-loaded livers. In autopsies of 78 persons who had died with AIDS, 25 had very high liver iron and 16 of these had hepatic tubercular infection.

Conditions Worsened by Iron-Loaded Liver
■ Alcoholic liver disease
■ Non-alcoholic liver steatohepatitis
■ Chronic viral hepatitis
■ Porphyria cutanea tarda
■ Alpha 1-antitrypsin deficiency
■ End-stage liver disease

Source. H. L Bonkovsky and R W Lambrecht

Viral hepatitis C is found in about half of the patients with porphyria cutanea tarda (PCT) and may influence porphyrin metabolism in these patients. Though the pathogenesis of PCT is not well understood, it is known that excess iron contributes to the overproduction of uroporphyrin.

PCT is a condition that manifests in blisters on the dorsal side of the hand. According to porphyrin metabolism expert Herbert Bonkovsky, iron participates in the development of PCT in three ways. The metal serves as a catalyst in the "formation of reactive oxygen species, which can enhance uroporphyrin formation by increasing the rate at which uroporphyrinogen is oxidized to urophophyrin. Iron may also act indirectly to inhibit uroporphyrinogen decarboxylase activity by enhancing the formation of nonporphyrin products of porphyrinogen oxidation that are themselves direct inhibitors of the enzyme. Finally, iron can act to increase urophorphyrin production by inducing delta-aminolevulinic acid synthase, thus increasing the amount of delta-aminolevulinic acid, the precursor to uroporphyrinogen, present in the cell." Persons with PCT can be helped with therapeutic phlebotomies to reduce iron levels.

Viral hepatitis C

Persons with hemochromatosis (HHC) plus viral hepatitis C (HCV) have been observed to develop advanced fibrosis/cirrhosis at a younger age and at a lower level iron concentration compared to HHC patients without hepatitis. In a recent study, the mean age of patients with either HHC or HCV was 57 years, whereas that of patients with both conditions was 43 years.

In two studies patients on low-iron diets had a reduction in serum transaminases (indicating liver recovery) as well as a lowering of serum ferritin and transferrin iron saturation. Hepatic iron deposits in chronic viral hepatitis patients are common and associated with activation of hepatic stellate cells. The activated hepatic stellate cell (HSC) is central to liver fibrosis.

Alcohol

Patients with iron overload have increased susceptibility to liver cell damage by alcohol. Hepatic cell uptake of iron may increase in the presence of alcohol. Twenty to 30 percent of alcoholics absorb twice the amount of iron from the diet as nonusers of alcohol. Furthermore, metabolism of alcohol can result in release of the metal from ferritin to result in enhanced production of reactive radicals.

The increased iron levels can cause hemochromatosis, a condition characterized by the formation of iron deposits throughout the body (e.g., in the liver, pancreas, heart, joints, anterior pituitary). Moreover, patients whose chronic alcohol consumption and alcoholic siderosis have led to liver cirrhosis are at increased risk for liver cancer.

Approximately 20–30 percent of alcohol misusers acquire up to twice the amount of dietary iron as do nonabusers of alcohol. These iron-loaded individuals are at increased risk for the same diseases as are persons with hemochromatosis.
—idInsight, *"Alcohol: How Much Is Safe?"*,
Third Quarter, 2000

Another complication in severe alcoholics is sideroblastic anemia. Approximately one-third of these patients contain ringed sideroblasts in their bone marrow. Alcohol may cause sideroblastic anemia by interfering with the activity of an enzyme that mediates a critical step in hemoglobin synthesis. Abstinence can reverse this effect. The ringed sideroblasts generally disappear from the bone marrow within 5–10 days, and RBC production resumes. In fact, excess numbers of young RBCs called reticulocytes can accumulate temporarily in the blood, indicating higher-than-normal RBC production.

A study conducted by Dr. Charles Lieber of Mr. Sinai School of Medicine in New York observed that drinking even moderate amounts of alcohol could lead to cirrhosis. In his study, participants were given diets supplemented with minerals (including iron) along with a daily dose of alcohol that was less than the amount needed to produce intoxication. After 18 days, subjects developed an eightfold increase in liver fat, a precondition of cirrhosis.

Non-alcoholic steatohepatitis (NASH)

Nearly half of the patients with NASH have iron-loaded livers. The majority of NASH patients are obese, hyperlipidemic, and insulin resistant (type II diabetes). Italian investigators studied 40 patients with hepatic steatosis and *HFE* mutations who neither abused alcohol nor had viral hepatitis or inflammation. They found that "NASH was significantly associated with the presence of metabolic alterations, the C282Y mutation, and severity of fibrosis." Unlike hereditary hemochromatosis, NASH patients present with elevated serum ferritin but normal transferrin iron saturation percentage and usually normal ceruloplasmin levels. These findings assist in the early diagnosis and treatment of NASH. Moreover, phlebotomy therapy has yielded improvement in insulin responsiveness and serum liver enzyme level.

The spleen

The spleen serves as the principle organ in the recycling of iron from spent red blood cells. In conditions of chronic hemolysis such as beta-thalassemia, sickle cell anemia, congenital dyserythropoietic anemia, or G6PD the spleen becomes overwhelmed and surgical removal may become necessary to stop chronic hemolysis.

In contrast, hereditary hemochromatosis spleens do not accumulate excessive iron because the tissue is mainly comprised of macrophages. Stainable iron is usually present in the spleen but in lesser amounts than in the liver and pancreas. The splenic capsule frequently contains iron deposits that are calcified. In autopsies of newborns with neonatal hemchromatosis, there is little stainable iron in the spleen, lymph, or bone marrow but significant amounts in the pancreas, thyroid, and the liver.

The gallbladder

The exact mechanism of how the gallbladder is affected in patients with iron overload is not widely studied. Gallbladders of HHC patients are often removed because of cholelithiasis. According to the Iron Disorders Institute Patient Database, some HHC patients who have had their gallbladders removed report that the stones are "variable in size and black in color," possibly indicating the presence of iron in the bile. In a 1996 US Centers for Disease Control and Prevention survey where 2851 hemochromatosis patients responded, liver and gallbladder disease was reported by 9.5 percent of males age 17–39 years and 5.2 percent in females of the same age range; 17.7 percent in males and 20.0 percent in females age 40–59, and 17.5 percent and 23.2 percent of females age 60–84. Thalassemic and CDAII patients likewise suffer from a high incidence of gallstones.

With specific attention to the sphincter of Oddi, French scientists examined 109 consecutive autopsies. These investigators concluded that chronic pancreatitis (which can be a consequence of excessive iron or chronic alcohol abuse) was more frequently associated with an abnormal sphincter of Oddi. At the University of Milan, 350 patients with alcoholic cirrhosis and hemochromatosis were studied. The incidence of cholelithiasis (gallstones) was 3 times higher in these patients than in nonalcoholic, iron-normal controls.

The pancreas

Iron deposits in the pancreas are predominantly localized in the tissue that secretes digestive enzymes. However, impairment of cells in this tissue rarely occurs. Rather, the accumulation of iron in the beta (insulin-producing cells) results in impaired glucose tolerance, as cited in chapter 5.

The normal pancreas secretes bicarbonate ions into the duodenum to result in elevation of the pH value with consequent cessation of excessive nonheme iron absorption into the bloodstream. However, persons whose pancreatic secretions are impaired, such as those with pancreatitis or cystic fibrosis, absorb increased quantities of iron.

References:

Ballas, S. K. "Iron Overload Is a Determinant of Morbidity and Mortality In Adult Patients with Sickle Cell Disease." *Seminars in Hematology* 38 (2001): 30–36.

Barton, J. C., and C. Q. Edwards, eds. *Genetics, Pathophysiology, Diagnosis and Treatment.* Cambridge: Cambridge University Press, 2000.

Barton, J. C., S. V. Rao, N. M. Pereira, T. Gelbart, E. Beutler, C. A. Rivers, and R. T. Acton. "Juvenile Hemochromatosis in the Southeastern United States: A Report of Seven Cases in Two Kinships." *Blood Cells, Molecules, and Diseases* 29 (2002): 104–15.

Beutler, E., T. Gelbart, and W. Miller. "Severe Jaundice in a Patient with a Previously Undescribed Glucose-6-Phosphate Dehydrogenase (G6PD) Mutation and Gilbert Syndrome." *Blood Cells, Molecules, and Diseases* 28 (2002): 104–7.

Blisard, K. S., and S. A. Bartow. "Neonatal Hemochromatosis." *Human Pathology* 17 (1986): 376–83.

Bonkovsky, H. L. "Iron and the Liver." *American Journal of Medical Science* 301 (1991): 32–43.

Bonkovsky, H. L., and G. F. Barnard. "The Porphyrias." *Current Treatment Options in Gastroenterology* 3 (2000): 487–500.

Bonkovsky, H. L., and R. W. Lambrecht. "Iron-induced Liver Injury." *Clinical Liver Disease* 4 (2000): vi–vii, 409–29.

Bothwell, T. H., R. W. Charlton, and A. G. Motulsky. "Hemochromatosis." In *Metabolic Basis of Inherited Diseases,* C. R. Scriver, A. L. Beaudet, W. S. Sly, and D. Valle, eds., 1433–62. 6th ed. New York: McGraw Information Sciences, 1989.

Bralet, M. P., J. M. Regimbeau, P. Pineau, S. Dubois, G. Loas, F. Degos, D. Valla, J. Belghiti, C. Degott, and B. Terris. "Hepatocellular Carcinoma Occurring in Nonfibrotic Liver: Epidemiologic and Histopathologic Analysis of 80 French Cases." *Hepatology* 32 (2000): 200–204.

Camaschella, C., A. Roetto, and M. De Gobbi. "Juvenile Hemochromatosis." *Seminars in Hematology* 39 (2002): 242–48.

Colombo, C., P. M. Battezzati, A. Crosignani, A. Morabito, D. Costantini, R. Padoan, A. Giunta. "Liver Disease in Cystic Fibrosis: A Prospective Study on Incidence, Risk Factors, and Outcome." *Hepatology* 36 (2002): 1374–82.

Conte, D., D. Barisani, C. Mandelli, S. Fargion, A. L. Fracanzani, L. Cesarini, P. Bodini, S. Pistoso, and P. A. Bianchi. "Prevalence of Cholelithiasis in Alcoholic and Genetic Haemochromatotic Cirrhosis." *Alcohol and Alcoholism* 28 (1993): 581–84.

DiBisceglie, A. M., H. L. Bonkovsky, S. Chopra, S. Flamm, R. K. Reddy, N. Grace, P. Killenberg, C. Hunt, C. Tamburro, A. S. Tavill, R. Ferguson, E. Krawitt, B. Banner, and B. R. Bacon. "Iron Reduction as an Adjuvant to Interferon Therapy in Patients with Chronic Hepatitis C Who Have Previously Not Responded to Interferon: A Multicenter, Prospective, Randomized, Controlled Trial." *Hepatology* 32 (2000): 135–38.

Diwakar, V., L. Pearson, and S. Beath. "Liver Disease in Children with Cystic Fibrosis." *Paediatric Respiratory Review* 2 (2001): 340–49.

Drobnik, J. R. Schwartz. *eMedicine Journal,* 2002. http://www.emedicine.com/derm/topic878.htm.

Ellervik, C., T. Mandrup-Poulsen, B. G. Nordestgaard, L. E. Larsen, M. Appleyard, M. Frandsen, P. Petersen, P. Schlichting,

T. Saermark, A. Tybjaerg-Hansen, and H. Birgens. "Prevalence of Hereditary Haemochromatosis in Late-Onset Type I Diabetes Mellitus: A Retrospective Study." *The Lancet* 358 (2001): 1405–9.

Evans, C. D., K. A. Oien, R. N. MacSween, and P. R. Mills. "Non-alcoholic Steatohepatitis: A Common Cause of Progressive Chronic Liver Injury?" *Journal of Clinical Pathology* 55 (2002): 689–92.

Facchini, F. S., N. W. Hua, and R. A. Stoohs. "Effect of Iron Depletion in Carbohydrate-Intolerant Patients with Clinical Evidence of Non-Alcoholic Fatty Liver Disease." *Gastroenterology* 122 (2002): 931–39.

Fargion, S., M. Mattioli, A. L. Fracanzani, M. Sampietro, D. Tavazzi, P. Fociani, E. Taioli, L. Valenti, and G. Fiorelli. "Hyperferritinemia, Iron Overload, and Multiple Metabolic Alterations Identify Patients at Risk for Nonalcoholic Steatohepatitis." *American Journal of Gastroenterology* 96 (2001): 2448–55.

Felitti, V. "Hemochromatosis: A Common, Rarely Diagnosed Disease." *The Permanente Journal* 3 (1999): 10–22.

Fleming, R. E., K. A. Ahmad, J. R. Ahmann, et al. 2003. "Decreased Liver Hepcidin Expression in the *HFE* Knockout Mouse." Poster #176 presented at the Bioiron World Congress, Washington, DC.

Fleming, R. E., and W. S. Sly. "Mechanisms of Iron Accumulation in Hereditary Hemochromatosis." *Annual Review of Physiology* 64 (2002): 663–80.

Ford, E. S., and M. E. Cogswill. "Diabetes and Serum Ferriitn Concentrations Among U.S. Adults." *Diabetes Care* 22 (1999): 1978–83.

Frazer, D. M., K. R. Bridle, S. J. Wilkins, et al. 2003. Failure of Hepcidin Upregulation in *HFE*-associated Haemochromatosis Implicates the Liver in the Regulation of Body Iron Homeostasis. Podium # 25 at the Bioiron World Congress, Washington, DC.

Ganz, T. "Hepcidin, a Key Regulator of Iron Metabolism and Mediator of Anemia of Inflammation." *Blood* 102 (2003): 783–88.

Guyader, D., C. Jacquelinet, R. Moirand, B. Turlin, M. H. Mendler, J. Chaperon, V. David, P. Brissot, P. Adams, and Y. Deugnier. "Noninvasive Prediction of Fibrosis in C282Y Homozygous Hemochromatosis." *Gastroenterology* 115 (1998): 929–36.

Israel, J. L., K. A. McGlynn, H. W. L. Hann, and B. S. Blumberg. "Iron-related Markers in Liver Cancer." In *Iron in Immunity, Cancer and Inflammation*, edited by M. de Sousa and J. H. Brock, 301–16. Chichester, NY: Wiley, 1989.

Iwasa, M., M. Kaito, J. Ikoma, Y. Kobayashi, Y. Tnaka, K. Higuchi, K. Takeushi, K. Iwata, S. Watanabe, and Y. Adachi. "Dietary Iron Restriction Improves Aminotransferase Levels in Chronic Hepatitis C Patients." *Hepato-Gastroenterology* 49 (2002): 529–31.

Katz R., A. Goldfarb, M. Muggia, and Z. Gimmon. "Unique Features of Laparoscopic Cholecystectomy in Beta-Thalassemic Patients." *Surgery Laparoscopic Endoscopy & Urcutaneous Technique* 13 (2003): 318–21.

Kew, M. D. "Pathogenesis of Hepatocellular Carcinoma in Hereditary Hemochromatosis Occurrence in Noncirrhotic Patients." *Hepatology* 11 (1990): 1086–87.

Lambrecht, R. W., and H. L. Bonkovsky. "Hemochromatosis and Porphyria." *Seminars in Gastrointestinal Disease* 13 (2002): 109–19.

Lamoril, J., C. Andant, L. Gouya, E. Malonova, B. Grandchamp, P. Martasek, J. C. Deybach, and H. Puy. "Hemochromatosis (*HFE*) and Transferrin Receptor-1 (TfR-I) Genes in Sporadic Porphyria Cutanea Tarda (PCT)." *Cell Molecular Biology* 48 (2002): 33–41.

Larson, A. M., S. L. Taylor, D. Bauermeister, L. Rosoff Jr, and K. V. Kowdley. "Pilot Study of the Relationship between Histologic Progression and Hepatic Iron Concentration in Chronic Hepatitis C." *Journal of Clinical Gastroenterology* 37 (2003): 406–11.

Lauret, E., M. Rodriguez, S. Gonzalez, A. Linares, A. Lopez-Vasquez, J. Martinez-Borra, L. Rodrigo, and C. Lopez-Larrea. "*HFE* Gene Mutations in Alcoholic and Virus-Related Cirrhotic Patients with Hepatocellular Carcinoma." *American Journal of Gastroenterology* 97 (2002): 1016–21.

Lieber, C. S. "Biochemical and Molecular Basis of Alcohol-Induced Injury to Liver and Other Tissues." *New England Journal Medicine* 319 (1988): 1639–50.

MacDonald, G. A., and L. W. Powell. "More Clues to the Relationship Between Iron and Steatosis: An Association with Insulin Resistance?" *Gastroenterology* 117 (1999): 1241–44.

Martin, E. D., P. Bedossa, and P. Oudinot. "Lesions of the Area of Oddi's Sphincter: Incidence and Association with Biliary and Pancreatic Lesions in a Series of 109 Autopsies." *Gastroenterology Clinical Biology* 11 (1987): 574–80.

Merryweather-Clarke, A. T., M. G. Zaahl, and E. Cadet, et al. 2003. "Heterozygosity for Novel Hepcidin Mutations May Modify the Phenotype of *HFE* C282Y Heterozygotes." Poster #50 presented at the Bioiron World Congress, Washington, DC.

Moyo, V. M., R. Makunike, I. T. Gangaidzo, V. R. Gordeuk, C. E. McLaren, H. Khumalo, T. Saungweme, T. Rouault, C. F. Kiire. "African Iron Overload and Hepatocellular Carcinoma." *European Journal of Haematology* 60 (1998): 28–34.

Muckenthaler, M., C. N. Roy, A. O. Custodio, B. Minana, J. deGraaf, L. K. Montross, N. C. Andrews, and M. W. Hentze. "Regulatory Defects in Liver and Intestine Implicate Abnormal Hepcidin and Cybrd1 Expression in Mouse Hemochromatosis." *Nature Genetics* 34 (2003): 102–27.

Nicolas, G., L. Viatte, M. Dennoun, et al. "Hepcidin, a New Iron Regulatory Peptide." *Blood, Cells, Molecules and Diseases* 29 (2002): 1327–35.

Nicolas, G., L. Viatte, D. Q. Lou, et al. "Constitutive Hepcidin Expression Prevents Iron Overload in a Mouse Model of Hemochromatosis. *Nature Genetics* 34 (2003): 97–101.

Niederau, C., R. Fischer, A. Sonnenberg, W. Stremmel, H. J. Trampisch, and G. Strohmeyer. "Survival and Causes of Death in Cirrhotic and in Noncirrhotic Patients with Primary Hemochromatosis." *New England Journal of Medicine* 313 (1985): 1256–62.

Nittis, T., and J. D. Gitlin. "The Copper-Iron Connection: Hereditary Aceruloplasminemia." *Seminars in Hematology* 39 (2002): 282–89.

Stremmel, W., H. D. Riedel, C. Niederau, and G. Strohmeyer. "Pathogenesis of Genetic Haemochromatosis." *European Journal of Clinical Investigation* 23 (1993): 321–29.

Tandon, N., V. Thakur, R. Kumar, C. Gupton, and S. K. Sarin. "Beneficial Influence of an Indigenous Low-iron Diet on Serum Indicators of Iron Status in Patients with Chronic Liver Disease." *British Journal of Nutrition* 83 (2000): 235–39.

Thakerngpol, K., S. Fucharoen, P. Boonyaphipat, K. Srisook, S. Sahaphong, V. Vathanophas, and T. Stitnimankarn. "Liver Injury Due to Iron Overload in Thalassemia: Histopathologic and Ultrastructural Studies." *BioMetals* 9 (1996): 177–83.

Thorburn, D., G. Curry, R. Spooner, E. Spence, K. Oien, D. Halls, R. Fox, E. A. B. McCruden, R. N. M. MacSween, and P. R. Mills. "The Role of Iron and Haemochromatosis Gene Mutations in the Progression of Liver Disease in Chronic Hepatitis C." *Gut* 50 (2002): 248–52.

Tonz, O., S. Weiss, H. W. Strahm, and E. Ross. "Iron Absorption in Cystic Fibrosis." *The Lancet* ii (1965): 1096–99.

Turlin, B., F. Juguet, R. Moirand, B. Turlin, F. Juguet, D. Le Quilleuc,

O. Loreal, J. P. Campion, B. Launois, M. P. Ramee, P. Brissot, and Y. Deugnier. "Increased Liver Iron Stores in Patients with Hepato-Cellular Carcinoma Developed on a Noncirrhotic Liver." *Hepatology* 22 (1995): 446–50.

von Herbay, A., H. de Groot, U. Hegi, W. Stremmel, G. Strohmeyer, and H. Sies. "Low Vitamin E Content in Plasma of Patients with Alcoholic Liver Disease, Hemochromatosis and Wilson's Disease." *Journal of Hepatology* 20 (1994): 41–46.

Weinberg, E. D. "Iron Withholding: A Defense Against Infection and Neoplasia." *Physiological Reviews* 64 (1984): 65–102.

———. "The Role of Iron in Cancer." *European Journal of Cancer Prevention* 5 (1996): 19–36.

Witte, D. L., W. H. Crosby, C. Q. Edwards, V. F. Fairbanks, and F. A. Mitros. "Hereditary Hemochromatosis." *Clinica Chimica Acta* 245 (1996): 139–200.

5

Endocrine System: Pituitary, Pancreas, Thyroid, Parathyroid

"Despite its frequency and effect on the endocrine system, haemochromatosis has attracted surprisingly little attention in endocrinology and
fertility textbooks."

—M. J. Tweed and J. M. Roland

In persons who have any of the three classical disorders of iron
overload (African siderosis, beta-thalassemia, hemochromatosis), the metal frequently accumulates in specific sites of various
endocrine glands. As cells in these sites acquire iron, they lose
their specialized functions and die. Most commonly attacked
by iron are those cells in the anterior pituitary gland that produce growth hormone and gonadal-stimulating hormones.

Anterior pituitary

Cells of the anterior pituitary gland are remarkably sensitive
to iron. In culture, as little as 1.0 µM iron can completely prevent growth. Even a moderate amount of iron deposition in the
gland, as detected by magnetic resonance imaging, interferes
with its endocrine functions. At autopsy of iron-loaded patients,
anterior pituitary tissue, especially the gonadotrophic region,
usually contains stainable iron, sometimes in massive amounts.
In contrast, the testis, even when atrophic, usually contains no
iron deposits. In thalassemia, in which iron accumulation begins
in childhood, patients commonly have pubertal and growth
delay or failure to thrive. In each of the iron-loading disorders,

young male adults often have impotence and bilateral testicular atrophy; young female adults have amenorrhea, infertility, and premature menopause.

In thalassemic children, an early start in chelation therapy is essential to enable the patients to attain normal pubertal development. In patients who have bone marrow transplants to remedy the thalassemic disorder (but whose pituitary functions had been depressed by iron), administration of gonadotrophins and growth hormone can be therapeutically useful.

When investigating endocrine causes of infertility in adults, hemochromatosis (HHC) must be included in the differential diagnosis. In HHC, an early diagnosis is important since aggressive phlebotomy therapy can restore some degree of pituitary gonadal and reproductive function. Patients with more established hemochromatosis may be helped with phlebotomy, plus testosterone in males and gonadotrophins in females.

Pancreas

In all disorders of iron overload, beta cells in the pancreas that function to produce insulin are assaulted by the metal. Thus diabetes mellitus is a common manifestation. For instance, in a group of 82 patients with beta-thalassemia, 16 (20 percent) had diabetes and 7 (9 percent) had impaired glucose tolerance. In 34 patients with HHC, 12 (35 percent) required exogenous insulin, 4 (12 percent) used oral hypoglycemic drugs, and 2 (6 percent) controlled the disease with diet. In hemochromatosis patients, the pancreas can acquire an iron load of as much as 50 times normal. The insulin-producing beta cells are especially sensitive to the metal. Thus it is not surprising that suppression of insulin synthesis is quite frequently observed. In fact, in an early description of the disorder, the term "bronze diabetes" was employed. Moreover, iron-induced insulin resistance often preceeds impaired secretion of the hormone. Diabetes is present in up to 60 percent of HHC patients, is often the initial manifestation of the HHC disorder, and, when present, almost always preceeds the diagnosis of HHC. In patients with ß-thalassemia, diabetes can also be a complication. In a set of 89 patients, impaired glucose tolerance was identified in 8.5 percent and diabetes in 19.5

percent. In African siderosis as well as in transfusional siderosis, the importance of iron loading as a risk factor for diabetes is well established.

In a study of a nonselected population of US adults, 714 had diabetes; 7861 were normal. Of the diabetics, 36 percent had elevated serum ferritin (>300 ng/mL in men, >150 ng/mL in women). Of the normal persons, only 12 percent had elevated ferritin levels. In a group of 716 Danish persons who developed type I diabetes after age 30, those homozygous for the C282Y gene mutation were 4.6 fold more likely to have developed the pancreatic disease than were the wild type normals.

In a set of 1013 middle-aged men in Finland, blood glucose and serum insulin concentration (a measure of insulin resistance) were elevated in persons with serum ferritin greater than 150 ng/mL. Iron also can be a risk factor for development of noninsulin-dependent type II diabetes. In one study, for example, 28 patients with increased serum ferritin (but negative for C282Y mutation) were split into two sets. One set served as the control; persons in the other set were phlebotomized 3 times during a 6-week period. In the de-ironed group, insulin resistance was significantly decreased.

Similarly, in a study of 30 vegetarians and 30 meat-eaters, mean serum ferritin and insulin resistance were nearly twice as high in those who ate meat. Phlebotomies of 6 of the meat eaters lowered serum ferritin and insulin resistance to the levels observed in the vegetarians. Moreover, in a set of 17 patients with non-alcoholic fatty liver disease, quantitative phlebotomy resulted in 40–55 percent reduction in plasma insulin concentration (an indication of lowered insulin resistance). In a 12-year study of 38,394 males aged 40–75, 1168 developed type II diabetes. Ingestion of heme iron from red meat was significantly associated with development of the disease.

Iron deposits in the pancreas are predominantly localized in the tissue that secretes digestive enzymes. However, impairment of cells in this tissue site rarely occurs. Rather, the accumulation of iron in the beta (insulin-producing) cells results in impaired glucose tolerance and, in many cases, a diabetic condition. The latter differs from type I and type II diabetes and might more correctly be termed "siderosis diabetes." Moreover,

FERRITIN

elevated in persons with diabetic conditions

Condition	Gender	Number of Persons	% with Elevated Serum Ferritin
Normal	Men	3,732	12.0
	Women	4,129	11.5
Impaired Glucose Tolerance	Men	416	17.8
	Women	285	29.7
Previously Diagnosed Diabetes	Men	252	35.9
	Women	362	34.9
Newly Diagnosed Diabetes	Men	160	46.3
	Women	144	51.1

Source: E. S. Ford and M. E. Cogswell

in siderosis, insulin resistance commonly occurs. In a group of 30 healthy vegetarians and 30 healthy meat-eaters, the mean serum ferritin of the former was 35 ng/mL, the latter 72 ng/mL. The mean fasting blood glucose level in the vegetarians was 74 mg/dL; in the meat-eaters, 124 mg/dL (values between 115 and 139 mg/dL indicate impaired glucose tolerance).

Thyroid and parathyroid

As in the pituitary and pancreas, iron loading occurs also in the thyroid gland. In HHC, accumulation of iron up to 25 times above normal has been observed and hypothyroidism is more common than in the general population. In patients with ß-thalassemia, exposure to iodide has been reported to result in development of subclinical hypothyroidism.

Damage to the parathyroid gland by excessive iron also has been noted in a set of 210 untreated hemochromatosis patients. One-third had an increase in serum parathyroid hormone fragments. The level of these fragments was correlated positively with elevated serum ferritin concentration. Furthermore, the extent of parathyroid damage was apparently associated with appearance of osteoarticular lesions.

References:

Alexandribes, T., N. Georgopoulus, S. Yarmenitis, and A. G. Vagenakis. "Increased Sensitivity to the Inhibitory Effect of Excess Iodide on Thyroid Function in Patients with Beta-Thalassemia Major and Iron Overload and the Subsequent Development of Hypothyroidism." *European Journal of Endocrinology* 143 (2000): 319–25.

Berkovitch, M., T. Bistritzer, S. D. Milone, K. Periman, W. Kucharczyk, and N. F. Olivieri. "Iron-Deposition in the Anterior Pituitary in Homozygous Beta-Thalassemia: MRI Evaluation and Correlation with Gonadal Function." *Journal of Pediatric Endocrinology and Metabolism* 13 (2000): 179–84.

Bothwell, T. H., R. W. Charlton, and A. G. Motulsky. "Hemochromatosis." In *The Metabolic Basis of Inherited Diseases,* C. R. Scriver, A. L. Beaudet, W. S. Sly, and D. Valle, eds., 1411–62. 6th ed. New York: McGraw Information Sciences, 1989.

Bronspiegel-Weintrob, N., N. F. Olivieri, B. Tyier, D. F. Andrews, M. H. Freedman, and F. J. Holland. "Effect of Age at the Start of Iron Chelation Therapy on Gonadal Function in ß-thalassemia Major." *New England Journal of Medicine* 323 (1990): 713–19.

Chern, J. P., K. H. Lin, M. Y. Lu, D. T. Lin, K. S. Lin, J. D. Chen, and C. C. Fu. "Abnormal Glucose Tolerance in Transferrin-Dependent Beta-Thalassemia Patients." *Diabetes Care* 24 (2001): 850–54.

DeSanctis, V. "Growth and Puberty and Its Management in Thalassemia." *Hormone Research* 58, suppl. 1 (2002): 72–79.

Eby, J. E., H. Sato, and D. A. Sirbasku. "Apotransferrin Stimulation of Thyroid Hormone Dependent Rat Pituitary Tumor Cell Growth in Serum-Free Chemically Defined Medium: Role of Fe(II) Chelation." *Journal of Cellular Physiology* 156 (1993): 588–600.

Edwards, C. Q., T. M. Kelly, G. Ellwein, and K. P. Kushner. "Thyroid Disease in Hemochromatosis: Increased Incidence in Homozygous Men." *Archives of Internal Medicine* 143 (1983): 1890–93.

Ellervik, C., T. Mandrup-Poulson, B. G. Nordestgaard, L. E. Larsen, M. Appleyard, M. Frandsen, P. Peterson, P. Schlichting, T. Saermark,

A. Tybjaerg-Hansen, and H. Birgens. "Prevalence of Hereditary Haemochromatosis in Late-Onset Type I Diabetes Mellitus: A Retrospective Study." *The Lancet* 358 (2001): 1405–9.

Facchini, F. S., N. W. Hua, and R. A. Stoohs. "Effect of Iron Depletion in Carbohydrate-Intolerant Patients with Clinical Evidence of Non-Alcoholic Fatty Liver Disease." *Gastroenterology* 122 (2002): 931–39.

Fernandez-Real, J. H., G. Penarroja, A. Castro, F. Garcia-Brigado, D. Hernandez-Aguado, and W. Ricart. "Blood-Letting in High-Ferritin Type 2 Diabetes—Effects on Insulin Sensitivity and Beta-Cell Function." *Diabetes* 51 (2002): 1000–1004.

Ford, E. S., and M. E. Cogswell. "Diabetes and Serum Ferritin Concentrations among U.S. Adults." *Diabetes Care* 22 (1999): 1978–83.

Hua, N. W., R. A. Stoohs, and F. S. Facchini. "Low Iron Status and Enhanced Insulin Sensitivity in Lacto-Ovo Vegetarians." *British Journal of Nutrition* 86 (2001): 515–19.

Jiang, R., J. Ma, A. Ascherio, M. J. Stampfer, W. C. Willett, and F. B. Hu. "Dietary Iron Intake and Blood Donations in Relations to Risk of Type II Diabetes in Men: A Prospective Cohort Study." *American Journal of Clinical Nutrition* 79 (2004): 70–75.

Pawlotsky, Y., P. LeDarter, R. Moirand, P. Guggenbuhl, A. M. Juanolle, E. Catheline, J. Meadeb, P. Brissot, Y. Deugnier, and G. Chales. "Elevated Parathyroid Hormone 44-68 and Osteoarticular Changes in Patients with Genetic Hemochromatosis." *Arthritis and Rheumatism* 42 (1999): 799–806.

Raiola, G., M. C. Galati, V. DeSanctis, M. C. Nicoletti, C. Pintor, M. DeSinore, and V. M. Acuri. "Anastasi, Growth and Puberty in Thalassemia Major." *Journal of Pediatric Endocrinology and Metabolism* 16, suppl. 2 (2003): 259–66.

Redrnon, J. B., and R. P. Robertson. "Iron and Diabetes." *Mayo Clinic Proceedings* 69 (1994): 90-2.

Siemens, L. J., and C. H. Mahler. "Hypogonadotrophic Hypogonadism in Human Hemochromatosis: Recovery of Reproductive Function after Iron Depletion." *Journal of Clinical Endocrinology and Metabolism* 65 (1987): 585–87.

Toumainen, T. P., K. Hyyssonen, R. Salonen, A. Terrahauta, H. Korpela, T. Lakka, G. A. Kaplan, and J. T. Saionen. "Body Iron Stores Are Associated with Serum Insulin and Blood Glucose Concentrations." *Diabetes Care* 20 (1997): 426–28.

Tweed, M. J., and J. M. Roland. "Hemochromatosis as an Endocrine Cause of Subfertility." *British Medical Journal* 316 (1998): 915–16.

Wilson, J. G., J. H. Lindquist, S. C. Grambow, E. D. Crook, and J. F. Maher. "Potential Role of Increased Iron Stores in Diabetes." *American Journal of Medical Science* 325 (2003): 332–39.

6

Central Nervous System

"The underlying pathogenic event in oxidative stress is cellular iron mismanagement."

—K. I. Thompson et al.

An association between brain iron and neurologic disease was made over 70 years ago with discovery of Hallervorden-Spatz disease. Abnormal accumulation of iron occurs in regions of the brain that undergo degeneration in illnesses such as Alzheimer's disease. Other brain areas such as the substantia nigra and basal ganglia that are affected in early onset are Parkinson's, Huntington's disease, Friedreick's ataxia, and HARP syndrome.

This maldistribution of brain iron contributes to the disease progression by accelerating the death of cells in the brain. In a recent report, the onset of Alzheimer's disease was found to occur as much as 5 years earlier if individuals carry the H63D mutation associated with hereditary hemochromatosis. Because excess iron is damaging to cells, there may be implications for iron in other neurologic diseases such as epilepsy and stroke. In a study of 51 patients with a diagnosis of acute stroke within 24 hours from onset of symptoms, serum ferritin was examined. Investigators found that serum ferritin levels were higher in patients with large lesions and concluded that increased serum ferritin levels correlate to severity of stroke and the size of the lesion.

Normal brain function is dependent on the correct amount

Selected examples of abnormal levels of iron in various neurologic diseases	
Disease	Observation
Aceruloplasminemia	Increased iron in retina and basal ganglia
Alzheimer's patients	Increased iron in amyloid plaques
Freidreich's Ataxia	Increased iron in mitochrondia of striatum and cerebellum
Hallervorden-Spatz	Increased iron in substantia nigra and globus pallidum
Hemochromatosis	Increased iron in basal ganglia and choroid plexus
Huntington's disease	Increased iron in striatum
Parkinson's disease	Increased iron in substantia nigra and striatum
Restless legs syndrome	Decreased iron in substantia nigra and putamen
Tardive dyskinesia	Increased iron in striatum
Multiple sclerosis	Increased iron in gray matter
HARP Syndrome	Increased iron in the pallidal nuclei

Source: J. R. Connor et al.

of iron because the metal is used both for energy production and for synthesis of many of the neurotransmitters that help cells communicate with each other. Thus, a brain iron imbalance without even causing cell death could contribute to other neurological disorders such as clinical depression, bipolar disease, and attention deficit disorders. In a retroactive study of 661 active outpatient psychiatric patients, a review of the charts of those who had iron overload revealed an unexpectedly high rate of bipolar affective disorder. Of these patients, without exception, it was noted that they were resistant to conventional psychiatric treatment.

As early as 1865, persons with advanced cases of hereditary hemochromatosis (HHC) began to be described in medical journals. The disorder was given such names as pigment cirrhosis, bronze diabetes, and, by 1935, hemochromatosis. The triad of liver disease, diabetes, and skin pigmentation continued to provide clues to the identification of the disorder. Most prominent of symptoms reported by HHC patients is a disabling fatigue, which has been observed in over 80 percent of hemochromatotics. During the past three decades, the very broad range of symptoms and organ systems that can be damaged by elevated iron finally has been recognized.

In 1980, in a thorough review of 34 cases of hemochromatosis, the authors noted that "neurologic symptoms have impressed us more than would be suggested by the general literature." Many of the patients had "marked lethargy, psychomotor retardation, and inability to think clearly." One patient said that he felt "mummified." Several patients were disoriented. Subsequent reports have extended these observations to include other neurologic manifestations such as dementia, depression, and a high rate of bipolar affective disorder.

Depression is a debilitating psychological disorder which may result from an imbalance in the neurotransmitters which nerve cells use to communicate with each other. Functional imaging studies have revealed that specific regions in the brain may also be involved in depression, supporting the idea that there is a biological explanation for this psychological disorder. There is strong evidence that depression associated with hemochromatosis may have similar biological underpinnings. Depression is also a symptom associated with hypothyroidism, a common condition experienced by hemochromatosis patients.

Indeed, excess iron can be a factor that prevents the patient from responding to conventional psychiatric treatment. Neurologic complaints of some patients are alleviated by therapeutic phlebotomy, the procedure used in de-ironing patients with body iron overload. Iron is required for synthesis of most of the chemical communicators in the brain. However, regions in the brain involved in motor skills and emotions are susceptible to iron toxicity. Although the dogma in neurology regarding hemochromatosis is that most of the brain is protected against iron overload, the studies upon which this dogma is built were performed prior to technological advances that are currently available, such as magnetic resonance imaging for living patients and enhanced ability to detect iron in autopsy samples. In addition, we now know there are two issues that are most important about iron in the brain; there must be a balance of iron (not too much or too little) and the timing of iron delivery is critical. Even the right amount of iron delivered at the wrong time can be harmful.

The brain has an exquisite system for maintaining a timely balance of iron. All organs have access to iron in the blood, but blood iron is not immediately available to the brain because the blood vessels coursing through the brain are modified to form a barrier between the brain and the blood. This barrier is important for keeping harmful substances in the blood out of the brain. To get required nutrients such as iron and glucose across this barrier, the endothelial cells that line blood vessels in the brain have carriers. For iron, the blood vessel cells use transferrin receptors to carry iron in from the blood. These receptors recognize the blood iron transport protein transferrin. In hemochromatosis (HHC), transferrin can be as high as 100 percent saturated with iron, unlike the normal saturation of roughly 30 percent. The high saturation of transferrin in HHC may fool the brain into thinking that plenty of iron is available and the levels of transferrin receptors on the brain blood vessels may decrease to keep too much iron from getting into the brain. The signals used between the brain and its blood vessels to determine how much (and when) iron should be transported into the brain must be discovered before we can directly test this idea.

At The Department of Neural and Behavioral Sciences, Pennsylvania State University College of Medicine, Dr. James Connor and his colleagues are investigating these signals. They have proposed that the amount and timely delivery of iron to the brain in HHC is disrupted as the brain tries to read signals regarding the amount of iron in the blood. Poorly timed or inappropriate amounts of iron delivery to the brain would directly affect the synthesis rates of the chemical communicators for nerve cells and inappropriate levels of chemical communicators could be associated with depression.

The data supporting the idea that the levels of iron or iron associated proteins (transferrin or ferritin) in blood can correlate

78

with depression and other psychological illnesses are growing. In one study, patients with varying psychiatric disorders had evidence of iron overload (high serum ferritin and high transferrin saturation) and this group of patients responded favorably to iron chelation therapy. In another study, a high percentage of patients with blood chemistry profiles consistent with iron overload suffered from bipolar affective disorder. Interestingly, the patients in this latter study were resistant to conventional treatment, which raises a separate but related question: How does iron status of the patient affect drug metabolism? A study which compared "jitteriness" in patients taking antidepressants found those patients with low serum iron were more likely to suffer the side effect of "jitteriness" than those with normal serum iron levels. Thus, a relationship between responsiveness to drug therapy and iron status may be worth considering during patient evaluations.

Specifically with regard to depression, there is evidence that low iron in blood can be associated with depression in some populations (i.e., iron-deficient women using the oral contraceptive pill) and depression was a reported side effect in a study using an iron chelator to treat individuals with thalassemia. In the brain, increased iron has been detected with MR imaging in specific regions in depressed patients. A popular therapeutic drug for depression, imipramine, can decrease the ability of a cell to obtain iron.

MR imaging is a powerful research tool for detecting levels of iron in the brains of living patients. It can be used diagnostically, as is currently the case for distinguishing some types of neurologic diseases in the brain from Parkinson's disease. Perhaps we should be arguing for increased use of MR imaging in hemochromatosis (HHC) to help us better understand the extent to which brain iron levels are affected in HHC and more specifically to determine the relationship between iron and depression. In this time of managed health care, the expensive imaging techniques must be thoroughly justified, and some centers which have a focus more on diagnosis than scientific understanding and advancement may need additional persuasion by their patients to help provide this tremendously necessary information.

Alzheimer's disease

Early onset of Alzheimer's disease (AD) may be associated with possession of HHC gene mutations. For instance, in one study, carriers of the H63D mutation had an earlier onset of AD than did noncarriers by about 5 years. Moreover, in persons who developed AD prior to age 70, the frequency of the H63D mutation was 5 times higher than in those persons who began to have AD symptoms after 80 years of age.

Many neurologic diseases show accumulation of iron at neuronal sites that specifically are disintegrating. In AD, iron staining of autopsy sections is associated with neuritic plaques. The metal can promote amyloid deposition in the diseased tissues. In AD brains, regions such as the hippocampus, the nuclear basalis of Meynert, and the superior temporal gyrus have elevated iron.

Moreover, transferrin levels generally are decreased throughout the cerebral cortex of AD patients. The Tf to iron ratio is lower in AD brains as compared with those of normal persons of similar age. Additionally, ferritin production is decreased, resulting in AD brain cells that lack ability to detoxify iron. These various observations suggest a relative decrease in iron mobility with a resulting increased incidence of free radical damage.

In an MRI examination of 31 patients with AD and 68 healthy controls, the ferritin iron content of several regions of the brain was compared. In AD patients, basal ganglia ferritin iron levels were significantly increased in the caudate and putamen regions (the possibility that the difference with the controls might have been caused by chance was less than 1:150), whereas no differences between patients and controls occurred in the white matter. Moreover, the duration of illness in the AD patients had no effect on the basal ganglia ferritin iron levels. This important observation indicates that elevated iron did not begin to accumulate after the tissue had become diseased but rather that the metal actually participates in the onset of the disease.

Furthermore, a SQUID magnetometry comparison of the quantity of magnetite iron in Alzheimer's disease brains with that of controls indicates that the iron-associated lesions may occur at an early preclinical age.

	Number	Transferrin-iron Saturation %	Serum Ferritin (ng/mL)
Mean iron values in normal persons, patients with Alzheimer's disease, and patients with Down syndrome			
Normal persons	15	39.0	63
Alzheimer's patients	10	50.9	133
Down syndrome patients	14	81.6	124

Source: G. Farrar et al.

Down syndrome

Patients with Down syndrome have neurochemical features similar to those with AD, and they also have a tendency to develop AD. In autopsy studies, more than 90 percent of Down syndrome patients who had lived at least 30 years had similar neuropathology to brains of AD persons.

Parkinson's disease, Huntington's disease, Friedreich's ataxia, aceruloplasminemia

In Parkinson's disease (PD), brain iron levels also are increased relative to ferritin levels. As with AD, a defect in iron management may result in excessive generation of free radicals. Elevated iron in PD is concentrated in dopaminergic neurons in the substantia nigra of the brain. The affected tissue also has a raised amount of lactoferrin, a protein whose principal function is that of scavenging free iron in sites of inflammation. However, the sequence of biochemical events that could lead to iron-induced free radical destruction of susceptible neurons has not yet been established. Nor is it at all certain that eventually drugs can be developed that could specifically prevent or remove iron loading from the substantia nigra.

Nevertheless, in a rat model of Parkinson's disease, injection of an iron chelator (5-14-(2-hydroxyethyl) piperazine-1-ylmethyl-quinoline–8-ol) (VK-28) completely protected against development of disease lesions. This pioneering study demonstrates that an iron chelator can pass from the bloodstream to the brain. The authors have proposed that the compound might also be useful in treatment of other neurodegenerative diseases in addition to Parkinson's.

Iron mismanagement likewise is involved in such neurologic diseases as Huntington's disease (HD) and Freidreich's ataxia (FA). In HD, iron accumulates in the basal ganglia early in the disease process, even before the onset of symptoms. In FA, a mitochondrial defect in the globus pallidus results in iron deposition in this organelle.

In aceruloplasminemia, massive iron deposits occur in liver, pancreas, brain, retina, and other tissues. The neurologic clinical features result from iron-associated progressive neurodegeneration of the retina and basal ganglia.

Epilepsy

Research with animal models indicates that iron accumulation may underlie the pathology of epilepsy. In a human study of 130 persons with epilepsy and 128 control subjects matched for sex and age, mean Tf iron saturation of the patients was 39.9 percent. This is significantly higher than the mean of the healthy subjects, which was 29.1 percent. Furthermore, abnormally high levels of Tf iron saturation (men greater than 60 percent; women greater than 48 percent) occurred in 10 of the persons with epilepsy, but in only 1 of the persons without epilepsy.

Schizophrenia and tardive dyskinesia

George Bartzokis, M.D., who invented the procedure for observing iron in the brain with high-resolution magnetic resonance imaging, examined the brains of 18 male schizophrenic patients with a cumulative exposure to neuroleptics of more than 1 year and 4 with less than 3 months of exposure. Calculated T2 relaxation time values were obtained for the basal ganglia. Patients with tardive dyskinesia (n = 9) had significantly shortened left caudate T2 relaxation times when compared to patients without tardive dyskinesia (n = 5). The group of four patients with fewer than 3 months' exposure to neuroleptics demonstrated a significantly greater variability of their left caudate T2 values. T2 relaxation time shortening may be related to iron levels in the basal ganglia and may be of predictive value in evaluating risk of tardive dyskinesia.

Tardive dyskinesia is a neurological syndrome caused by the long-term use of neuroleptic drugs (or antipsychotics). Neuroleptic drugs are generally prescribed for psychiatric disorders, as well as for some gastrointestinal and neurological disorders. Tardive dyskinesia is characterized by repetitive, involuntary, purposeless movements. Features of the disorder may include grimacing, tongue protrusion, lip smacking, puckering and pursing, and rapid eye blinking. Rapid movements of the arms, legs, and trunk may also occur. Impaired movements of the fingers may appear as though the patient is playing an invisible guitar or piano.

Restless legs syndrome

Restless legs syndrome (RLS), although until recently little recognized, is a prevalent disorder affecting between 5 and 15 percent of the adult population. The accepted diagnostic criteria for RLS is based on the clinical findings in the illustration.

Characteristics of Restless Legs Syndrome

- A strong urge to move the extremities, usually the legs, frequently accompanied by dysesthesias (abnormal sensations on the skin, such as a creeping or crawling sensation, numbness, prickliness, burning or cutting feeling).

- Restless movements of the extremities made to relieve the urge to move and sometimes occurring spontaneously.

- Onset or exacerbation of symptoms when at rest and relief with movement, particularly walking. The onset may occur after some period of rest, but the relief is almost immediate with movement and persists as long as the movement continues.

- Symptoms have a marked circadian pattern becoming worse at night with a peak severity usually in the middle of the night.

While much of the clinical intervention for RLS has focused on the dopaminergic system (caused by dopamine), there is a growing body of literature that suggests a significant role for iron.

In an investigation of RLS, brains from 7 individuals who had been diagnosed with RLS were compared with brains from 5 normal persons. In the RLS brains, iron was markedly decreased in the substantia nigra. Furthermore, in neuromelanin-containing cells, transferrin was increased but transferrin receptor content was decreased in the RLS brains as compared with the normal brains. The authors have proposed that RLS may be caused by a defect in regulation of synthesis of the transferrin receptor.

Multiple sclerosis

Maldistribution of iron is prominent also in brains of patients with multiple sclerosis (MS). Excessive accumulation of iron in the gray matter, as detected by MRI, is associated with brain atrophy and is a strong predictor of disability and disease progression. On the other hand, in the normally iron-rich white matter, the metal is delivered by ferritin rather than transferrin; however, in MS, ferritin is absent in the plaque lesions. In a mouse model of MS, parenteral injection of iron-free ferritin resulted in a reduction in disease progression. Possibly the protein was able to deliver iron from body stores into the affected brain tissue. In brain tissue from MS patients, the normal pattern of transferrin and ferritin binding distributions is disrupted. This suggests that loss of ferritin binding is involved in or is a consequence of demyelination associated with MS.

In a study of eating habits of patients with multiple sclerosis, investigators found that diets of the MS patient was higher than recommended levels in saturated fat, protein, vitamin A, vitamin C, folate, and iron.

An iron chelating anthracycline-based drug, mitoxantrone (MITOX), recently has been approved for treatment of very active MS patients. Unfortunately, when anthracyclines combine with iron, cardiomyopathy may develop. To prevent this undesirable side effect in cancer patients, a second iron chelator, dexrazoxane (DZR), is given. In an animal model of MS, concurrent administration of MITOX and DZR has been shown to be an effective therapy. Moreover, to the surprise of the authors, DZR by itself is likewise effective. Thus the authors are recommending that DZR, a drug safe and effective in cancer patients, be placed in clinical trials for patients with MS.

Acquired Immunodeficiency Syndrome (AIDS) dementia

During the advanced stages of AIDS, severe iron loading occurs in bone marrow, liver, spleen, muscle, and brain. The principal cause of iron accumulation is the chronic inflammatory response that involves iron withholding (see chapter 14). At least one-third of AIDS patients have excessive accumulation in the brain of hemosiderin-loaded macrophages, most evident in gyral white matter. Iron mismanagement in the central nervous system may underlie the dementia that occurs in some AIDS patients.

Memory

Still another manifestation of neurodegeneration is loss of memory. In a recently reported study, rat pups 10–12 days old were given doses of iron comparable to those in high-iron milk formula fed to human infants. The iron-exposed rats exhibited "longlasting detrimental effects upon performance of both appetitively and negatively reinforced tests of memory." Autopsy of iron-exposed rats showed significant increased iron in the substantia nigra.

References:

Bartzokis, G., D. Sultxer, J. Cummings, L. E. Hold, D. B. Hance, V. W. Henderson, and J. Mintz. "In Vivo Evaluation of Brain Iron in Alzheimer's Disease Using Magnetic Resonance Imaging." *Archives of General Psychiatry* 57 (2000): 47–53.

Bartzokis, G., H. J. Garber, S. R. Marder, and W. H. Olendorf. "MRI in Tardive Dyskinesia: Shortened Left Caudate T2." *Biological Psychiatry* 28 (1990): 1027–36.

Bartzokis, G., J. Cummings, S. Perlman, D. R. Hance, and J. Mintz. "Increased Basal Ganglia Iron Levels in Huntington Disease." *Archives of Neurology* 56 (1999): 569–74.

Ben-Shachar, D., N. Kahana, V. Kampel, A. Warshawsky, M. B. Youdim II. "Neuroprotection by a Novel Brain Permeable Iron Chelator, VK-28, against 6-Hydroxydopamine Lesion in Rats." *Neuropharmacology* 46 (2004): 254–63.

Burdo, J. R., and J. R. Connor. "Brain Iron Uptake and Homeostatic Mechanisms: An Overview." *BioMetals* 16 (2003): 63–75.

Connor, J. R. "Iron in Central Nervous System Disorders." In *Key Topics in Brain Research*, edited by P. Riederer and M. B. H. Youdim. Vienna: Springer-Verlag, 1993.

Connor, J. R., E. A. Milward, S. Moalem, M. Sampietro, P. Boyer, M. E. Percy, C. Vergani, R. J. Scott, and M. Chorney. "Is Hemochromatosis a Risk Factor for Alzheimer's Disease?" *Journal of Alzheimer's Disease* 3 (2001): 471–77.

Connor, J. R., P. J. Boyer, S. L. Menzies, B. Dellinger, R. P. Allen, W. G. Ondo, and C. J. Early. "Neuropathological Examination Suggests Impaired Brain Iron Acquisition in Restless Legs Syndrome." *Neurology* 61 (2003): 304–9.

Connor, J. R., and S. A. Benkovic. "Iron Regulation in the Brain: Histochemical, Biochemical, and Molecular Considerations." *Annals of Neurology* 32 (1992): S51–S61.

Cutler, P. "Iron Overload and Psychiatric Illness." *Canadian Journal of Psychiatry* 39 (1994): 8–11.

Davis, J. D., R. A. Stern, and L. A. Flashman. "Cognitive and Neuropsychiatric Aspects of Subclinical Hypothyroidism: Significance in the Elderly." *Current Psychiatry Reports* 5 (2003): 384–90.

Erdemoglu, A. K., and S. Ozbakir. "Serum Ferritin Levels and Early Prognosis of Stroke." *European Journal of Neurology* 9 (2002): 633–37.

Farrar, G., P. Altmann, S. Welch, O. Wyschrij, B. Ghoso, J. Lejeune, J. Corbett, V. Prasher, and J. A. Blair. "Defective Gallium-Transferrin Binding in Alzheimer Disease and Down Syndrome: Possible Mechanism for Accumulation of Aluminum in Brain." *The Lancet* 335 (1990): 747–50.

Feifel, D., and C. W. Young. "Iron Overload among a Psychiatric Population." *Journal of Clinical Psychiatry* 58 (1997): 74–78.

Gelman, B. "Iron in CNS Disease." *Journal of Neuropathy & Experimental Neurology* 54 (1995): 477–86.

Hautot, D., Q. A. Pankhurst, N. Khan, and J. Dobson. "Preliminary Evaluation of Nanoscale Biogenic Magnetite in Alzheimer's Disease Brain Tissue." *Proceedings of Royal Society London B* 270, suppl. (2003): S62–S64.

Higgins, J. J., M. C. Patterson, N. M. Papadopoulos, R. O. Brady, P. G. Pentchev, and N. W. Barton. "Hypoprebetalipoproteinemia, Acanthocytosis, Retinitis Pigmentosa, and Pallidal Degeneration (HARP Syndrome)." *Neurology* 42 (1992): 194–98.

Hirsch, E. C., and B. A. Faucheux. "Iron Metabolism and Parkinson's Disease." *Movement Disorders* 13, suppl. 1 (1998): 39–45.

Hulet, S. W., S. Powers, and J. R. Connor. "Distribution of Transferrin and Ferritin Binding in Normal and Multiple Sclerotic Brains." *Journal of Neurologic Science* 165 (1999): 48–55.

Hulet, S. W., S. O. Hetliger, S. Powers, J. R. Connor. "Oligodendrocyte Progenitor Cells Internalize Ferritin Via Clathrin-Dependent Receptor Mediated Endocytosis." *Journal of Neuroscience Research* 61 (2000): 52–60.

Ikeda, M. "Iron Overload without the C282Y Mutation in Patients with Epilepsy." *Journal of Neurology & Neurosurgical Psychiatry* 70 (2001): 551–53.

Levine, S. M., S. Maiti, M. R. Emerson, and T. V. Pedchenko. "Apoferritin Attenuates Experimental Allergic Encephalomyelitis in SJL Mice." *Developmental Neuroscience* 24 (2002): 177–83.

Milder, M. S., J. Cook, S. Stray, and C. A. Finch. "Idiopathic Hemochromatosis, an Interim Report." *Medicine* 59 (1980): 34–49.

National Institute of Neurological Disorders and Stroke. http://www.ninds.nih.gov/health_and_medical/disorders/tardive_doc.htm

Sampietro, M., L. Caputo, A. Casatta, M. Meregalli, A. Pellagatti, J. Tagliabue, G. Annoni, and C. Vergani. "The Hemacromatosis Gene Affects the Age of Onset of Sporadic Alzheimer's Disease." *Neurobiology and Aging* 22 (2001): 563–68.

Schroder, N., A. Fredriksson, P. I. R. M. Vianna, R. Roesler, I. Izquierdo, and T. Archer. "Memory Deficits in Adult Rats Following Postnatal Iron Administration." *Behavioral Brain Research* 124 (2001): 77–85.

Thompson, K. I., S. Shoham, and J. R. Connor. "Iron and Neurologic Disorders." *Brain Research Bulletin* 55 (2001): 155–64.

Timmerman, G. M., and A. K. Stuifbergin. "Eating Patterns in Women with Multiple Sclerosis." *Journal of Neuroscience Nurse* 31 (1999): 152–58.

Weilbach, F. X., A. Chan, K. V. Toyka, and R. Gold. "Cardioprotector Dexrazoxane Augments Therapeutic Efficacy of Mitoxantrone in Experimental Autoimmune Encephalomyelitis." *Clinical Experimental Immunology* 135 (2004): 49–55.

Weinberg, G. A., J. R. Boelaert, and E. D. Weinberg. "Iron and HIV Infection." In *Micronutrients and HIV Infection*. Edited by H. Friis, 135–57. Boca Raton, FL: CRC Press, 2002.

Zivadinov, R., and R. Bakshi. "Role of MRI In Multiple Sclerosis II: Brain and Spinal Cord Atrophy." *Bioscience* 9 (2004): 647–64.

7

Cardiovascular System

"Regardless of whether iron overload in human beings results from transfusions in patients with thalassemia major, hereditary hemochromatosis, or other causes, it (iron overload) impairs cardiac function and is a major cause of death."

—*Yang et al.*

In both females and males who have inherited iron-loading disorders, accumulation of the metal results most noticeably in progressive loss of function of the liver, joints, endocrine glands, and the heart. In beta-thalassemia, an inherited disorder in which hemoglobin is produced incorrectly, patients absorb as much as 2–5 grams/year of excess iron in a futile attempt to produce useful hemoglobin. Moreover, blood transfusions, which are often needed to give the patient adequate red blood cells, increase the iron burden because each pint transfused delivers one-fourth gram of iron. Unfortunately, excessive quantities of iron cannot be excreted, but are deposited in various body sites.

The deleterious effects of iron accumulation in thalassemic patients begin to appear as early as the first decade of life. Heart muscle is a prime target for iron deposition. Even with a small quantity of extra iron deposition in the heart, the muscle cells degenerate to result in loss of electrical conductivity (heart fluttering) and muscle function. Capillary bleeding also occurs. Indeed, survival of patients with ß-thalassemia is determined by the extent of iron loading within the heart. In a set of 1087 beta-thalassemic patients born after 1960 and who died before 1989, heart disease had developed in 77 percent and was by far the most common cause of death.

Normal heart and normal iron

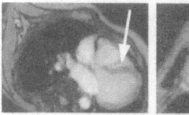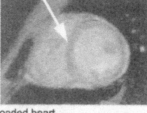

Severe iron-loaded heart

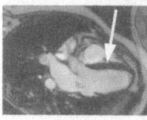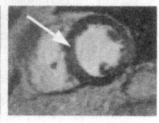

Images courtesy of Dr. D.J. Pennell, Cardiovascular Magnetic Resonance Unit, Royal Brompton Hospital, London

To better understand iron overload induced cardiomyopathy (disease of the heart muscle), investigators at The Rammelkamp Center for Education and Research, Cleveland, began to study the hearts of Mongolian gerbils. This animal model was chosen because accumulated iron in the heart of the Mongolian gerbil is similar to that observed in patients with thalassemia major.

As part of their study, the Rammelkamp scientists induced iron into the gerbils with daily subcutaneous injections of iron dextran. They performed various tests on the gerbils, including electrocardiograms (EKGs). Tests tracked the response over more than 70 weeks while iron injections continued to be administered. Among their observations, these investigators found that the Q-T interval prolongation was of utmost significance.

The "Q-T" wave is the one that follows the "P" wave on an electrocardiogram and is usually not prominent on EKGs of persons with normal healthy hearts. However, in patients with iron-induced cardiomyopathy, the Q-T wave is extended or elongated. An elongated Q-T wave frequently accompanies congestive heart failure.

AP*, ECG, Ventricular Currents and Common Gene Names

*Ventricular action potential

Image courtesy of Rammelkamp Research
Center, Cleveland, Ohio

Autopsies of these experimental animals revealed iron deposits that were mostly in the left ventricle and epicardium (outer layer of the wall of the heart). Smaller amounts of iron were present in the right ventricle and atria and within the cells of the heart, but not the interstitium (fluid space between heart cells). These investigators showed for the first time that the iron content of gerbil ventricular cardiomyocytes was increased to amounts similar to those of patients with iron-induced cardiomyopathy.

In subsequent studies the Rammelkamp investigators gave daily subcutaneous injections of the iron chelator deferoxamine

(DF). DF prevented most of the electrocardiographic changes and prolonged survival of the gerbils. However, DF was unable to remove significant amounts of cardiac iron.

Iron-induced cardiomyopathy is the main cause of death in patients with ß-thalassemia (thalassemia major). ß-thalassemia occurs mainly in native persons in tropical and semi-tropical countries where malaria is endemic. A second widespread disorder of iron loading, hereditary hemochromatosis (HHC), is seen in persons of northern European descent. In HHC, hemoglobin synthesis is normal. However, a serum protein (*HFE*) that ordinarily combines with the transferrin receptor protein to prevent entry of excessive iron into body cells is distorted because of either one or two gene mutations.

Thus in HHC, about 2–4 times the normal amount of iron is absorbed from the diet by the intestinal cells. The two gene mutations responsible for HHC are designated CY and HD. The normal gene is designated wt/wt (wild type). Persons with HHC can have CY/CY, HD/HD, or CY/HD mutations. The first two are called homozygotes; the third is called a compound heterozygote and often is considered to indicate a carrier of the disorder. Simple carriers are designated as CY/wt or HD/wt. Many, but not all, HHC homozygotes as well as some carriers load iron. Of persons who do accumulate the metal, some will develop deterioration of heart, liver, endocrine glands, or other organs.

About 0.3–0.5 percent of persons of European descent are homozygous for HHC. About 5–15 percent are carriers of one or two of the gene mutations. It has been difficult to estimate the percent of untreated HHC patients who die of heart disease because often a diagnosis of HHC had not been considered nor had body iron values been obtained. In a recent study, HHC carriers were observed to have increased risk of dying prior to age 65, but the causes of the premature mortality were not ascertained. In a 1996 Centers for Disease Control and Prevention survey of 2851 living HHC patients, 24 percent reported symptoms of heart fluttering.

In several studies of large groups of persons, some of those identified as CY/wt or CY/HD were found to have increased body iron burden and some of the carriers were observed to have increased risk of heart disease. For example, 12,239 women, aged 51–69 years, were followed for 16–18 years; in this group, 4 percent were CY/wt.

Cardiovascular disease in wt/wt women was elevated 1.6 fold by smoking, but in CY/wt women smokers, the elevation in risk was 3.5 fold. The induction of iron loading by tobacco smoking is described in chapter 8. If, additionally, the CY/wt smokers had high blood pressure, the increased risk for cardiovascular disease was 19 fold. Similarly, in a study of 1150 men aged 42–60 years, the risk of myocardial infarction was increased by 2.3 fold in the 6.7 percent of the group who were CY/wt carriers.

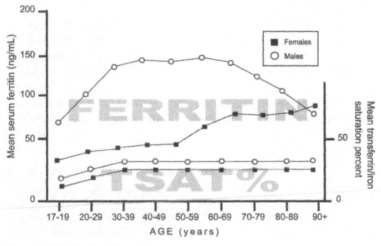

Source: L. R. Zacharski et al.

General population studies

The possible association of cardiovascular disease with elevated body iron burden has been studied in numerous groups of persons that contained an unknown mix of normal persons and HHC carriers. Twenty-four studies were evaluated in 1999. In half of these, a positive association was found. In half, no association was observed.

Generally, the positive studies had employed serum ferritin as the measure of body iron burden. In episodes of inflammation, serum ferritin can be elevated, but investigators who employed the ferritin test usually were aware of this confounding effect and they excluded subjects with inflammation from their analyses. The negative studies tended to employ hemoglobin, hematocrit, serum iron or transferrin iron saturation percent. These four tests do not accurately indicate body iron burden. Note in the illustration on the previous page that the percent of iron saturation of transferrin normally remains independent of the increased body iron burden that occurs with aging.

Contributing factors

Many factors that can contribute to positive or negative effects on body iron burden are being discovered and will be discussed further in chapters 13 and 15. Various combinations of these factors could markedly affect the outcome of health or disease in individual persons. In theory, for instance, CY/wt carriers who are nonsmokers, not hypertensive, and who exercise vigorously and take a daily aspirin could greatly lower their risk of heart disease. More-over, mutations of genes other than *HFE* that perhaps have not yet been discovered could have a strong impact on the action of the *HFE* gene protein product. As cited earlier, a mutation in the transferrin receptor gene results in lowered efficiency of the transferrin receptor protein whose function is to control, together with the *HFE* protein, the amount of iron allowed into our body cells.

In several studies,

Factors that Contribute to Iron Damage of the Cardiovascular System
■ Cellular iron uptake gene mutations (hemochromatosis)
■ Hemoglobin synthesis gene mutations (thalassemia)
■ High LDL cholesterol
■ Hypertension
■ Ingestion of high amounts of heme iron
■ Tobacco smoking

94

investigators have noted that ingestion of heme iron (in red meats) contributes to the risk of iron loading and heart disease. Nonheme iron (in plant foods) tends not to increase risk because its absorption in the intestine is inhibited by iron deposits already in the body. Thus a vegetarian diet helps to prevent accumulation of iron in men and in nonmenstruating women. Men who donate blood and women who menstruate can consume heme iron and yet avoid excessive iron buildup.

The powerful oxidant activity of iron may damage not only heart muscle cells but also arterial walls. In the latter case, the level of cholesterol is important. A well-controlled study in rabbits has demonstrated that iron loading significantly increases the formation of aortic wall lesions in animals that have high, but not low, cholesterol. Iron catalyzes the oxidation of LDL cholesterol to lipofuscin that results in formation of foam cells, a component of arterial wall plaque. Endothelial function of the brachial artery has been shown to be suppressed by iron loading via increased oxidative stress. Function of the endothelium could be restored by iron depletion. Moreover, iron loading also can accelerate clot formation after arterial injury, apparently by increasing vascular oxidative stress. In a study of 13,932 adults (NHANES III), the risk of elevated C-reactive protein (a marker of inflammation) was not affected by elevated ferritin alone but was significantly raised in persons with high ferritin plus elevated low density lipoprotein (LDL) or with high ferritin plus deficient high density lipoprotein (HDL). Thus prevention and/or treatment of iron loading might decrease CRP and cardiovascular disease in high risk patients.

Some women and men inherit a disorder in which cholesterol buildup occurs early in adulthood. As the men accumulate excessive iron, their heart disease risk rises promptly. In contrast, the young women who have high cholesterol do not have an accompanying increased risk of heart disease, provided that they continue to menstruate.

Cardiovascular disease and iron

One of the many functions of the white blood cells called macrophages is to scavenge excessive iron. Persons who inhale iron, as cited in chapter 8, develop iron-loaded alveolar macrophages. Some of these cells migrate to blood vessels such as the coronary arteries and aorta, where they become dangerous for either of two reasons. First, the heavily iron-loaded cells may lose some of the metal which would then become available to oxidize LDL cholesterol. Second, some of the macrophages might have become infected in the lungs with inhaled bacteria. Two important examples are *Chlamydia pneumoniae* and *Coxiella burnetti*, which not only cause pneumonia but also can participate in the development of infectious lesions within the coronary arteries. As cited in chapter 12, growth of these bacteria is stimulated in iron-loaded macrophages.

However, in untreated homozygotic HHC persons macrophages have below-normal quantities of iron. Accordingly, these persons will tend to be protected from both noninfectious and infectious causes of coronary artery disease. Nevertheless, as cited earlier, untreated HHC persons will have myocardial deterioration inasmuch as iron accumulates in their heart muscle cells.

As will be more fully described in chapter 18, men of all ages can prevent excessive accumulation of iron by blood donation. Several studies have demonstrated that male blood donors have significantly lower rates of heart attacks than those of male nondonors. In a group of 468 nonsmoking males who had LDL cholesterol levels greater than 160 mg/dl, the risk of a cardiovascular event among the blood donors was only 62 percent of that experienced by the nondonors. Not surprisingly, among 429 nonsmokers with LDL cholesterol levels less than 130 mg/dl, essentially no benefit was obtained by blood donation. In a different study over a 12-year period of men who had relatively high serum cholesterol, one of 153 blood donors (0.7 percent) and 316 of 2529 nonblood donors (12.5 percent) had an acute myocardial infarction. The probability that this remarkable outcome would have occurred simply by chance is less than 1 in 10,000.

Researchers at Cleveland Clinic found that high levels of myeloperoxidase or low levels of glutathione peroxidase 1 can be helpful in predicting myocardial infarction in patients with chest pain. These investigators concluded a single initial measurement of plasma myeloperoxidase independently predicts the early risk of myocardial infarction, as well as the risk of major adverse cardiac events in the ensuing 30-day and 6-month periods.

"There is little doubt that an excessive amount of stored iron is cardiotoxic."

—J. Sullivan

The iron hypothesis

In 1981, Dr. Jerome L. Sullivan proposed that the lower incidence of heart disease in premenopausal women as compared with men and postmenopausal women is due to the lower amount of body iron in the former group. In the Framingham heart study investigators found that "men had significantly higher serum ferritin concentrations than females." This finding tends to support the hypothesis that females who are still menstruating and therefore losing iron are somewhat protected by this process against heart attack.

Menstruation, estrogen, and iron

In the Framingham Heart Study the health status of several thousand men and women was monitored biannually for several decades, starting in 1948. By the time of the thirteenth examination, it had become apparent that premenopausal women rarely develop myocardial infarction or die of heart disease (HD). Indeed, in persons of similar age, the male-to-premenopausal-female ratio for heart attack was 15:1. However, protection from heart disease by premenopausal status was lost to women who had an early hysterectomy.

That the protective factor is not estrogen was shown by the observation that women who had an early hysterectomy with retention of functional (estrogen-synthesizing) ovaries lost the same degree of protection as did those whose ovaries were removed. Furthermore, postmenopausal women who take exogenous estrogen fail to regain the protective factor enjoyed by premenopausal women.

Moreover, premenopausal women who used original formulations of oral contraceptive agents (OCA) that contained a high amount of estrogens (30–80 micrograms/tablet) absorbed higher than normal quantities of dietary iron, had lower menstrual flow, and had as much as a 3.5 fold increased risk of heart disease as compared with nonOCA users.

During pregnancy, with cessation of menstruation, the placental tissue synthesizes continually increasing amounts of estrogen. Thus in the second and third trimesters, respectively, there is a fivefold and ninefold increase in absorption of dietary iron. Fortunately, the pregnant person does not become iron loaded. Instead, the additional iron supplies the needs of the placenta, fetus, and blood loss at the time of delivery.

In normal menstruation, about one pint of blood is lost annually. Each pint contains approximately one-fourth gram of iron. Men begin to accumulate excessive iron deposits in their early twenties and, by age 40, have about 4 times as much of the metal as do women who have not yet proceeded through natural or surgical menopause.

In addition to the factors shown on page 94, contributing factors reported to lower the incidence of heart disease include exercising, taking aspirin, and drinking tea. Proposed mechanisms for these beneficial items will be discussed in greater detail in

Blood donation	■
Menstruation	■
Exercise	■
Iron chelation	■
Drinking tea	■
Use of aspirin	■
Factors that Lower Body Iron Burden	

chapter 18. During the past score of years, evidence has accumulated that prompt removal of iron by specific iron chelators can protect against myocardial injury.

In summary, it is now quite apparent that excessive iron in either arteries or heart muscle cells is detrimental to a properly functioning cardiovascular system.

References:

Araujo, J. A., E. L. F. Romano, B. E. Brito, V. Parthe, M. Romano, M. Bracho, B. F. Montano, and J. Cardier. "Iron Overload Augments the Development of Atherosclerotic Lesions in Rabbits." *Arteriosclerosis, Thrombosis & Vascular Biology* 15 (1995): 1172–80.

Asherio, A., W. C. Willett, E. B. Rimm, E. L. Giovannucci, and M. I. Stampfer. "Dietary Iron and Risk of Coronary Diseases among Men." *Circulation* 89 (1994): 969–74.

Barrett, J. F. R., P. G. Whittaker, J. G. Williams, and T. Lind. "Absorption of Non-heme Iron from Food during Normal Pregnancy." *British Medical Journal* 309 (1994): 79–82.

Barrett-Connor, E. "Looking for the Pony in the HERS Data." *Circulation* 105 (2002): 902–3.

Bartolini, G., F. F. Italia, G. Ferraro, T. Lombardo, C. Tamburino, and S. Cordaro. "Histopathology of Thalassemie Heart Disease: An Endomyocardial Biopsy Study." *Cardiovascular Pathology* 6 (1997): 205–11.

Bathum, L., L. Christiansen, H. Nybo, K. A. Ramberg, D. Gaist, B. Jeune, N. E. Petersen, I. Vaupel, and K. Christensen. "Association of Mutations in the Hemochromatosis Gene with Shortened Life Expectancy." *Archives of Internal Medicine* 61 (2001): 2441–44.

Blankenberg, S., H. J. Rupprecht, C. Bickel, M. Torzewski, G. Hafner, L. Tiret, M. Smieja, F. Cambien, J. Meyer, and K. J. Lackner. "Glutathione Peroxidase 1 Activity and Cardiovascular Events in Patients with Coronary Artery Disease." *New England Journal of Medicine* 23 (2003): 1605–13.

Brennan, M. L., M. S. Penn, F. Van Lente, V. Nambi, M. H. Shishehbor, R. J. Aviles, M. Goormastic, M. L. Pepoy, E. S. McErlean, E. J. Topol, S. E. Nissen, S. L. Hazen. "Prognostic Value of Myeloperoxidase in Patients with Chest Pain." *New England Journal of Medicine* 349 (2003): 1595–1604.

Day, S. M., D. Duqaine, L. V. Mundada, R. G. Menon, B. V. Khan, S. Rajogopalan, and W. P. Fay. "Chronic Iron Administration Increases Vascular Oxidative Stress and Accelerates Arterial Thrombosis." *Circulation* 107 (2003): 2601–6.

de Valk, B., and J. Marx. "Iron, Atherosclerosis, and Ischemic Heart Disease." *Archives of Internal Medicine* 159 (1999): 1542–8.

Fleming, D., K. Tucker, P. Jacques, G. Dallal, P. Wilson, and R. Wood. "Dietary Factors Associated with the Risk of High Iron Stores in the

Elderly Framingham Heart Study Cohort 1–4." *American Journal of Clinical Nutrition* 76 (2002):1375–84.

Frassinelli-Gunderson, E. P., S. Morgan, and J. R. Brown. "Iron Stores in Users of Oral Contraceptive Agents." *American Journal of Clinical Nutrition* 41 (1985): 703–12.

Gaenzer, H., P. Marschang, W. Sturm, G. Neumayr, W. Vogel, J. Patsch, and G. Weiss. "Association between Increased Iron Stores and Impaired Endothelial Function in Patients with Hereditary Hemochromatosis." *Journal of American College of Cardiology* 40 (2002): 2189–94.

Geleijnse, J. M., L. J. Launer, A. Hofman, H. A. P. Pols, and J. C. M. Witteman. "Tea Flavonoids May Protect against Atherosclerosis." *Archives of Internal Medicine* 159 (1999): 2170–74.

Gordon, T., W. B. Kannel, C. Hjortland, and P. M. McNamara. "Menopause and Coronary Heart Disease." *Annals of Internal Medicine* 89 (1978): 157–61.

Gum, P. A., M. Thamilarasan, J. Watanabe, E. H. Blackstone, and M. S. Lauer. "Aspirin Use and All-Cause Mortality among Patients Being Evaluated for Known or Suspected Coronary Artery Disease." *Journal of the American Medical Association* 286 (2001): 1187–94.

Kiechi, S., G. Egger, M. Mayr, C. J. Wiedermann, E. Bonou, F. Ovberhollenzer, M. Muggeo, Q. Xu, G. Wick, W. Poewe, and J. Willett. "Chronic Infections and the Risk of Carotid Atherosclerosis." *Circulation* 103 (2001):1064–70.

Kuryshev, Y. A., G. M. Brittenham, H. Fujioka, P. Kannan, C. C. Shieh, S. A. Cohen, and A. M. Brown. "Decreased Sodium and Increased Transient Outward Potassium Currents in Iron-Loaded Cardiac Myocytes: Implications for the Arrhythmogenesis of Human Siderotic Heart Disease." *Circulation* 100 (1999): 675–83.

Mainous, A. G. III, B. J. Wells, C. J. Everett, J. M. Gill, and D. E. King. "Association of Ferritin and Lipids with C-reactive Protein." *American Journal of Cardiology* 93 (2004): 559–62.

McDonnell, S. M., B. L. Preston, S. A. Jewell, J. C. Barton, C. Q. Edwards, P. C. Adams, and R. Yip. "Survey of 2,851 Patients with Hemochromatosis Symptoms and Response to Treatment." *American Journal of Medicine* 106 (1999): 619–24.

Meyers, D. G., D. Strickland, P. A. Maloley, J. J. Seburg, J. E. Wilson, and B. F. McManus. "Possible Association of a Reduction in Cardiovascular Events with Blood Donation." *Heart* 78 (1997): 188–93.

Obejero-Paz, C., T. Yang, W. Q. Dong, M. N. Levy, G. M. Brittenham, Y. A. Kuryshev, and A. M. Brown. "Deferoxamine Promotes Survival and Prevents Electorcardiographic Abnormalities in the Gerbil Model of Iron-Overload Cardiomyopathy." *Journal of Laboratory Clinical Medicine* 141 (2003): 121–30.

Olivieri, N. F. "The Beta-Thalassemias." *New England Journal of Medicine* 341 (1999): 99–109.

Roest, M., Y. T. von der Schouw, B. de Valk, J. J. Marx, M. I. Tempelman, P. G. de Groot, J. J. Sixma, and J. D. Banga. "Heterozygosity for a Hereditary Hemochromatosis Gene Is Associated with Cardiovascular Death." *Circulation* 100 (1999): 1268–73.

Salonen, J. T., T. P. Tuomainen, R. Salonen, T. A. Lakka, and K. Nyyssonen. "Donation of Blood Is Associated with Reduced Risk of Myocardial Infarction." *American Journal of Epidemiology* 148 (1998): 445–61.

Salonen, J. T., K. Nyssonen, H. Korpela, J. Tuomilehto, R. Seppanen, and R. Salonen. "High Stored Iron Levels Are Associated with Excess Risk of Myocardial Infarction in Eastern Finnish Men." *Circulation* 86 (1992): 803–11.

Slone, D., S. Shapiro, D. W. Kaufman, L. Rosenberg, O. F. Miettinen, and P. D. Stolley. "Risk of Myocardial Infarction in Relation to Current and Discontinued Use of Oral Contraceptives." *New England Journal of Medicine* 305 (1981): 420–4.

Sullivan, J. L. "Iron and the Sex Difference in Heart Disease Risk." *The Lancet* (1981): 1293–94.

———. "The Iron Paradigm of Ischemic Heart Disease." *American Heart Journal* 117 (1989): 1177–89.

———. "Blood Donation May Be Good for the Donor." *Vox Sanguinis* 61 (1991): 161–64.

Sullivan, J. L., and E. D. Weinberg. "Iron and The Role of *Chlamydia Pneumoniae* in Heart Disease." *Emerging Infectious Diseases* 5 (1999): 724–26.

Surber, R., H. H. Sigusch, H. Kuehnert, and H. R. Figulla. "Haemochromatosis (*HFE*) Gene C282Y Mutation and the Risk of Coronary Artery Disease and Myocardial Infarction: A Study in 1279 Patients Undergoing Coronary Angiography." *Journal of Medical Genetics* E58 (2003): e58.

Toumainen, T. P., K. Kontula, K. Nyssonen, T. A. Lakka, T. Helio, and J. T. Salonen. "Increased Risk of Acute Myocardial Infarction in Carriers of the Hemochromatosis Gene Cys282Tyr Mutation." *Circulation* 100 (1999): 1274–79.

Tzonou, A., P. Ligiou, A. Trichopoulou, V. Tsoutsos, and D. Trichopoulos. "Dietary Iron and Coronary Heart Disease Risk: A Study from Greece." *American Journal of Epidemiology* 147 (1998): 161–66.

United States Preventive Services Task Force. "Routine Iron Supplementation During Pregnancy." *Journal of the American Medical Association* 270 (1993): 2846–54.

Weinberg, E. D. "Iron and the Role of *Coxiella Burnetii* in Heart Disease." *Journal of Trace Elements and Experimental Medicine* 14 (2001): 409–10.

————. "Do Some Carriers of Hemochromatosis Gene Mutations Have Higher Than Normal Rates of Disease and Death?" *BioMetals* 15 (2002): 347–50.

Yang, T., W. Q. Dong, Y. A. Kuryshev, C. Obejero-Paz, M. N. Levy, G. M. Brittenham, S. Kiatchoosakun, D. Kirkpatrick, B. D. Hoit, and A. M. Brown. "Bimodal Cardiac Dysfunction in an Animal Model of Iron Overload." *Journal of Laboratory Clinical Medicine* 140 (2002): 263–71.

Yuan, X. M., W. Li, A. G. Olsson, and U. T. Brunk. "Iron in Human Atheroma and LDL Oxidation by Macrophages Following Erythrophagocytosis." *Atherosclerosis* 124 (1996): 61–73.

Zacharski, L. R., D. L. Ornstein, S. Woloshin, and L. M. Schwartz. "Association of Age, Sex, and Race with Body Iron Stores in Adults: Analysis of NHANES III Data." *American Heart Journal* 140 (2000): 98–104.

Zurlo, M. G., P. de Stefano, C. Borgna-Pignatti, A. di Palma, A. Piga, C. Melevendi, F. di Gregorio, M. G. Burattini, and S. Terzoli. "Survival and Causes of Death in Thalassemia Major." *The Lancet* ii (1989): 27–30.

8

Pulmonary System

"There are increased airway concentrations of total iron and ferritin-bound iron in patients with chronic bronchitis and, to a greater extent, in patients with cystic fibrosis. Particularly in cystic fibrosis patients who also demonstrated decreased airway concentrations of transferrin, ferritin-bound iron in airways may promote oxidative injury and enhance bacterial growth."

—S. W. Stites et al.

All systems of the body can become iron loaded by ingestion of excessive quantities of the metal. Uniquely, the respiratory system can, as well, accumulate dangerous amounts by inhalation. Especially hazardous is inhalation of such iron-contaminated materials as urban air particulates, tobacco smoke, silica, and various kinds of asbestos.

Several components of the iron withholding defense system attempt to scavenge inhaled iron. Lung epithelial lining fluid contains transferrin, a powerful iron chelator that can convey the metal to safe storage sites. The alveolar (lung) macrophages can increase their production of ferritin to sequester the metal. Moreover, as ferritin molecules become engorged with iron, they are converted to insoluble hemosiderin. Unfortunately, macrophages loaded with iron become impaired in their normal function of exerting antimicrobial and anti-neoplastic cell activity.

The earliest studies on iron loading and cancer began with inhalation. In the 1930s, physicians started to report that industrial workers who inhale iron are at increased risk for cancers of the respiratory tract. In December 1936, Swiss physician Julian Dreyfus reported what was considered at the time to be a bizarre account of two siblings who developed lung cancer as a result of inhaled iron oxide. The first of the two siblings to be seen by Dr. Dreyfus was the 44-year-old female. She was admitted to Hospital de La Chaux de Fords, Switzerland, because she was experiencing shortness of breath and chest pain. Her family history of illness was not unusual, but the attending physician found a nodule, which he determined to be cancerous; so, he removed it surgically. Shortly after the operation, the woman's condition worsened. She complained of pain in the left side of her chest; a lung tap produced over a liter of red liquid. Three weeks later, another tap produced a liter of yellow reddish-brown fluid. Now feeble, barely able to breathe, and with a faint heartbeat, the woman was admitted to the hospital. More lung taps were done, and tumor tissue was found in the fluid; she was diagnosed with metastasis of lung carcinoma—and died three weeks later.

Barely 9 months after her death, her 36-year-old brother was admitted to the same hospital for prolonged bronchitis. He was diagnosed with pleurisy. Four months later he returned to the hospital complaining of bronchial pain. An x-ray showed in the lower third of the right lung, directly above the diaphragm, a poorly defined shadow. He was treated, but developed a severe cough and eventually returned to the hospital. A pleuropuncture (tap) brought forth the same yellow reddish-brown, cloudy liquid as that of his now-deceased sister.

Fluid extracted from his lungs also contained tumor tissue; he was diagnosed with metastasis of a lung carcinoma, just as his older sister had been diagnosed. He was given radiotherapy, which seemed to have favorable effects.

Rarely had Dreyfus seen lung cancer in patients so young, and its occurrence within relatively young individuals from the same family prompted him to ask more detailed questions about the family's history. Conversations with the patient revealed that when he was a child, his mother worked at home, polishing screws for a watch factory. She used a rotating steel disk onto which she continuously dusted a red polishing powder.

From their birth until the boy was 12, and his sister 20, both siblings were always in the room where the mother worked with this powder. Initially, they were present as spectators, then as helpers. Curious, Dreyfus contacted the watch factory and was told the powder was iron oxide. He obtained a sample of the powder and had it analyzed to be certain. Indeed, the polishing dust contained the metal, iron.

Both siblings had been exposed to prolonged inhalation of iron dust. That they died of lung cancer would be no surprise to someone who knows about hemochromatosis and iron overload. An interesting epilogue to this story is that a third sibling, a female, had been sent away to live elsewhere at a very young age for some unknown reason. She was therefore spared inhaling the iron oxide dust. This sibling lived a normal life span with no evidence of lung cancer.

In England, studies of iron miners substantiated that these workers were twice as likely to die of lung cancer as were coal miners. Iron miners in Slovakia had a three- to fourfold increased chance of incurring lung cancer as compared with nonminers. In France, an increased risk of lung cancer, as much as five- to twelvefold, was reported in iron miners.

Cell Types of Lung Cancer and Smoking Habits in Iron Ore Miners		
Histological Description	Smokers	Nonsmokers
Small cell carcinoma	23	3
Squamous cell carcinoma	9	1

Source: C. Edling

Moreover, death due to cancers of the larynx, bronchial tubes, and lungs was seen also among steel foundry and metal finishing workers. In the British steel industry in Sheffield, in 1926–35, the risk for these diseases was reportedly increased by 2.5 fold. Pennsylvania steel workers in the 1970s were found to have nearly a twofold increase in cancer over workers in non-steel industries, and the risk in steel foundry workers in Ontario

105

was increased nearly fivefold. Especially in danger are those men who have been employed in iron industries for several decades.

The carcinogenic hazard of inhaled iron also is observed in animals. For instance, mice exposed to ferric oxide dust during their early months of life develop malignant lung tumors as they age. Control mice exposed to dust without ferric oxide develop only a small number of nonmalignant tumors.

Working in the iron and steel industry is by no means the only way in which humans are exposed to inhaled iron. Industrial sand workers can be exposed to inhalation of iron contained in crystalline silica. In a 22-year study in 18 plants of 4027 domestic industrial sand workers exposed to crystalline silica, investigators Steenland and Sanderson observed a 60 percent excess of lung cancer mortality in the exposed cohort compared with the US male population. According to the International Agency for Research of Cancer, inhaled crystalline silica from occupational source is a carcinogen. Indeed, as early as 1940, inhaled silica was shown to induce lung cancers in mice. However, the International Agency for Research on Cancer noted that the epidemiologic evidence was not entirely consistent and that different forms of silica might vary in carcinogenic efficacy. A possible cause of fluctuation in potency might be variable contamination of silica with a known carcinogen, such as iron. Additionally, inconsistency could reflect different levels of tissue iron in persons who inhale silica.

Another dangerous source of the metal is that found in varieties of asbestos, primarily crocidolite and amosite. Exposure to these varieties of asbestos can result in carcinoma of lungs, esophagus, and stomach, as well as mesothelioma (membrane cancer) of pleural, pericardial, and peritoneal linings. Cigarette smoking and crocidolite exposure have synergistic effects that promote ferritin release by alveolar macrophages, which could catalyze oxidative injury to other alveolar cells.

According to Dr. Ann Aust, Utah State University, an expert in inhaled environmental particulates, "Two properties of the asbestos fibers that appear to affect their carcinogenicity are size and durability. . . . Generally the longer the fiber resides in the lung, the more likely it is to be carcinogenic." Asbestos fiber, once inhaled, remains in the lung for a lifetime. These fibers can actually acquire iron from the cells in the lung. Lungs can become quite burdened with iron just from the amount of this metal present in one's body. Because these fibers can accumulate iron from the body, it was originally thought that this was a protective mechanism. Thus, it becomes of great significance that these fibers remain in the lung forever after the individual is exposed to the asbestos, and that the iron these individuals accumulate becomes bioavailable and potentially life threatening. Within the past 50 years, it has become well established that exposure to varieties of asbestos that contain iron silicates can result in malignancies of the lungs and lung lining. The cancers usually appear about 20 or more years after the initial contact with the iron fiber. Varieties of asbestos that consist of magnesium silicate without iron contamination are far less dangerous.

Other perilous varieties of asbestos include tremolite, which has a very high content of iron. A form of asbestos that is composed of magnesium rather than iron silicate (chrysotile) is dangerous mainly because it contains pure veins of tremolite. Indeed, the risk of inhaling tremolite has been reported from areas in the Mediterranean region and in the South Pacific, where local residents scrape the mineral from hillsides and employ it as whitewash for the interior and exterior of homes. Inhabitants of these homes have a greatly increased chance of developing respiratory tract cancers.

Aust and her colleagues continue to examine the extent to which bioavailable iron in the urban environment causes acute death. When particle levels in the urban environment rise above a certain level, epidemiologists can predict what percentage of the population will die in the next 24 hours from cardiopulmonary problems. Dr. Aust and her team of scientists examined three particular types of coal fly ash: one from Utah, one from Illinois, and one from North Dakota. It turns out that these combustion particles are very capable of releasing iron and inducing an inflammatory mediator; the smaller the particle of iron, the greater the amount of the inflammatory mediator released. The smaller the particles, the more damaging to the lung. When iron was removed from the particles using Desferal, a chemical that binds with and removes iron, the particles' ability to induce this inflammatory mediator was completely eliminated.

Perhaps most troubling is the role of inhaled iron in causing lung cancer in tobacco smokers. Compared with nonsmokers, moderate smokers have a tenfold increased risk of dying from lung cancer, and heavy smokers incur a fifteen- to twenty-five-fold increased risk.

We don't typically think of iron as something we inhale; actually, it may seem odd that a heavy metal such as iron can be inhaled. But for 50 years (1925–1975), an even heavier metal, lead, was inhaled in large quantities from automobile exhaust fumes.
—*E. D. Weinberg and C. D. Garrison,*
idInsight, *First Quarter, 2001*

Tobacco leaves incorporate a great amount of iron. Usually iron is gotten from food we eat, where the amount of iron that we absorb is regulated. This highly sophisticated system assures that we get adequate amounts of iron to function. When iron is inhaled, it bypasses this system. Instead, the iron is taken directly into the lungs, completely uncontrolled. When metals are ingested the intestinal lining permits only 5–10 percent absorption, whereas the lung allows 30–50 percent entry into the circulatory system. The lower respiratory tract of cigarette smokers contains an increased amount of iron that is predominantly sequestered within alveolar macrophages, but is also present in alveolar epithelial fluid. Alveolar macrophages are white blood cells of the lungs with a defense purpose. When iron inhalation is chronic, as it is for smokers or for those constantly exposed to secondhand smoke, iron in the lungs eventually reach levels that cannot be contained by the alveolar macrophages. Overwhelmed with iron, these defense cells are unable to defend the lungs against opportunistic infection or disease such as cancer.

As little as 4 picograms of iron in a single defense white blood cell renders it unable to kill cancer cells. The alveolar macrophages attempt to scavenge the inhaled iron and render the iron insoluble, but about one-fourth of it remains active as a destructive oxidizing agent. Such agents cause disruptions

Iron Content of Alveolar Cells in Smokers Versus Nonsmokers

	Total (n=43)	Nonsmokers (n=19)	Smokers (n=24)
Fe μg X 10⁻⁶ cells			
Mean± SD	0.45 ± 0.35	0.33 ± 0.21	0.55 ± 0.40
Range	0.039 — 1.79	0.039 — 0.84	0.095 — 1.79

Source: J. L. Corhay et al.

and mutations of cell DNA as well as inactivation of cell membranes that are essential for good health. Furthermore, as cancer cells emerge from the damaged tissue lesions, they use the excessive iron to grow and multiply. To make matters worse, the tar and gas phases of cigarette smoke contain chemicals that promote the release of stored iron from the macrophages. The amount of sequestered iron in these cells is a measure of the number of cigarettes smoked daily or recently. Similar increases in lung macrophage iron are noted in iron and asbestos workers as well as in persons who inhale iron-contaminated air particulates.

Inhaled iron increases risk not only of respiratory tract cancers and infections but also of cardiovascular disease. Increased risk of developing rheumatoid arthritis (RA) also has been reported. In a recent study, 31,336 postmeno-pausal women who had no history of RA were monitored for 11 years. During that period, 158 cases of RA developed. The patients were twice as likely to be current smokers or nearly twice as likely to have stopped smoking within the past decade as they were to be never smokers or women who had quit smoking more than 10 years earlier.

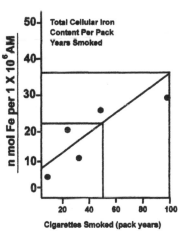

Source: S. McGowan and S. Henley

This study indicates that at least a decade or more of non-smoking apparently is required for the body's defenses to safely dispose of the previously inhaled iron. The metal must not only be packaged into ferritin, but the iron-engorged ferritin must also be gradually converted to insoluble hemosiderin. The latter cannot be excreted; rather it is placed in burial sites throughout the body, where hopefully it will cause no interference with normal tissue functions.

Unfortunately, macrophage defense against inhaled asbestos iron is even less adequate than against tobacco iron. Persons who stopped inhaling asbestos for as long as 20 years remain at risk for development of respiratory tract cancers.

Tuberculosis

Excessive iron in pulmonary tissues is associated not only with increased risk of neoplastic disease but also with that of microbial cell growth. For instance, 10 patients with pulmonary fungal infection caused by *Pneumocystis carinii* had a sevenfold increase in iron concentration in acellular bronchoalveolar lavage fluid, compared with 5 healthy controls.

Legionella pneumophila and *Mycobacterium tuberculosis* require iron-loaded macrophages for bacterial multiplication. The risks of legionellosis and of tuberculosis are strongly increased in cigarette smokers.

Pulmonary hemosiderosis

Pulmonary hemosiderosis is characterized by accumulation of iron in the form of hemosiderin in the lungs. The condition can be present in adults as a result of pancreatic insufficiency or cardiac or collagen vascular disease but is primarily seen in children due to Heiner's syndrome, which is a group of symptoms, including allergies to cow's milk, that can result in blood loss. Children with this condition will have repeated respiratory problems, coughing, sometimes coughing up blood, and iron-deficiency anemia due to the blood loss from the lung. They might display symptoms of anemia, such as fatigue, heart arrhythmia, or pallor, and also run a fever or vomit.

Dorr G. Dearborn, Ph.D., M.D., Pediatric Pulmonary Division, Case Western Reserve University School of Medicine, who is an expert in pulmonary hemosiderosis (PH), recommends that if a physician should encounter "an infant or child [who] has a chronic cough and chest congestion and who is anemic, . . . the physician might consider the possibility of pulmonary hemosiderosis among all the other more common diagnostic possibilities."

Cystic fibrosis

Investigators Stites, Plautz, Bailey, O'Brien-Ladner, and Wesselius examined the iron levels of patients with chronic bronchitis or cystic fibrosis. Sputum was obtained from 33 patients, including 10 patients with cystic fibrosis (CF) and 18 with chronic bronchitis (CB). Compared with controls, concentrations of iron in sputum were increased in both patient groups, with the greater amounts of iron in the cystic fibrosis patients. Ferritin content of sputum was also increased in each group, with cystic fibrosis patients higher than patients with chronic bronchitis. Compared with control subjects, sputum transferrin was decreased in the CF patients but not in the CB patients.

Reactive oxygen species (ROS) may contribute to airway injury in patients with cystic fibrosis. Iron catalyzes oxidant injury by promoting generation of highly reactive hydroxyl radicals. Iron in the lower respiratory tract may be free, ferritin bound (from which iron can be reductively mobilized), or transferrin bound (which generally prevents iron mobilization).

Liver disease in CF patients usually presents at puberty, but the clinical signs of liver disease appear late, by which time cirrhosis may be established. In a set of 16 young cystic fibrosis patients and 13 normal children, nonheme iron absorption was increased sixfold in the CF patients. In a different study of 10 young adults with CF and 5 normal controls, no detectable iron was found in control sputum. In CF mean sputum, on the other hand, iron content was 242 ng/mL.

More than 800 different mutations are estimated to be associated with cystic fibrosis disease. Investigators Rohlfs, Shaheen, and Silverman, University of North Carolina, Chapel Hill, studied 89 CF patients and found an association between the frequency of *HFE* genes in patients with cystic fibrosis, especially those with meconium ileus.

111

These investigators determined the frequency of the C282Y and H63D mutations in a group of 89 CF patients with meconium ileus. The carrier frequency of C282Y among the CF patients with meconium ileus was 19.4 percent versus 7.7 percent in the unaffected control group. Their findings are suggestive of a relationship between the development of meconium ileus or other gastrointestinal diseases in CF and the *HFE* gene.

References:

Aust, A., L. Lund, C. Chao, S. Park, and R. Fang. "Role of Iron in the Cellular Effects of Asbestos." *Inhalation Toxicology* 12 (2000): S75S–80S.

Campbell, J. A. "Effects of Precipitated Silica and of Iron Oxide on the Incidence of Primary Lung Tumours in Mice." *British Medical Journal* 2 (1940): 275–80.

Colombo, C., P. M. Battezzati, A. Crosignani, A. Morabito, D. Costantini, R. Padoan, and A. Giunta. "Liver Disease in Cystic Fibrosis: A Prospective Study on Incidence, Risk Factors, and Outcome." *Hepatology* 36 (2002): 1374–82.

Corhay, J. L., G. Weber, T. H. Bury, S. Mariz, I. Roelandts, and M. F. Radermecker. "Iron Content in Human Alveolar Macrophages." *European Respiration Journal* 5 (1992): 804–9.

Criswell, L. A., L. A. Merlino, J. R. Cerhan, T. R. Mikuls, A. S. Mudano, M. Burma, P. Folsom, A. R. Folsom, and K. G. Saag. "Cigarette Smoking and the Risk of Rheumatoid Arthritis among Postmenopausal Women: Results from the Iowa Women's Health Study." *American Journal of Medicine* 112 (2002): 465–71.

Diwakar, V., L. Pearson, and S. Beath. "Liver Disease in Children with Cystic Fibrosis." *Paediatric Respiratory Review* 2 (2001): 340–9.

Dreyfus, J. "Lung Carcinoma among Siblings Who Have Inhaled Dust Containing Iron Oxides during Their Youth." *Clinical Medicine* 30 (1936): 256–60.

Edling, C. "Lung Cancer and Smoking in a Group of Iron Ore Miners." *American Journal of Industrial Medicine* 3 (1982): 191–99.

Ghio, A., R. Pritchard, K. Dittrich, and J. Samet. "Non-heme (Fe 3+) in the Lung Increases with Age in Both Humans and Rats." *Journal of Laboratory Clinical Medicine* 129 (1997): 53–61.

Luce, D., et al. "Environmental Exposure to Tremolite and Respiratory Cancer in New Caledonia: A Case Control Study." *American Journal of Epidemiology* 151 (2000): 259–65.

McGowan, S., and S. Henley. "Iron and Ferritin Contents and Distribution in Human Alveolar Macrophages." *Journal of Clinical Medicine* 111 (1988): 611–17.

Plautz, M. W., K. Bailey, and L. J. Wesselius. "Influence of Cigarette Smoking on Crocidolite-Induced Ferritin Release by Human Alveolar Macrophages." *Journal of Laboratory Clinical Medicine* 136 (2000): 449–56.

Rohlfs, E. M., N. J. Shaheen, and L. M. Silverman. "Is the Hemochromatosis Gene a Modifier Locus for Cystic Fibrosis?" *Genetic Testing* 2 (1998): 85–88.

Silica, Some Silicates, Coal Dust and Para-aramid Fibrils. Monograph 68. "Elevation of Carcinogenic Risks to Humans." International Agency for Research on Cancer, Lyon, France, 1997.

Smith, K. R., and A. E. Aust. "Mobilization of Iron from Urban Air Particulates Leads to the Generation of Reactive Oxygen Species in Vitro and Induction of Ferritin Synthesis in Human Lung Epithelial Cells." *Chemical Research in Toxicology* 10 (1997): 828–34.

Steenland, K., and W. Sanderson. "Lung Cancer among Industrial Sand Workers Exposed to Crystalline Silica." *American Journal of Epidemiology* 153 (2001): 695–703.

Stites, S. W., B. Walters, A. R. O'Brien-Ladner, K. Bailey, and L. J. Wesselius. "Increased Iron and Ferritin Content of Sputum from Patients with Cystic Fibrosis or Chronic Bronchitis." *Chest* 114 (1998): 814–19.

Weinberg, E. D. "Iron, Asbestos, and Carcinogenicity." *The Lancet* i (1989): 1399–1400.

———. "The Role of Iron in Cancer." *European Journal of Cancer Prevention* 5 (1996): 19–36.

———. "The Development of Awareness of the Carcinogenic Hazard of Inhaled Iron." *Oncology Research* 11 (1999): 109–13.

Wesselius, L. J., M. E. Nelson, and B. S. Skikne. "Increased Release of Ferritin and Iron by Iron-Loaded Alveolar Macrophages in Cigarette Smokers." *American Journal of Respiratory Critical Care Medicine* 150 (1994): 690–95.

9
Joints

"Besides chronic fatigue, joint pain is a leading complaint of hemochromatosis patients."
                                    —Joanne Jordan, M.D., M.P.H., Associate Professor of Medicine and
                                              Orthopedics, University of North Carolina, Chapel Hill

It is now well established that in persons with hereditary hemochromatosis (HHC) arthritis is a quite common condition. But this recognition is relatively recent. Early descriptions of HHC emphasized possible development of diabetes, liver cirrhosis, and skin darkening (due to melanin deposition) but completely overlooked joint pain. Not until 1964 was arth-ropathy described as a potential complication of HHC.

Besides fatigue and impotence, arthritis is a very early symptom of HHC. Tenderness, pain, and loss of function can occur in any of several joints. Pain or aching in joints of the hands (especially the first two metacarpal-phalangeal joints), the knees, and ankles are most commonly associated with

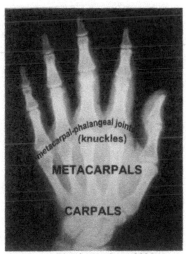

Source: Iron Disorders Institute, 2004

hemochromatosis arthritis. Involvement of joints of the fingers may cause the patient to keep the hand clenched; this condition is termed "iron fist." Many persons who need hip or knee replacements, especially at younger ages, have unrecognized HHC. The joint lesions usually are degenerative rather than inflammatory, but often the patient is misdiagnosed as having rheumatoid arthritis (RA) without the serum rheumatoid factor. HHC arthropathy is often mistaken for RA.

One recent study compared arthritis symptoms in individuals with *HFE* mutations, newly identified through a large screening program, with individuals lacking such mutations from the same population. Individuals with hemochromatosis genotypes reported a higher frequency of some arthritis symptoms than did controls.

Even carriers of the C282Y mutation may be at increased risk for osteoarthritis. For instance, in a group of 176 patients with arthritic lesions in the hand, the prevalence of carriers was 12.5 percent; of noncarriers, 7.8 percent. Among the older patients, the percentages were 36 percent for carriers and 26 percent for noncarriers.

Both RA and hemochromatosis arthritis are symmetrical but each has distinctive characteristics. In HHC arthritis there is bone enlargement, joint narrowing, and joint damage (erosion, pitting); whereas in RA, inflammation and synovial thickening is more prominent. In HHC arthritis, the second and third metacarpals, wrists, shoulders, hips, knees, and ankles are the joints most typically affected, whereas in RA, the joint involvement is more global.

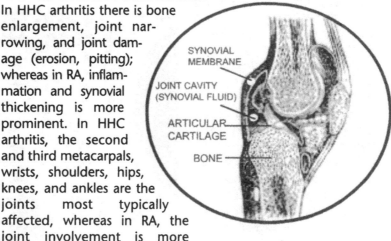

SYNOVIAL MEMBRANE

JOINT CAVITY (SYNOVIAL FLUID)

ARTICULAR CARTILAGE

BONE

Source: Iron Disorders Institute, 2004

Rheumatoid arthritis

Rheumatoid arthritis (RA) occurs in non–iron loaded persons. Unlike HHC arthritis, RA is an autoimmune condition characterized by inflammation of joints. About 1 percent of all populations are affected, women 2–3 times more commonly than men. Disease symptoms usually begin between 25 and 50 years of age. In about 70 percent of cases, an altered serum protein is formed. It is a gamma globulin called rheumatoid factor.

An indicator of inflammation, elevation of the erythrocyte sedimentation rate, is present in 90 percent of cases. In RA, about 25 percent of the cells of the synovial linings of the diseased joints have iron deposits. Even though the RA patient exhibits iron in the synovium, the iron is there more from inflammation in the joint rather than classic iron overload.

Synovial macrophages attempt to scavenge the toxic iron deposits by packaging the metal in ferritin and hemosiderin. In fact, in RA, synovial fluid ferritin is much higher than the level of ferritin in serum. Unfortunately, a portion of the joint iron remains "free" to catalyze oxidative radical reactions that cause extensive disruption of cell membranes and promote inflammatory tissue damage.

Patients with such chronic inflammatory diseases as RA tend to have a mild anemia called the anemia of chronic disease (ACD). Features of ACD include lowered values of hemoglobin, serum iron, and transferrin iron saturation; high normal or elevated serum ferritin; and ample iron deposits in bone marrow. These patients have lowered "functional" iron but are not iron deficient. The mechanism of production of ACD and its role in defense against disease are described in chapter 14.

There is accumulating evidence that tobacco smoking is a risk factor for development of RA, but it is not presently known if the high iron contamination of the smoke is the causative agent. For instance, in a population of 31,336 middle-aged women, the risk of developing RA was doubled in current smokers and nearly doubled in those who had quit smoking within the past decade (as compared with nonsmokers for over 10 years, who no longer were at increased risk).

Some persons with RA who do not form rheumatoid factor

AGES	DIAGNOSED WITH HHC	ONSET OF JOINT SYMPTOMS
17-24	1	6
25-34	13	12
35-44	20	23
45-54	46	34
55-64	41	27
65-78	29	5
unknown	9	22

Source: H. R. Schumacher

have a complicating skin condition called psoriatic arthritis. Elevated iron is present in their skin lesions. Another misleading diagnosis is pseudogout. It is not fully understood how excessive iron initiates and promotes joint destruction.

Patients with a chronic inflammatory disease such as rheumatoid arthritis (RA) are considered by some clinicians to be anemic and often are prescribed oral iron supplements. However, an important feature of ACD is the natural physiologic blocking of intestinal iron absorption. Thus, injection of iron is sometimes considered. Unfortunately, and not surprisingly, injected iron induces a flareup of joint inflammation.

The patients are not allergic to iron, as seen by the lack of increase in serum immune complexes. Rather, upon injection, the iron-binding capacity of both serum and synovial fluid becomes saturated with the result that low-molecular-weight iron complexes accumulate. These "free" iron compounds are the actual agents that cause the oxidative damage.

Indeed, even super-large doses of oral iron (given by some clinicians to overcome the intestinal absorption block) can activate the inflammatory condition. For instance, an RA patient was fed 200 mg of ferrous sulfate three times per day for three days (a total amount of two-thirds of a gram of iron!). She experienced a severely increased intensity of symptoms. Her pain index rose from 0 up to 5. Her morning stiffness increased, and her grip strength declined. Also increased was production

	Women		Men	
Age in years	General Population	HHC	General Population	HHC
17-38	5.9	10.3	5.2	8.9
40-59	23.4	34.9	14.7	22.2
60-84	51.1	42.8	33.8	31.5

Percentage of persons in general population and in those with HHC who reported arthritic symptoms

Source: S. M. McDonnell et al.

of rheumatoid factor and, not surprisingly, ferritin.

In agreement with these observations in humans are studies in animals. For example, two groups of rats were maintained on diets that contained, respectively, 20 and 300 parts per million of iron. There was no difference in the two sets in growth or body weight. However, injection of inflammatory substances caused a far greater chronic arthritic response in the rats that had received the excessive amount of oral iron. Ironically, the excessive amount actually is employed in the formulation of animal feeds in the United States!

In 36–72 percent of patients with HHC arthritis, calcification of joint cartilage can be detected by x-ray. The deposits consist of crystals of calcium pyrophosphate. However, de-ironing procedures often do not lead to amelioration of joint pain.

In a 1996 US Centers for Disease Control and Prevention Patient Survey of 2851 respondents, 1241 reported arthritis pain. Of these patients only 9.2 percent reported improvement following phlebotomy, whereas 34 percent reported their pain was worse. In an earlier study of 300 hemochromatosis patients the response was similar; 42 percent felt worse after phlebotomy. Perhaps benefit might fail to occur, especially

JOINT PAIN AFTER INITIAL PHLEBOTOMY	
WORSE	42 %
SAME	32
BETTER	27
PAIN DURING	15
PAIN AFTER	13

Source: H. R. Schumacher

119

in those individuals who have the calcium salt deposits. In the same 300 patients, hot compresses provided the greatest pain relief.

Possible therapy

Scientists in Glasgow studied the effects of human lactoferrin on arthritis caused by infection. Mice given *Staphylococcus aureus* developed septic arthritis. Joints of these mice with established inflammation were injected peri-articularly with 0.5 mg or 1 mg of human lactoferrin, and arthritis was monitored for 3 days. Mice injected with the lactoferrin showed significantly suppressed local inflammation for up to 3 days, achieving up to 71 percent of the effect of corticosteroid. Human lactoferrin may have clinical utility in reducing articular inflammation, particularly in septic arthritis.

EFFECTS OF THERAPY ON JOINT PAIN		
	HELPED	DID NOT HELP
ASPIRIN	57	6
NSAIDS	32	10
HOT APPLICATION	154	5
COLD APPLICATION	33	109 WORSENED

Source: H. R. Schumacher

Osteoporosis

Osteoporosis has been described in hemochromatosis and, as well, is a prominent feature of African siderosis. Involvement of the spine and the head of the femur often are seen. It has been postulated that iron loading leads to chronic deficiency of vitamin C and that this, in turn, causes the decay of the skeletal system. Injection of animals with iron dextran has resulted in marked decline in the quantity of vitamin C in the liver and diminished bone mineral density. The degeneration of the skeletal system due to dietary lack of vitamin C in humans (i.e., scurvy) has been recognized for several centuries.

References:

Blake, D., and P. A. Bacon. "Iron and Rheumatoid Disease." *The Lancet* i (1982): 623.

Bothwell, T. H., R. W. Charlton, and A. G. Motulsky. "Hemochromatosis." In *Metabolic Basis of Inherited Diseases,* C. R. Scriver, A. L. Beaudet, W. S. Sly, and D. Valle, eds., 1433–62. 6th ed. New York: McGraw Information Sciences, 1989.

Criswell, L. A., L. A. Merlino, J. R. Cerhan, T. R. Mikuls, A. S. Mudana, M. Burma, A. R. Folsom, and K. G. Saag. "Cigarette Smoking and the Risk of Rheumatoid Arthritis among Postmenopausal Women: Results from the Iowa Women's Health Study." *American Journal of Medicine* 112 (2002): 465–71.

Drews, F. J. A., C. J. Morris, E. J. Lewis, and D. R. Blake. "Effect of Nutritional Iron Deficiency on Acute and Chronic Inflammation." *Annals of Rheumatic Disease* 46 (1987): 859–65.

Felitti, V. "Hemochromatosis: A Common Rarely Diagnosed Disease." *Permanente Journal* 3 (1999): 10–20.

Guillen, C., I. B. McInnes, D. Vaughan, A. B. Speekenbrink, and J. H. Brock. "The Effects of Local Administration of Lactoferrin on Inflammation in Murine Autoimmune and Infectious Arthritis." *Arthritis Rheumatology* 43 (2000): 2073–80.

Jordan, J. M. "Arthritis in Hemochromatosis or Iron Storage Disease." *Current Opinion in Rheumatology* 16 (1) (2004): 62–66.

McCurdie, I., and J. D. Perry. "Haemochromatosis and Exercise Related Joint Pains." *British Medical Journal* 318 (1999): 449–51.

McDonnell, S. M., B. L. Preston, S. A. Jewell, J. Barton, C. Q. Edwards, P. C. Adams, and R. Yip. "A Survey of 2851 Patients with Hemochromatosis: Symptoms and Response to Treatment." *American Journal of Medicine* 106 (1999): 619–24.

Morris, C. J., J. R. Earl, C. W. Trenam, and D. R. Blake. "Reactive Oxygen Species and Iron—A Dangerous Partnership in Inflammation." *International Journal of Biochemistry Cell Biology* 27 (1995): 109–22.

Ross, J. M., R. M. Kowalchuk, J. Shaulinsky, L. Ross, D. Ryan, and P. D. Phatak. "Association of Heterozygous Hemochromatosis C282Y Gene Mutation with Hand Osteoarthritis." *Journal of Rheumatology* 30 (2003): 121–25.

Schumacher, H. R. "Hemochromatosis and Arthritis." *Arthritis and Rheumatology* 7 (1964): 41–50.

Schumacher, H. R., P. C. Straka, M. A. Krikker, and A. T. Dudley. "The

Arthropathy of Hemochromatosis." *Annals of New York Academy of Sciences* 526 (1988): 224–33.

Vaiopoulos, G., G. Papanikolaou, M. Politou, I. Jibreel, N. Sakellaropoulos, and D. Loukopoulos. "Arthropathy in Juvenile Hemochromatosis." *Arthritis and Rheumatology* 48 (2003): 227–30.

Weinberg, E. D. "Iron Therapy and Cancer." *Kidney International* 55, suppl. 69 (1999): S131–S134.

10

Skin, Nails, Oral Cavity, Hearing, and Vision Abnormalities

"Skin hyperpigmentation is characteristic of iron overload and present in about 50–70 percent of the patients with hemochromatosis."
—Jacek Drobnik, M.D., Ph.D., Assistant Professor of
Physiology and Medicine, Department of Pathophysiology,
Medical University of Lodz, Poland

Emerging evidence supports a relationship of excess body iron with diseases of skin such as psoriasis, cellulitis, porphyria cutanea tarda (PCT), and leprosy, as well as with conditions such as hyperpigmentation, premature aging, loss of body hair and premature balding, ichthyosis, platonychia, and koilonychia (spoonlike indention in the fingernails). The latter condition may also be present in patients with chronic iron deficiency.

Excessive iron in skin promotes growth of various bacterial and fungal pathogens; among the most dreaded is the leprosy bacterium. This very slow-growing microbe requires iron-loaded macrophages in order to multiply. Dermal tissues high in iron are associated with active cases of leprosy. During recovery and in arrested cases, the iron level becomes similar to that of healthy persons.

Human skin in body parts normally exposed to sunlight contains about 3 times more iron and 10 times more ferritin than occurs in those areas that usually remain clothed. A similar threefold elevation in skin iron content was produced in mice by ultraviolet irradiation of the animals for 6 weeks. Further elevations of fivefold, tenfold, and fifteenfold, respectively, were observed after 12, 18, and 24 weeks of irradiation.

Absorption of iron through the skin of barefoot farmers underlies the development of sarcomas of the lower extremities. This disease is highly prevalent in those parts of African nations that conform geographically to continental rifts where the soil is rich in iron oxide volcanic clays. Soils high in iron oxide in Iceland and in the Faroe Islands also are associated with a very high incidence of the sarcoma. The disease mainly occurs in men because of their occupational involvement with iron-rich soil and because their body iron burden generally is higher than that of women.

Photoaging of skin is associated with wrinkling and sagging due to general alteration of the epidermal and dermal components. The process involves iron-catalyzed formation of destructive oxidant radicals. In tests with cells of human skin fibroblasts, the toxicity of ultraviolet irradiation was shown to be directly correlated with the amount of iron added to the cultures.

Skin hyperpigmentation, called "bronze diabetes" due to the bronze color of the skin with concurrent diabetes mellitus, is characteristic of iron overload and present in about 50–70 percent of the patients with hemochromatosis. The color differs and is reported to be ashen-gray in about 50 percent and brown or mixed in about 50 percent. The presentation is generally over the entire body and especially prominent on the face, the palms of the hands, bottoms of the feet, within creases, and under the eyes. In a study of 100 patients, "approximately one-half had metallic gray pigmentation, one-fifth had a frankly brown pigmentation, and the remainder had an intermediate shade. External genital hyperpigmentation was seen in one-third of patients, and one-fifth had hyperpigmentation of flexural folds, scars, and nipple areolae," according to Jacek Drobnik.

Hyperpigmentation is generally thought to be caused by increased melanin, but this condition may also be due to excessive amounts of cutaneous iron. Hairless mice injected with iron had "hemosiderin granules extracellularly between collagen

124

bundles as well as within dermal macrophages, Langerhans cells and indeterminate dendritic cells of the epidermis. A larger amount of iron was deposited in the facial than in the dorsal skin, resulting in darker pigmentation of the former. This study suggests that brownish discoloration of skin in hemochromatosis might be attributable in some degree to accumulation of hemosiderin and that pronounced hyperpigmentation of the face in hemochromatosis might be due to increased activation of melanocytes by a high content of hemosiderin."

Hemosiderin is believed to increase activation of melanocytes, yet one study found normal levels of beta-melanocyte-stimulating hormone (beta-MSH) in patients with hemochromatosis. The authors concluded that an elevated level of beta-MSH was not significant in the development of hyperpigmentation in HHC patients.

Other skin changes in hemochromatotics are dry, atrophied, and scaly skin, koilonychia, and hair loss, especially in the pubic area and outermost region of the eyebrow, and vary according to gender. Total body hair loss can be experienced by some patients with iron overload. Causes of total body hair loss could be due to abnormal hormones such as in hypothyroidism, a possible consequence of iron overload.

Koilonychia, also called spoon nails, is most often associated with iron deficiency. This condition, however, is also seen in patients with iron overload, especially on the first three digits: the thumb, pointing finger, and middle finger. High levels of iron interfere with the absorption of zinc, which can be confirmed by testing serum zinc levels. Iron removal therapy will generally correct koilonychia.

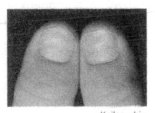

Koilonychia

Porphyria cutanea tarda (PCT) is another skin condition seen in patients with elevated body iron. PCT is characterized by blisters on the dorsal part of the hand. About 40 percent of patients with PCT carry the C282Y mutation of *HFE*, the gene for hemochromatosis. The high iron levels serve to catalyze the formation of reactive oxygen species (ROS). According to metabolic experts Bonkovsky and Lambrecht,

"ROS can enhance uroporphyrin formation by increasing the rate at which uroporphyrinogen is oxidized to urophophyrin. Iron may also act indirectly to inhibit uroporphyrinogen decarboxylase activity by enhancing the formation of nonporphyrin products of porphyrinogen oxidation that are themselves direct inhibitors of the enzyme. Finally, iron can act to increase urophorphyrin production by inducing delta-aminolevulinic acid synthase, thus increasing the amount of delta-aminolevulinic acid, the precursor to uroporphyrinogen, present in the cell."

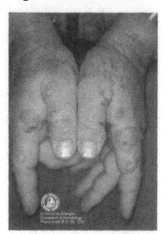

Note the blistering and koilonychia in this patient example. PCT may accompany hemochromatosis; therefore, patients with skin discoloration, blisters, or complaints of skin pain when exposed to the sun should be further evaluated for iron loading.

Oral cavity

In periodontal disease, iron levels are higher in the gingival fluid and saliva, which can enhance growth of pathogens and increased

Photo courtesy of: Professor of medicine Dr. M. Simon, Dermatologische Universitatsklinik Erlangen, Germany

free radical activity. These effects contribute to the deterioration of the gingiva.

In studies of the effects of iron on pathological and non-pathological strains of *P. gingivalis*, investigators found that under iron-limiting conditions, the pathogenic strains of *P. gingivalis* had a much lower requirement for human iron-loaded transferrin and hemin than the nonpathogenic strains.

The study provided evidence that the ability of *P. gingivalis* to multiply in vitro under iron-limiting conditions may be correlated with its ability to induce infections in an animal model. Isolates of *P. gingivalis* possessing a low requirement for iron are likely to have a higher potential for initiating periodontal infections.

Lactoferrin (Lf), a protein that binds with free iron in serum, withholds iron from harmful pathogens, and reduces oxidative stress by suppressing free radical production. In a study of juveniles with "localized gingivitis," investigators found that the level of bound iron in Lf is significantly reduced in these patients compared to controls. Their data suggest that Lf in this context has a reduced capacity to bind iron and that Lf iron levels may play an important role in this type of disease.

According to summary reports of the Iron Disorders Institute Patient Registry, over one-third of hemochromatosis patients report problems with their gums, including swollen, spongy, or bleeding gums. Physicians might recommend to their patients Oralbalance® products, such as biotène (Laclede, Inc.). The biotène products contain lactoferrin, which traps free (unbound) iron, depriving harmful bacteria and fungi access to the metal. These products also contain lysozyme, which is an antibacterial.

"These results provide further evidence of the recently reported intrinsic role of iron in aminoglycoside ototoxicity, and highlight a potential risk of aminoglycoside administration in patients with elevated serum iron."

—B. J. Conlon and D. W. Smith

Hearing loss

Aminoglycoside drugs have been widely used since 1945, but the extent of hearing impairment in iron-loaded humans that might have been triggered by use of these antibiotics is not yet known. During the past half century, it has become apparent that the majority of useful antibiotics can combine with various metals, often specifically with iron. In a few cases, iron helps the drugs to heal illnesses; in others, it may interfere with the useful action of the drugs; in still others, iron might have no noticeable effect.

The antibiotic action of the aminoglycosides (amikacin, gentamicin, kanamycin, neomycin, netilmicin, streptomycin, tobramycin) is not altered by iron. However, the metal strongly increases toxicity of these drugs for the infected host. Elevated body iron increases the risk of hearing loss and possibly deafness. In the series of hemochromatosis/iron overload cases reported in 1980, about 30 percent had hearing impairment.

The tissues most likely to be harmed by iron-activated aminoglycosides are the proximal tubules of the kidney and the hair cells of the inner ear. Kidney injury has been reported in 10–20 percent of patients receiving these drugs. Moreover, of the 4 million patients in the United States treated with aminoglycosides each year, nearly half may suffer some hearing impairment. The drug-iron combination is thought to be dangerous because of its ability to catalyze formation of free (i.e., hydroxyl) radicals which are very powerful cell-damaging oxidants.

Accordingly, damage to hosts could be predicted to be increased if the drugs are given with iron and to be decreased if they are given with iron chelators. Evidence from several research groups indicates that this is indeed what happens. When fed iron-enriched diet and injected with gentamicin, rats had increased tubular damage and guinea pigs had elevated hearing injury. The amount of iron enrichment in each study was comparable to that consumed by some humans who take iron supplements.

When the iron chelator deferoxamine (DF) was injected along with gentamicin, rats had lowered renal toxicity and guinea pigs had lowered ototoxicity. Similarly, ototoxicity in guinea pigs due to injection of neomycin was decreased in animals injected with DF. An iron chelator with fewer side effects than DF, namely dihydroxybenzoate (DHB), was even more efficient than DF in protecting guinea pigs from hearing damage due to gentamicin, kanamycin, and streptomycin. Furthermore, another iron chelator, salicylate, also successfully protected guinea pigs from gentamicin-induced hearing loss. Drugs commonly ingested by humans, such as aspirin and ibuprofen, are iron chelators, but it is not known if these could prevent the aminoglycosides from combining with iron in body tissues.

A possibly more reliable method of protection against kidney damage and hearing loss than use of iron chelators would be avoidance of acquisition of excessive iron. Unless prescribed by a clinician for medical reasons, dietary iron supplements should be eliminated. Another important source of excessive iron is tobacco smoking. Due to the large quantity of iron in tobacco leaves, a one-pack-per-day cigarette smoker is esti-

128

mated to inhale over one million picograms of iron per day. Indeed, in a recent study of nearly 4000 persons, active as well as passive inhalation of cigarette smoke itself was observed to significantly contribute to hearing loss. Thus it would seem prudent for cigarette smokers to be especially cautious in using aminoglycoside antibiotics.

"Iron retinotoxicity leads to a dysfunction of all layers but the changes may be reversible in the early period of the disease. The late period iron toxicity produces more severe damage to the inner retina than the outer retina."

—M. Imaizumi et al.

Vision

Iron can damage vision in several ways. In a study in rats, exposure to cigarette smoke (which is high in iron contamination) was found to be cytotoxic to lens tissue. The iron was deposited in the lenses of the animals. Cigarette smoking has also been observed to increase development of cataracts.

In another investigation, iron accumulation was correlated with retinal neurodegeneration. In aceruloplasminemia, an inherited condition in which there is an absence or abnormally low amount of circulating ceruloplasmin, peripheral retinal degeneration is a consequence. Iron depends upon ceruloplasmin for normal transport, and when the protein is absent or insufficient iron delivery is flawed.

Candida albicans, a fungus responsible for candidiasis infections has been detected in the eyes of patients with cataracts. *Candida* is suppressed by lactoferrin, an iron-binding protein found in human secretions such as tears. In Sjogren's Disease, body fluids such as saliva and tear production are diminished. Since lactoferrin is contained in these fluids, patients with Sjogren's can have less lactoferrin and possibly have an increased incidence of candidiasis infection on the lens of the eyes. To date, there are no scientific studies to substantiate the increased incidence of ocular candidiasis.

In age-related macular degeneration (AMD), increased iron levels have been found upon autopsy in AMD-affected maculas as compared with normal maculas. The difference is significant and the authors have proposed that treatment of AMD with iron chelators should be evaluated.

References:

Bissett, D. L., R. Chatterjee, and D. P. Hannon. "Chronic Ultraviolet Radiation Induced Increase in Skin Iron and the Protective Effect of Topically Applied Iron Chelators." *Photochemical Photobiology* 54 (1991): 215–23.

Brady, J. J., H. A. Jackson, A. G. Roberts, R. R. Morgan, S. D. Whatley, G. L. Rowlands, C. Darby, E. Shudell, R. Watson, J. Paiker, M. W. Worwood, and G. H Elder. "Co-Inheritance of Mutations in the Uroporphyrinogen Decarboxylase and Hemochromatosis Genes Accelerates the Onset of Porphyria Cutanea Tarda." *Journal of Investigative Dermatology* 115 (2000): 868–74.

Brittenham, G. M., G. Weiss, P. Brissot, F. Laine, A. Guillygomarch, D. Guyader, R. Moirand, and Y. Deugnier. "Clinical Consequences of New Insights in the Pathophysiology of Disorders of Iron and Heme Metabolism." *Hematology* (American Society of Hematology Education Program) (2000): 39–50.

Chevrant-Breton, J., M. Simon, M. Bourel, and B. Ferrand. "Cutaneous Manifestations of Idiopathic Hemochromatosis: Study of 100 Cases." *Archives of Dermatology* 113 (1977): 161–65.

Conlon, B. J., B. P. Perry, and D. W. Smith. "Attenuation of Neomycin Ototoxicity by Iron Chelation." *The Laryngoscope* 108 (1998): 284–87.

Conlon, B. J., and D. W. Smith. "Supplemental Iron Exacerbates Aminoglycoside Toxicity In Vivo." *Hearing Research* 115 (1998): 1–5.

Cruickshanks, K. J., R. Klein, B. E. Klein, T. L. Wiley, D. M. Nondahl, and T. S. Tweed. "Cigarette Smoking and Hearing Loss." *Journal of the American Medical Association* 279 (1998): 1715–19.

Drobnik, Jacek. "Hemochromatosis." http://www.emedicine.com/derm/topic878.htm.

Dupond, A. S., N. Magy, P. Humbert, and J. L. Dupond. "Nail Manifestations of Systemic Diseases." *Review Practices* 50 (2000): 2236–40.

Fausti, S. A., J. A. Henry, H. I. Schaffer, D. J. Olson, R. H. Frey, and W. J. McDonald. "High-Frequency Audiometric Monitoring for Early Detection of Aminoglycoside Ototoxicity." *Journal of Infectious Diseases* 165 (1992): 1026–32.

Fine, D. H., D. Furgang, and F. Beydouin. "Lactoferrin Iron Levels Are Reduced in Saliva of Patients with Localized Aggressive Periodontitis." *Journal of Periodontology* 73 (2002): 624–30.

Forge, A., and J. Schacht. "Aminoglycoside Antibiotics." *Audiology and Neurootology* 5 (2000): 3–22.

Grenier, D., V. Goulet, and D. Mayrand. "The Capacity of Porphyromonas Gingivalis to Multiply under Iron-Limiting Conditions Correlates with Its Pathogenicity in an Animal Model." *Journal of Dental Research* 80 (2001): 1678–82.

Hahn, P., A. H. Milam, and J. L. Dunaief. "Maculas Affected by Age-Related Macular Degeneration Contain Increased Chelatable Iron in the Retinal Pigment Epithelium and Bruch's Membrane." *Archives of Ophthalmology* 121 (2003): 1099–1105.

Imaizumi, M., C. S. Matsumoto, K. Yamada, Y. Nanba, Y. Takaki, and K. Nakatsuka. "Electroretinographic Assessment of Early Changes in Ocular Siderosis." *Ophthalmologica* 214 (2000): 354–59.

Lambrecht, R. W., and H. L. Bonkovsky. "Hemochromatosis and Porphyria." *Seminars in Gastrointestinal Disease* 13 (2002): 109–19.

Marklova, E. "Microelements and Inherited Metabolic Diseases." *Acta Medica* (Hradec Kralove) 45 (2002): 129–33.

McDonnell, S. M., B. L. Preston, S. A. Jewell, J. Barton, C. Q. Edwards, P. C. Adams, and R. Yip. "A Survey of 2,851 Patients with Hemochromatosis: Symptoms and Response to Treatment." *American Journal of Medicine* 106 (1999): 619–24.

Moirand, R., P. C. Adams, V. Bicheler, P. Brissot, and Y. Deugnier. "Clinical Features of Genetic Hemochromatosis in Women Compared with Men." *Annals of Internal Medicine* 127 (1997): 105–10.

Momotani, E., N. Wuscher, P. Ravisse, and N. Rastogi. "Immunohisto-chemical Identification of Ferritin, Lactoferrin and Transferrin in Leprosy Lesions of Human Skin Biopsies." *Journal of Comparative Pathology* 106 (1992): 213–20.

Morliere, P., S. Salmon, M. Aubailly, A. Risler, and R. Santus. "Sensitization of Skin Fibroblasts to UVA by Excess Iron." *Biochimica Biophysica Acta* 1334 (1997): 283–90.

Niederau, C., G. Strohmeyer, and W. Stremmel. "Epidemiology, Clinical Spectrum and Prognosis of Hemochromatosis." *Advances in Experimental Medicine and Biology* 356 (1994): 293–302.

Petrovich, I. U. A., R. P. Podorozhnaia, T. I. Genesina, and G. F. Beloklitskaia. "Iron in Oral Cavity Fluid in Gingival Inflammation."

Patol Fiziol Eksp Ter. Patologicheskaia Fiziologiia Eksperimentalnaia Terapiia 3 (1996): 22–24.

Priuska, E. M., and J. Schacht. "Formation of Free Radicals by Gentamicin and Evidence for an Iron/Gentamicin Complex." *Biochemical Pharmacology* 50 (1995): 1749–52.

Sha, S. H., and J. Schacht. "Salicylate Attenuates Gentamicin-Induced Ototoxicity." *Laboratory Investigation* 79 (1999): 807–13.

Sheskin, J., and R. Zeimer. "In Vivo Study of Trace Elements in Leprous Skin." *Dermatologia* 16 (1977): 745–47.

Simonart, T., J. C. Noel, G. Andre, D. Parent, J. P. Van Vooren, P. Hermans, Y. Lunardi-Yskandar, C. Lambert, T. Dieye, C. M. Farber, C. Liesnard, R. Snoeck, M. Heenen, and J. R. Boealaert. "Iron as a Potential Co-Factor in the Pathogenesis of Kaposi's Sarcoma." *International Journal of Cancer* 78 (1998): 720–26.

Smith, A. G., S. Shuster, A. Bomford, and R. Williams. "Plasma Immunoreactive Beta-Melanocyte-Stimulating Hormone in Chronic Liver Disease and Fulminant Hepatic Failure." *Journal of Investigative Dermatology* 70 (1978): 326–27.

Song, B. B., D. J. Anderson, and J. Schacht. "Protection from Gentamicin Ototoxicity by Iron Chelators in Guinea Pig in Vivo." *Journal of Pharmacology & Experimental Therapeutics* 282 (1997): 369–77.

Song, B. B., S. H. Sha, and J. Schacht. "Iron Chelators Protect from Aminoglycoside Induced Cochleo- and Vestibulo-Toxicity." *Free Radical Biology & Medicine* 25 (1998): 189–95.

Tsuji, T. "Experimental Hemosiderosis: Relationship between Skin Pigmentation and Hemosiderin." *Acta Derma Venerology* 60 (1980): 109–14.

Walker, P. D., and S. V. Shah. "Evidence Suggesting a Role for Hydroxyl Radical in Acute Renal Failure in Rats." *Journal of Clinical Investigation* 81 (1988): 334–41.

Weinberg, E. D. "The Mutual Effects of Antimicrobial Compounds and Metallic Cations." *Bacteriological Reviews* 21 (1957): 46–68.

———. "The Development of Awareness of the Carcinogenic Hazard of Inhaled Iron." *Oncology Research* 11 (1999): 109–13.

Yefimova, M. G., J. C. Jeanny, N. Keller, C. Sergeant, X. Guillonneau, C. Beaumont, and Y. Courtois. "Impaired Retinal Iron Homeostasis Associated with Defective Phagocytosis in Royal College of Surgeons Rats." *Investigative Ophthalmology Visual Science* 43 (2002): 537–45.

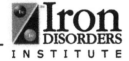

PART TWO

Pathology, Iron, and Our Natural Defense Mechanisms

11
Cancer

"Four epidemiological studies have been performed that are generally consistent with the hypothesis that increased available body iron stores increase the risk of cancer or of general mortality."

—*Richard G. Stevens, Ph.D., cancer epidemiologist*

For more than 70 years, evidence has been accumulating that elevated iron initiates and promotes cancer cell growth. Among the first observations of iron-related cancer were those of Dreyfus in the early 1930s where inhalation of iron dust resulted in lung cancer for two young children who polished watch screws with iron oxide.

We don't think of iron as a carcinogen, but as an essential nutrient to sustain life. Though it is true that all life would cease to exist without iron, the metal has the potential to become toxic and free, where its lethal capabilities come into play.

How iron is carcinogenic

Iron can be carcinogenic in three ways. First, ferric ions are reduced by superoxide and the ferrous product is reoxidized by peroxide to regenerate ferric ions and hydroxyl radicals. Reactive oxidants such as hydroxyl radicals, when generated in close proximity to DNA, cause mutations, cross linking of DNA, and strand breaks in DNA. The radicals also can cause structural changes in nuclear and cytoplasmic cell membranes. Additionally, cellular permeability is increased.

Secondly, in addition to initiating the cancer process, iron can bolster the growth of cancer cells by suppressing host white blood cell defenses. For instance, tumorcidal activity of macrophages has been found to be abolished by iron dextran, carbonyl iron, or iron-loaded ferritin, but not by plain dextran, carbon particles, or iron-poor ferritin.

The third way in which iron can be carcinogenic is that of providing an essential nutrient for unrestricted tumor cell multiplication. Although normal and cancer cells have a similar growth requirement for iron, the unrestricted proliferation and spread of cancer cells would be expected to require an enhanced and probably diversified supply of the metal. Indeed, cancer cells have a much greater ability than normal cells to take in the growth-essential iron.

For example, in normal human type B lymphocytes, expression of transferrin receptor protein is a multistep, tightly regulated process that requires the presence of several regulatory substances. In contrast, malignant B type lymphocytes express transferrin receptor proteins constantly and therefore can absorb iron continuously. Similarly, transferrin receptors are expressed in greater amounts by leukemic cells than by normal white blood cells. Moreover, human melanoma cells and small cell lung cancer cells can produce their own transferrin-like molecules in order to efficiently obtain elevated amounts of iron.

Even in the absence of transferrin, some varieties of leukemic cells can obtain the metal from inorganic forms of iron! Normal and cancer cells differ not only in how they obtain iron but also in how they use it. Normal cells divert much of their iron intake into intracellular storage in ferritin, whereas cancer cells consign a higher proportion to tasks involving metabolism and further cell multiplication.

Inhalation

The earliest studies on iron loading and cancer began with inhalation as described in detail in chapter 8 on the pulmonary system and iron.

Ingestion

Since 1988, a number of studies in animals that either (a) produce spontaneous tumors, (b) are inoculated with tumor cells, or (c) are exposed to chemical carcinogens have shown that excess iron in the diet enhances development of liver, colorectal, and mammary-gland cancers. In humans, these types of studies would be unethical. However, in large groups of humans such as 0.5 percent of persons of European descent and 10 percent of sub-Saharan Africans, genetic mutations can result in assimilation of excessive dietary iron.

In the European disorder, hereditary hemochromatosis (HHC), the resulting increased tissue iron load is associated with markedly elevated risk of liver cancer, usually but not always subsequent to development of liver cirrhosis. Excessive frequency of esophageal cancer, thyroid cancer, and malignant melanoma also has been reported.

The carrier rate of HHC is about 10–15 percent among persons of European descent. Some of these carriers of the HHC gene mutations can also become iron loaded with ensuing increased risk of various cancers. Of special concern are those carriers who have two HHC gene mutations (compound heterozygotes) and who also have a double (homozygote) mutation in a gene that determines the structure of the transferrin receptor protein. In one study, these persons were observed to have an increased risk of sevenfold for multiple myeloma and for breast cancer and a ninefold increased risk for colorectal cancer. The compound mutations in the HHC gene plus the double mutation in the transferrin receptor gene alter the HHC protein and the transferrin receptor protein. These alterations render the combination inefficient in its normal task of preventing body cells from accumulating excessive iron.

"HFE gene mutations are associated with an increased risk of colon cancer. Cancer risk is greatest in mutation carriers who are older or consume high quantities of iron."

—N. J. Shaheen et al.

In African siderosis, the amount of liver cancer likewise is quite high. In a study of 601 autopsies of adults from seven countries of central and southern Africa, 20 percent of the males and 15 percent of the females had very marked liver iron loading. These persons had an eighteenfold increase in death from hepatoma as compared with those whose livers showed slight or no iron loading.

In persons who lack known genetic disorders of intestinal iron assimilation, an association between elevated body iron values and increased risk of malignancy also has been reported. For instance, in a set of 3345 men, 6.9 percent developed cancers during a 10-year period. The patients had a mean transferrin iron saturation value of 33.1 percent at least 4 years prior to diagnosis, whereas the men who remained free of cancer had a mean transferrin iron saturation value of 30.7 percent. The probability that this difference might have occurred simply by chance is less than 1 in 500.

In another group of 41,276 women and men followed for 14 years, 6 percent developed cancers. Among persons in this group whose initial transferrin iron saturation value was more than 60 percent, the risk for colorectal cancer was increased more than threefold.

In persons with or without mutations in the HHC gene, consumption of excessive amounts of red meat (beef, lamb, venison) or of alcohol can result in increased absorption of iron from the diet. Nonheme iron is the predominant form of the metal in plant foods. Animal foods contain a much larger amount of heme iron. Unlike absorption of nonheme iron, absorption of the heme content of red meat is relatively unaffected by the level of iron deposits already in the body. Indeed, the percentage of heme iron absorbed is 5–10 times greater than that of nonheme iron. The ability of alcohol to enhance intestinal absorption of nonheme iron has often been demonstrated. During intake of alcohol, stomach acid secretion is enhanced. The increased acidity helps to maintain iron ions in solution as they reach the duodenum where absorption into the bloodstream takes place.

Injection

As mentioned above, iron loading can also occur by injection through the skin. As with inhalation and ingestion, animal studies have found that injected iron is associated with such malignant diseases as hepatomas, colorectal cancers, mesotheliomas and kidney tubular cell carcinomas. In humans given iron intramuscularly, some cases of sarcomas have resulted at the sites of injection. Persons who walk barefoot over volcanic clay that is rich in iron oxide likewise are at risk of developing sarcomas. In fact, in specific geographic areas of Cameroon, Zaire, Rwanda, Burundi, and Uganda, this sarcoma comprises as much as 20 percent of adult malignancies.

"One might worry about the iron-injectable compounds which are being tested and used. One could almost guess that someone is going to find iron dextran carcinogenic."

—A. Furst, 1960

A large quantity of iron (200–250 mg) is present in red blood cells in a 1-pint blood transfusion. Thus injection of multiple pints of whole blood in patients at the time of cancer surgery might be associated with enhanced recurrence of malignant growth. A survey of 27 published reports on this unresolved matter found that 14 groups of investigators recorded an increased risk; 13 groups did not.

Fifteen to 20 percent of adults who are long-term survivors of acute leukemia develop transfusional iron overload. This hazardous complication is so common that routine evaluation of all patients is recommended and therapeutic phlebotomy should be performed as necessary.

Decompartmentalization

Still another possible danger of iron loading results from the release of the metal from normal body sites. Iron can escape from normal cells by mechanical, chemical, or infectious injury. Thus persons with intestinal mucosal bleeding due to untreated Crohn's disease or ulcerative colitis have, respectively, a four- to sevenfold or a ten- to twentyfold increased risk of developing colorectal cancer. Patients with bleeding in the urinary bladder wall due to schistosomal bladder worms have an elevated risk of bladder cancer. Patients with chronic forms of viral hepatitis leak iron from damaged liver cells, and they have greatly increased risk of liver cancer.

139

References:

Aust, A., L. Lund, C. Chao, S. Park, and R. Fang. "Role of Iron in the Cellular Effects of Asbestos." *Inhalation Toxicology* 12 (2000): S75S–80S.

Barton, J. C., and L. F. Bertoli. "Transfusion Iron Overload in Adults with Acute Leukemia: Manifestations and Therapy." *American Journal of Medical Sciences* (2000) 319: 73–78.

Bilello, J. P., E. E. Cable, and H. C. Ison. "Expression of E-cadherin and Other Paracellular Junction Genes Is Decreased in Iron-Loaded Hepatocytes." *American Journal of Pathology* 162 (2003): 1323–38.

Criswell, L. A., L. A. Merlino, J. R. Cerhan, T. R. Mikuls, A. S. Mudano, M. Burma, P. Folsom, A. R. Folsom, and K. G. Saag. "Cigarette Smoking and the Risk of Rheumatoid Arthritis among Postmenopausal Women: Results from the Iowa Women's Health Study." *American Journal of Medicine* 112 (2002): 465–71.

Dreyfus, J. "Lung Carcinoma among Siblings Who Have Inhaled Dust Containing Iron Oxides during Their Youth." *Clinical Medicine* 30 (1936): 256–60.

Furst, A. *Metal Binding in Medicine.* See "Metals in Tumors," p. 346. Philadelphia, PA: J. B. Lippincott, 1960.

Luce, D., et al. "Environmental Exposure to Tremolite and Respiratory Cancer in New Caledonia: A Case Control Study." *American Journal of Epidemiology* 151 (2000): 259–65.

Shaheen, N. J., L. M. Silverman, T. Keku, L. B. Lawrence, E. M. Rohlfs, C. F. Martin, J. Galanko, and R. S. Sandler. "Association Between Hemochromatosis (*HFE*) Gene Mutation Carrier Status and the Risk of Colon Cancer." *Journal of National Cancer Institute* 95 (2003): 154–59.

Stevens, R. G. "Iron and the Risk of Cancer." *Medical Oncology and Tumor Pharmacotherapy* 7 (1990): 177–81.

Weinberg, E. D. "Iron, Asbestos, and Carcinogenicity." *The Lancet* i (1989): 1399–1400.

———. "The Role of Iron in Cancer." *European Journal of Cancer Prevention* 5 (1996): 19–36.

———. "The Development of Awareness of the Carcinogenic Hazard of Inhaled Iron." *Oncology Research* 11 (1999): 109–13.

———. "Do Some Carriers of Hemochromatosis Gene Mutations Have Higher Than Normal Rates of Disease and Death?" *Biometals* 15 (2002): 347–50.

12

Infection

"Iron is the metallic ion that presently appears to be most critical in determining whether an infectious agent is to be permitted to multiply in mammalian host tissues."

—E. D. Weinberg, 1966

By 1966, medical microbiologists had learned that infections due to bacteria, fungi, and protozoa are greatly intensified by the presence of excessive iron. Nearly all pathogenic micro-organisms need iron for survival, growth, and multiplication. None are able to bring in to the body of the host an adequate supply of the metal for their further multiplication. Accordingly, the microbial invaders either must acquire iron from the host or die. As is the case for cancer cell invaders, the preferred tissue sites for microbial cell multiplication are those that contain elevated or easily acquired iron. The table on page 147 contains a list of microbial genera whose growth in humans or animals is stimulated by excess iron.

Pathogens use one of four strategies to acquire iron from their hosts:

• *Heme receptor:* A very direct (and quite alarming) way is that some pathogens can break open our red blood cells and extract the iron from the extruded hemoglobin. This is why such highly virulent strains of streptococcal and staphylococcal bacteria are able to cause life-threatening infections. A variation on this method is for the pathogen to enter the intact red blood cells and extract iron from the internal hemoglobin. For this reason, such a dangerous protozoan as the malarial pathogen is able to cause so much deadly disease.

• *Transport protein receptors:* Another way for invaders to obtain iron is by attaching themselves to host proteins that contain iron, such as transferrin in blood serum and lactoferrin in other body fluids. Human meningococcal meningitis bacteria can pull iron directly from our transferrin molecules. That is why this pathogen, when it enters the bloodstream, can so quickly cause a fatal infection. However, these bacteria are not able to extract iron from transferrin molecules of animals. Thus the human meningococcus cannot cause disease in dogs or cows or horses. On the other hand, some pathogens can obtain iron from animal but not from human transferrin. For instance, *Actinobacillus pleuropneumonia* binds only to swine transferrin and thus causes a serious pneumonia only in hogs.

At least one pathogen, the spirochete that causes Lyme disease, has evolved to bypass the need for iron and uses manganese instead. Apparently the spirochete is able to withdraw manganese from human transferrin.

The human bacterial pathogen that causes most of our stomach ulcers, *Helicobacter pylori*, can withdraw iron from human lactoferrin. This iron-binding protein is a normal component of our stomach secretions. However, the human pathogen cannot use iron that is bound to cow or horse lactoferrin and thus is not the cause of ulcers in those animals.

• *Siderophore receptors:* A third method of microbial iron acquisition involves production by the invaders of small molecules called siderophores. These small molecules can remove iron from transferrin. The pathogens then proceed to extract the iron atoms from the siderophores. Some invaders are quite dangerous because they not only form siderophores but also break open red blood cells. Examples include highly pathogenic strains of *Escherichia coli*.

Also life threatening are invaders that can use various host small molecules as siderophores. For instance, listerial bacteria, a cause of some cases of animal and human septicemias and meningitis, produce no siderophores of their own. However, they can employ a host molecule, such as adrenaline, as a siderophore.

• *Cryptic receptors:* A fourth category of methods of microbial iron acquisition involves entrance of the pathogen into the host cells and then forcing the cells to pull in extra iron for use by the invader. Examples include such serious human pathogens as an airborne bacterium called *Coxiella* that results in Q fever and the cause of a tick-borne bacterial disease called ehrlichiosis. Some human pathogens, such as the bacteria that cause tularemia (sometimes called deer-fly fever or rabbit fever) and Legionnaire's pneumonia, are unable to extract iron from body fluids. Instead, they grow only inside host macrophages that provide readily available iron. The mycobacterium that causes tuberculosis can develop slowly in body fluids but grows best when inside iron-loaded host macrophages.

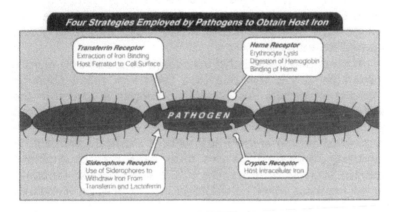

How microbes impaired in iron acquisition succeed as pathogens

Still other potential pathogens have so little ability to acquire host iron that they are dangerous only in persons who have severely iron-loaded body sites. A good example is a bacterium called *Vibrio vulnificus* that lives in coastal, marshy areas and which often is a contaminant of shellfish. This pathogen can obtain growth-essential iron from transferrin only if the protein is burdened with an abnormally high amount of iron.

In normal persons, the transferrin iron saturation percentage is 25–35 percent. In untreated hemochromatosis (HHC), it can rise to 100 percent. In one study, none of eight strains of *V. vulnificus* could grow in the presence of transferrin with 30 percent saturation; nearly all could grow with transferrin at 100 percent saturation. In normal mice, an injection of one million bacterial cells of *V. vulnificus* was needed to cause a lethal infection. In mice injected with iron, only one injected bacterial cell resulted in death!

Accordingly, persons who develop septicemia due to *V. vulnificus* are found to have either a wound associated with coastal seawater or to have eaten raw shellfish, plus are found to have an iron-loading condition. The latter includes alcoholism, African siderosis, chronic hepatitis, hemochromatosis, and thalassemia. Even some carriers of HHC gene mutations have elevated iron values and are susceptible to lethal infections due to *V. vulnificus*. As we will see in chapter 18, all persons in danger of iron loading are warned to avoid ingestion of raw shellfish. Moreover, if wounded in coastal waterways, they must obtain immediate antibiotic therapy.

Another potentially lethal infection that occurs only in iron-loaded persons is that due to a bacterium called *Capnocytophaga canimorsis*. This impaired pathogen is carried in the saliva of about 15–25 percent of healthy dogs and cats. Persons with normal iron values who are nipped or bitten by the contaminated healthy animals heal without medical treatment. In contrast, iron-loaded persons must have prompt antibiotic therapy to avoid development of a fatal septicemia. Especially at risk are those who have disorders such as HHC or alcoholism.

Iron loading of healthy persons lowers resistance to microbial infection

Healthy persons who become iron loaded either by injection, ingestion, inhalation, or decompartmentalization of iron develop marked susceptibility to microorganisms that normally are present in their environment. For example, in New Zealand in the early 1970s, all healthy Maori infants were injected with iron dextran. It was assumed, with absolutely no evidence, that the diet of Maori mothers was low in iron. In the same hospital nurseries, Caucasian infants received no iron injection and thus served as controls. The children who received the injection had a sevenfold increase in septicemias and meningitis caused by normally nonpathogenic strains of

E. coli and related environmental bacteria. When these appalling results were recognized, the iron injections were halted and the epidemic promptly disappeared.

In a study in a malarial area in Africa, pregnant women were injected with iron. It was not realized that they had latent (non-multiplying) malarial protozoa as a sequel to having recovered from the disease during childhood. The iron injections triggered clinical relapses, which then had to be treated with chloroquine.

Many instances of overloading diets with iron have resulted in an increase in bacterial infections. In young infants, for example, botulism spores may be present in the intestine but usually are unable to germinate and are harmless. Germination, however, can cause infant botulism. The germinated bacteria multiply in the intestine and secrete a neurotoxin into the child's nervous system. In a series of 69 cases in California, 39 had been breast-fed, 30 formula fed. Ten cases were fatal; each had been fed formula with added iron. Of the 59 survivors, the mean age of onset of the disease was 7.6 weeks in formula-fed infants and 13.8 weeks in breast-fed infants. Of the latter group, the median age of onset of those who had received supplemental iron was 8.3 weeks; of those receiving no extra iron, 15.6 weeks.

In an outbreak in infants of systemic (invasive) salmonellosis in Guam, formula-fed infants less than 6 months of age had an increased risk over breast-fed infants of ninefold for this serious bacterial disease. Moreover, among the 200 formula-fed infants, the 75 ill babies were 3 times more likely than the 125 healthy infants to have received formula with an iron content greater than 179 micromolar. Note that this quantity is 22 times the natural amount of iron in breast milk!

As early as 1870, A. Trousseau, a noted Parisian professor of clinical medicine, warned his medical students against feeding iron preparations to patients with quiescent (latent) tuberculosis. He was certain that this procedure could trigger clinical episodes of the disease. In recent years, numerous studies in animals have validated Trousseau's judgment. In 2001, moreover, in a study in humans, elevated dietary iron was associated with a 3.5 fold increase in cases of active tuberculosis. The

145

probability that this result might have occurred by chance is less than 1 in 1000.

Persons who inhale excessive iron are at greatly increased risk of developing such serious infections as streptococcal and Legionnaire's pneumonias, Q fever, and pulmonary tuberculosis. Especially at risk are smokers of iron-loaded tobacco and workers in various iron and steel industrial jobs.

Cystic fibrosis (CF) patients have elevated iron in sputum. The increased risk for iron-dependent *Pseudomonas* infection of the respiratory tract of CF patients is well established.

Decompartmentalized Iron can promote Infection

Patients who release iron deposits from liver cells in episodes of viral hepatitis or hemoglobin iron from red blood cells in episodes of malaria, sicklemia, Oroya fever, and other hemolytic diseases become very susceptible to invasive salmonella infections. So frequently does this happen that, in the early decades of the twentieth century, it was mistakenly believed that viral hepatitis was actually caused by salmonella bacteria. Furthermore, although quinine does not inhibit salmonella, the use of the drug to successfully treat malarial patients would at the same time cause their associated salmonella infection to clear up.

Still another type of altered iron metabolism associated with an infectious disease has become apparent during the past quarter of a century. In human immunodeficiency virus (HIV) infection, particularly in its more advanced stages, iron consistently has been observed to accumulate in bone marrow, muscle, liver, spleen, and brain white matter. The main cause of this form of iron loading is the patient's chronic recurrent inflammatory response that attempts to withhold iron from invading "opportunistic" bacterial, fungal, and protozoan pathogens. (The iron withholding defense system is described in chapter 14.)

Unfortunately, the severe buildup of iron in specific cells and tissues promotes the growth of unusual microorganisms that ordinarily are unable to acquire the metal in normal persons. Examples include normally nonpathogenic mycobacteria; candidal, cryptococcal, and pneumocystic fungi; and leishmanial protozoa. We will see in chapter 14 that well regulated iron withholding defense is essential for host victory over microbial

146

Microbial genera with strains whose growth in body fluids, cells, tissues, or intact vertebrate hosts is stimulated by excess iron.

Pathogenic growth
stimulated by excess iron

	Genera
FUNGI	Candida, Cryptococcus, Histoplasma, Paracoccidioides, Pneumocystis, Pythium, Rhizopus, Trichosporon
PROTOZOA	Entamoeba, Leishmania, Naegleria, Plasmodium, Toxoplasma, Trichomonas, Tritrichomonas, Trypanosoma
GRAM-POSITIVE & ACID FAST BACTERIA	Bacillus, Clostridium, Corynebacterium, Erysipelothrix, Listeria, Mycobacterium, Staphylococcus, Streptococcus, Tropheryma
GRAM-NEGATIVE BACTERIA	Acinetobacter, Aeromonas, Alcaligenes, Campylobacter, Capnocytophaga, Chlamydia, Coxiella, Ehrlichia, Enterobacter, Escherichia, Helicobacter, Klebsiella, Legionella, Moraxella, Neisseria, Pasteurella, Proteus, Pseudomonas, Salmonella, Shigella, Vibrio, Yersinia

Source: E. D. Weinberg, 1999

invaders. In contrast, saturation of the iron withholding defense coupled with deficiency of immune cellular resistance can lead to host demise.

Humans deprived of protein nutrition can develop such conditions as kwashiorkor, in which levels of transferrin can be as low as 10 percent of normal. Even with low iron intake, this defense protein can become completely (100 percent) iron sat-

147

urated. Such individuals have greatly increased risk of infection. In fact, some have developed lethal infections when health workers unknowingly gave them iron without first feeding protein to ensure their rebuilding of transferrin.

An important component of our inflammatory defense is haptoglobin. This protein, produced by the liver during inflammatory episodes, combines with hemoglobin that has leaked into serum. The combination prevents iron buildup in serum and it is filtered out of the bloodstream by macrophages. Humans have one of three phenotypes of haptoglobin: Hp-1, Hp-2, or Hp-2-2. In the United States, the approximate distribution, respectively, is 15 percent, 48 percent, and 37 percent.

Unfortunately, Hp-2-2 is less efficient than either of the other two phenotypes in maintaining low serum iron values. In a study in Belgium of 653 patients with AIDS, transferrin iron saturation in Hp-1, Hp-2, and Hp-2-2, respectively, was 29, 32, and 38 percent. Serum ferritin was, respectively, 92, 154, and 270 nanograms/mL. Not surprisingly, median survival of Hp-1 and Hp-2 patients was 11 years, whereas mean survival of Hp-2-2 patients was only 7.33 years. Moreover, in a set of 526 Zimbabwe pregnant women with AIDS, the viral load of Hp-2-2 patients was double that of Hp-1. Furthermore, women with serum ferritin greater than 24 ng/mL had 4 times the viral load of those with serum ferritin less than 6 ng/mL. In a different study of rural patients in Zimbabwe who had tuberculosis, the odds of death were 6 times greater in Hp-2-2 patients than in those whose phenotype was Hp-1.

Hypersplenism is often seen in patients with infection, chronic hemolysis, and iron overload diseases. In some cases, such as thalassemia or conditions of dyserythropoiesis, a splenectomy, the surgical removal of the spleen, is the only way to slow hemolysis and iron loading.

Once the spleen has been removed, the patient is more susceptible to infections with germs such as *pneumoccoci*, *meningococci*, *H. influenzae* and some protozoan infections. Among other pathogens that thrive on the extra iron in the sera of splenectomized persons are strains of *Hemophilus* and of *Capnocytophaga*.

References:

Delanghe, J. R., and M. R. Langlois. "Haptoglobin Polymorphism and Body Iron Stores." *Clinical Chemistry Laboratory Medicine* 40 (2002): 212–16.

Friis, H., E. Gomo, N. Nyazema, P. Ndhlovu, H. Karup, P. H. Madsen, and K. F. Michaelsen. "Iron, Haptoglobin Phenotype, and HIV-1 Viral Load: A Cross Sectional Study among Pregnant Zimbabwe Women." *Journal of Acquired Immune Deficiency Syndrome* 33 (2003): 74–81.

Gangaidzo, I. T., et al. "Association of Pulmonary Tuberculosis with Increased Dietary Iron." *Journal of Infectious Disease* 184 (2001): 936–39.

Posey, J. R., and F. C. Gherardini. "Lack of a Role for Iron in the Lyme Disease Pathogen." *Science* 288 (2000): 1651–53.

Vasil, M. L., and U. A. Ochsner. "The Response of Pseudomonas Aeruginosa to Iron: Genetics, Biochemistry and Virulence." *Molecular Microbiology* 34 (1999): 399–413.

Weinberg, E. D. "Roles of Metallic Ions in Host-Parasite Interactions." *Bacteriological Reviews* 30 (1966): 1336–51.

———. "Iron and Susceptibility to Infectious Disease." *Science* 184 (1974): 952–56.

———. "Iron Withholding: A Defense against Infection and Neoplasia." *Physiological Reviews* 64 (1984): 65–102.

———. "Patho-Ecological Implications of Microbial Acquisition of Host Iron." *Reviews in Medical Microbiology* 9 (1998): 171–78.

———. "The Development of Awareness of the Carcinogenic Hazard of Inhaled Iron." *Oncology Research* 11 (1999): 109–13.

———. "Iron Loading and Disease Surveillance." *Emerging Infectious Diseases* 5 (1999): 346–52.

———. "The Role of Iron in Protozoan and Fungal Infectious Diseases." *Journal of Eukaryotic Microbiology* 46 (1999): 231–36.

———. "Microbial Pathogens with Impaired Ability to Acquire Host Iron." *BioMetals* 13 (2000): 85–89.

———. "Modulation of Intra-Macrophage Iron Metabolism During Microbial Cell Invasion." *Microbes & Infection* 2 (2000): 85–89.

———. "Human Lactoferrin: A Novel Therapeutic with Broad Spectrum Potential." *Journal of Pharmacy & Pharmacology* 53 (2001): 1303–10.

———. "Iron, Infection and Sudden Infant Death." *Medical Hypotheses* 56 (2001): 730–33.

Weinberg, G. A, J. R. Boelaert, and E. D. Weinberg. "Iron and HIV Infection." In *Micronutrients and HIV Infection*. Edited by H. Friis, 135–58. Boca Raton, FL: CRC Press, 2002.

13
Sudden Infant Death Syndrome (SIDS)

"Liver iron concentrations have been shown to be higher in victims of SIDS than in postmortem controls, suggesting that high levels of tissue iron may be implicated in SIDS."

—R. Raha-Chowdhury et al.

Sudden infant death syndrome (SIDS) is the term used for infants between one-half and 12 months of age who die unexpectedly and for which a thorough autopsy fails to show an obvious cause of death. In this age group, SIDS accounts for 30–60 percent of all deaths. The syndrome occurs worldwide; the reported rate varies from 0.1 to 2.2 per thousand infants. In the United States, the rate is 1.7 per thousand. The peak incidence of SIDS occurs between 2 and 4 months of age.

Gastrointestinal and respiratory tract pathogens associated with infant deaths.								
	Microorganism	SIDS		Non-SIDS Deaths		Live-Healthy Controls	
Specimen	Name	Number	%	Number	%	Number	%
Feces	Clostridium perfringens	164	80	57	2	29	20
Feces	Cl. perfringens type A type	164	77	57	2	29	3
Feces	Escherichia coli 025;HI;02;H7;04;H2	246	66	17	5	180	23
Lung	Pneumocystis carinii	177	31	342	3	Not Available	

Source: T. G. C. Murrell et al. and S. I. Vargas et al.

Three risk factors for SIDS are well established: non–breast feeding, maternal smoking, and prone sleeping position. Two additional risk factors have been proposed: microbial infection in the gastrointestinal or respiratory tracts and postnatal iron loading. These five risk factors have been incorporated into a single unifying concept.

Infection as an underlying factor in SIDS

The newborn infant has passively acquired maternal protein antibodies to a variety of common microbial pathogens and toxins. Within a few weeks, however, these proteins begin to be broken down. The infant must quickly learn to actively produce its own antibodies. The critical time period during which maternal immune protection has diminished and infant immunity to a spectrum of microbes and their toxins has yet to fully mature is 2–4 months. This period corresponds quite well to the peak incidence of SIDS as well as to such infectious diseases as infant botulism and salmonellosis.

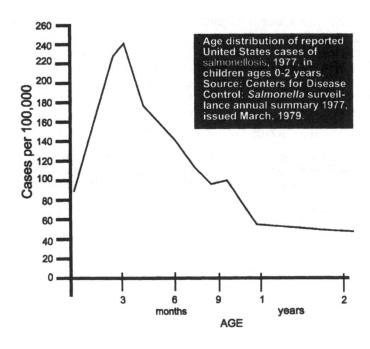

Age distribution of reported United States cases of salmonellosis, 1977, in children ages 0-2 years. Source: Centers for Disease Control: *Salmonella* surveillance annual summary 1977, issued March, 1979.

During the past several decades, a considerable variety of microbial pathogens have been reported to be resident in either the respiratory or the gastrointestinal tracts of infants who die of SIDS. Most prominent in the respiratory tract are *Bordetella pertussis*, *Hemophilus influenzae*, *Pneumocystis carinii*, *Staphylococcus aureus*, and *Streptococcus pyogenes*. In the gastrointestinal tract, most commonly cited are *Clostridium botulinum*, *Clostridium perfringens*, *Escherichia coli*, and *Helicobacter pylori*.

In cases of SIDS, the microbial invaders are not observed in the deeper tissues of the child, such as bloodstream, brain, liver, etc. Were the microbes to have been found in such tissues, they would be considered the primary cause of death and the diagnosis of SIDS would be excluded.

In addition to growing in the gastrointestinal or respiratory

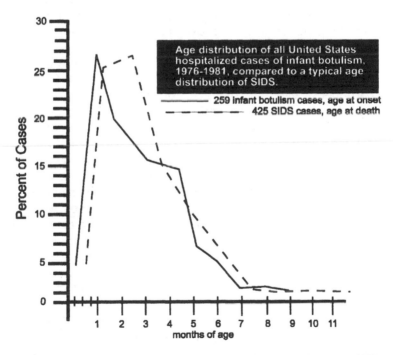

Age distribution of all United States hospitalized cases of infant botulism, 1976-1981, compared to a typical age distribution of SIDS.

259 infant botulism cases, age at onset
425 SIDS cases, age at death

Source. S. S. Arnon, 1980

tracts, some pathogens produce endotoxin or specific exotoxins that could cause a series of biochemical events leading to death. For example, growth of *Clostridium botulinum* in the intestine of young infants can result in sufficient exotoxin to cause respiratory paralysis. Moreover, combinations of intestinal *Escherichia coli* endotoxin with nasopharyngeal *Staphylococcus aureus* exotoxins are significantly more toxic than are each of the single toxins. The toxins are absorbed into the bloodstream where the dangerous combination would occur.

Iron as a risk factor for infection and toxin formation

As described in chapter 12, the vast majority of pathogenic microorganisms must obtain iron from their hosts. The metal is required not only for growth in the host but also for toxin formation. Indeed, the same quantity of iron that promotes optimal microbial growth permits maximal toxin formation. However, the iron content in human milk of 5–10 µM allows excellent growth and development of the full-term infant but is not adequate for growth of toxigenic bacteria. Breast milk contains about 23 µM of the iron-binding protein lactoferrin. Ninety-five percent of lactoferrin molecules are iron-free and thus function effectively to withhold the metal from the pathogens, even at the acid pH value of the stomach. Accordingly, the gastrointestinal tracts of healthy breast-fed infants who are not given iron supplements are free from toxigenic pathogens. Instead, these tracts contain the natural flora of nonpathogenic *Lactobacillus* and *Bifidobacterium*.

Lactobacillus species abstain from all use of iron. They employ manganese and cobalt to activate those enzymes that are iron dependent in pathogens. Growth of lactobacilli results in an infant gut pH value of 5.1–5.4, whereas the pH of infant intestines colonized by toxigenic bacteria is in the more alkaline range of 5.9–8.2. Bifidobacterial species do require iron, but they have developed a unique iron acquisition system that functions at pH 5 and which is not suppressed by lactoferrin.

As compared with breast-fed infants, episodes of acute respiratory tract infection and of diarrhea are significantly elevated in non–breast-fed infants less than 6 months of age. In a different study of nearly 10,000 infants, failure to initiate or to continue breast-feeding resulted in an eight- to tenfold increase in the rate of diarrheal mortality.

In a well-studied outbreak of salmonellosis, formula-fed infants less than 6 months of age had an increased risk over breast-fed infants of ninefold. Moreover, among the 200 formula-fed infants, the 75 cases of infection were 3 times more likely than the 125 healthy infants to have received formula with an iron content greater than 179 μM. In a different survey of 60 cases of infant botulism, dietary iron from formula or other sources contributed to the fulminant form of the disease.

Iron as a risk factor for SIDS

Breast milk substitutes lack human lactoferrin and contain various amounts of added iron. Non–breast-feeding has usually, but not always, been identified as a possible risk factor for SIDS. In a study of 128 cases of SIDS compared with 503 live infants, the bottle-fed children had a 2.45 fold increased chance of SIDS. Similarly, in a set of 98 SIDS cases and 196 live infants, non–breast-feeding increased the chance for SIDS by 3.7 fold. In an extensive review of epidemiological studies on SIDS, the authors stated that "reasonably strong" evidence exists for the recognition of non–breast-feeding as a risk factor.

Infants who die of SIDS appear to have been burdened, during postnatal life, with a higher load of iron than infants who die of non-SIDS causes. In a series of 112 cases of SIDS compared with 115 deaths from other causes, the risk of SIDS was increased 6.4 fold by giving iron drops 2 days before death and 9.2 fold by giving iron 2 weeks before death.

In another study of 63 cases of SIDS, the median liver nonheme iron concentration was 3 times that of the median concentration in 15 non-SIDS deaths. That this clear difference might have occurred by random chance was less than 1 in 499. Furthermore, the median blood ferritin value in SIDS infants was likewise 3 times that of infants who died of other causes. The investigators ruled out hereditary hemochromatosis as a cause of the difference and also showed that ferritin levels at birth did not differ between infants who were to die of SIDS from those who were to die of other causes. Apparently, SIDS infants are not born with abnormally high iron burdens.

Rather, they accumulate the metal during their few months of postnatal life.

Smoke inhalation and prone sleeping position associated with SIDS

Babies in households in which mothers smoke have a much increased chance of developing SIDS. In the study of 128 cases of SIDS compared with 503 live infants, the heavier the smoking, the higher was the risk. In a different investigation, infants whose mothers smoked more than 10 cigarettes daily had a 3.6 fold increased risk of SIDS as compared with infants whose mothers did not smoke.

Tobacco contains about 84 micrograms of iron per gram; approximately 0.1 percent is present in mainstream smoke. Active smokers have a markedly elevated level of iron in their respiratory tract and fluids. Passive inspiration of tobacco smoke would be expected to increase the infant's respiratory tract iron burden. Infants of parents who smoke have higher admission rates for respiratory tract infection in the first year of life. Those infants under 6 months of age whose immune systems are not yet fully developed and who are exposed to passive smoke would especially be subject to increased growth and toxigenesis of respiratory tract pathogens.

Prone sleeping position interferes with normal drainage of nasopharyngeal secretions into the esophagus. Thus the bacterial load in the upper respiratory tract would be greater in infants placed in the prone position as compared with the supine position. The microbes apparently grow in secretions that have pooled in the upper airways of infants who sleep in the prone position. In fact, in the study cited earlier, infants placed in the prone sleeping position had a 5.74 fold increased risk of SIDS.

Progress in encouragement of breast-feeding as well as in lowering the quantity of iron added to milk formulas are important steps in lowering the risk of iron-related sudden death in infants.

When mothers are not able to breast-feed their infants, formulas fortified with at least 4.5 but not more than 10 milligrams of iron per liter (4.5–10 mg/L) of formula are recommended. The attending family physician or pediatrician can determine an individual child's needs within this range. There are milk-based and soy-based formulas from which to choose. Again, individual needs must be assessed based on circumstances, such as whether the formula is the only source of food, the formula is supplemental to some amount of breast milk, the child is being raised as a vegetarian, or the child has allergies. All of these factors along with general health and growth rate of the child will help the physician to determine the right formula.

References:

Arnon, S. S. "Infant Botulism." *Annual Review of Medicine* 31 (1980): 541–60.

———. "Breast Feeding and Toxigenic Intestinal Bacteria: Missing Links in SIDS?" *Reviews in Infectious Disease* 6 (1984): S193–S201.

Dwyer, T., and A. L. Ponsoby. "Sudden Infant Death Syndrome—Insights from Epidemiological Research." *Journal of Epidemiology and Community Health* 46 (1992): 98–102.

Gilbert, R. E., R. E. Wigfield, P. J. Fleming, P. J. Berry, and P. T. Rudd. "Bottle Feeding and the Sudden Infant Death Syndrome." *British Medical Journal* 310 (1995): 88–90.

Griffin, I. J., and S. A. Abrams. "Iron and Breastfeeding." *Pediatric Clinics of North America* 48 (2001): 401–13.

Haddock, R. L., S. N. Cousens, and C. C. Guzman. "Infant Diet and Salmonellosis." *American Journal of Public Health* 81 (1991): 887–l000.

Haglund, R., and S. Cnattingius. "Cigarette Smoking as a Risk Factor for Sudden Infant Death Syndrome: A Population-Based Study." *American Journal of Public Health* 80 (1990): 29–32.

Lindsay, J. A., A. S. Mach, M. A. Wilkinson, L. M. Martin, F. M. Wallace, A. M. Keller, and L. M. Wojciechowski. "Clostridium Perfringens Type A Cytotoxic Enterotoxin(s) as Triggers for Death in the Sudden Infant Death Syndrome: Development of a Toxico-Infection Hypothesis." *Current Microbiology* 27 (1993): 51–59.

Lopez-Alarcon, M., S. Villalpando, and A. Fajardo. "Breast-Feeding Lowers the Frequency and Duration of Acute Respiratory Infection and Diarrhea in Infants under Six Months of Age." *Journal of Nutrition* 127 (1997): 436–43.

Mitchell, E. A., A. W. Stewart, D. M. O. Becroft, B. J. Taylor, R. P. K. Ford, D. M. J. Barry, E. M. Allen, and A. P. Roberts. "Results from the First Year of the New Zealand Cot Death Study." *New Zealand Medical Journal* 104 (1991): 71–76.

Moore, C. A., R. Raha-Chowdbury, D. G. Fagan, and M. Worwood. "Liver Iron Concentrations in Sudden Infant Death Syndrome." *Archives of Diseases of Childhood* 70 (1994): 295–98.

Murphy, M., J. Nicholl, and A. O'Callahan. "Iron and the Sudden Infant Death Syndrome." *British Medical Journal* 298 (1989): 1643.

Murrell, T. G. C., W. G. Murrell, and J. A. Lindsay. "Sudden Infant Death Syndrome (SIDS): Are Common Bacterial Toxins Responsible, and Do They Have Vaccine Potential?" *Vaccine* 12 (1994): 365–68.

Peterson, D. R. "Epidemiological Comparisons of the Sudden Infant Death Syndrome with Other Major Components of Infant Mortality." *American Journal of Epidemiology* 110 (1979): 699–709.

Raha-Chowdbury, R., C. A. Moore, T. Bradley, and R. Henley. "Blood Ferritin Concentrations in Newborn Infants and the Sudden Infant Death Syndrome." *Journal of Clinical Pathology* 49 (1996): 168–70.

Sayers, N. M., D. B. Drucker, J. A. Morris, and D. R. Telford. "Significance of Endotoxin in Lethal Synergy Between Bacteria Associated with Sudden Infant Death Syndrome: Follow Up Study." *Journal of Clinical Pathology* 49 (1996): 365–68.

Vargas, S. I., C. A. Ponce, and W. T. Hughes. "Association of Primary Pneumocystis Carinii Infection and Sudden Infant Death Syndrome." *Clinical Infectious Disease* 29 (1999): 1489–93.

Vege, A., and T. O. Rogmum. "Inflammatory Responses in Sudden Infant Death Syndrome." *FEMS Immunology Medical Microbiology* 25 (1999): 67–78.

Weinberg, E. D. "Acquisition of Iron and Other Nutrients in Vivo." In *Virulence IT Mechanisms of Bacterial Pathogens*. Edited by J. A. Roth, C. A. Bolin, K. A. Brogdon, and M. J. Wannemuehler, 79–94. Washington, DC: American Society of Microbiology, 1995.

———. "The Lactobacillus Anomaly: Total Iron Abstinence." *Perspectives in Biology & Medicine* 40 (1997): 578–83.

———. "The Development of Awareness of the Carcinogenic Hazard of Inhaled Iron." *Oncology Research* 11 (1999): 109–13.

————. "Iron, Infection and Sudden Infant Death." *Medical Hypotheses* 56 (2001): 730–34.

Worwood, M., R. Raha-Chowdbury, D. Eagen, and C. A. Moore. "Postmortem Blood Ferritin Concentrations in Sudden Infant Death Syndrome." *Journal of Clinical Pathology* 48 (1995): 763–67.

Yoon, P. W., R. E. Black, R. H. Moulton, and S. Becker. "Effect of Not Breastfeeding on the Risk of Diarrheal and Respiratory Mortality in Children under Two Years of Age in Metro Cebu, the Philippines." *American Journal of Epidemiology* 143 (1996): 1142–48.

14

Iron Withholding Defense System (IWDS)

"The invaded host plays an active part in the depletion of utilizable iron."
—I. Kochan

In *King Lear*, a tragedy written by William Shakespeare in 1605, the Earl of Gloucester is assaulted by the enemies of the king. In act 3, scene 7, they gouge out the earl's eyes. Gloucester's servant cries out: "I'll fetch some flax and whites of eggs to apply to his bleeding face."

Shakespeare and his contemporaries were apparently aware of the beneficial properties of the described concoction. It is unlikely, however, that they knew that the raw egg white used to treat the earl's injury contains an anti-infection factor. Microbial pathogens were not to be discovered for another two and one-half centuries, and the exact anti-infective factor in the whites of eggs not until 1944.

Indeed, egg-laying creatures have been employing the anti-infection factor for countless thousands of years. Finally, in 1944, microbiologists Arthur Schade and Leona Caroline discovered that the active ingredient is a protein whose function is to remove and bind "free" iron from the egg white. The two scientists were trying to develop a dysentery bacterial vaccine for the US Army. To enhance bacterial growth in culture, they tried adding raw egg white. To their surprise, the egg white completely prevented bacterial growth. Intrigued, Schade and Caroline pursued investigation and determined that an iron-binding protein prevented the white from becoming contaminated with microorganisms.

Birds' eggs are inherently subject to spoilage. Each egg is enclosed by a semi-permeable membrane within a fragile porous shell. The pores are needed for exchange of oxygen and carbon dioxide as the embryo develops, but microbes can invade through the pores. In nature, eggs are deposited in nests heavily laden with bacteria and molds. The birds employ iron withholding defense to protect their priceless embryos from infectious rot. They place an ample quantity of iron in the yolk for the rapidly developing chick to use for its growth. To prevent potential spoilage microbes that have migrated through the shell from multiplying or even from surviving, the birds place no iron in the white. They include the iron binding protein as 12 percent of the egg white solids. Moreover, since the protein functions best at alkaline pH values, our biochemically astute birds have raised the pH of the white to a value of 9.5.

When Schade and Caroline recognized the immense, broad spectrum antimicrobial power of the protein (which they termed "siderophilin" or "iron loving" in Greek), they predicted that it might be useful also in blood. Within 2 years, they showed that siderophilin is indeed the key factor that prevents most microbial invaders from growing in blood. We now know that the protein has a similar function in lymph and in cerebrospinal fluid (CSF). The protein comprises 3.5 percent of serum proteins and is active at pH 7.4, the normal pH value of blood.

One year after this momentous discovery, other scientists demonstrated that the protein has a second function, namely, to transport iron to host cells. They renamed the protein "transferrin" ("transporter of iron" in Latin). In healthy humans, 25–30 percent of the iron binding capacity of transferrin (Tf) is employed to transport the metal; 70–75 percent to withhold the iron from microbial invaders and to prevent blood, lymph, and CSF from accumulating "free" iron. During periods of infection and inflammation, the potential iron withholding capacity of transferrin can increase to as much as 90–95 percent. However, in iron-loaded humans, transferrin is encumbered with an excessive amount of the metal. As the percent-

162

age of saturation rises above normal, the anti-infective function correspondingly declines.

Partners in defense: transferrin, lactoferrin, ferritin

Unfortunately, to successfully accomplish its iron transport function, transferrin must be able to release the metal readily. The release is accomplished when the protein enters a host cell, encounters an endosome that has an acid pH value, and unloads the iron atoms. In fact, were the pH of our blood to become even slightly acidic, transferrin would lose its iron-binding capacity.

In tissue sites of microbial invasion, the pH does decline because of acids released from the invaders as well as from the defending white blood cells. Fortunately, animals and humans have available a protein partner to transferrin that specifically is designed to retain iron in body sites that have acid as well as neutral pH values. This compound is called "lactoferrin" (Lf) because it was first discovered in human milk in which it comprises 20 percent of the total protein. The class of proteins that contains transferrin, lactoferrin, and a few other similar compounds are now called "siderophilins."

Lactoferrin and transferrin are similar in size and structure. Each can tightly bind two atoms of iron per molecule. Unlike transferrin, lactoferrin has a single assignment, that of scavenging "free" iron. Also, unlike transferrin, the iron that lactoferrin acquires is not used for healthy cells. Eventually iron is deposited in ferritin-hemosiderin that is contained in cells of the liver (hepatocytes) and other cells that function to permanently sequester the metal.

Ferritin, present in all host cells, is a cylindrical protein nearly 6 times larger than siderophilins. Each ferritin molecule can retain up to 4500 atoms of iron. As ferritin molecules become engorged with iron, they are converted to hemosiderin, which functions as a highly insoluble iron burial site. Ferritin molecules discharged from decaying cells are found in blood serum but do not scavenge iron in this location.

The two circulating partners, transferrin and lactoferrin, act in a complementary manner to continuously purge body fluids and tissues of nonprotein bound "free" iron. Whereas transferrin is

Examples of Quantities of Lactoferrin in Human Fluids

The amount of lactoferrin in human fluids is directly related to the condition.

FLUID	Concentration (micromolar)	Underlying Condition
Colostrum	100	Normal
Breastmilk	20-60	Normal
Tears	25	Normal
Saliva	0.11	Normal Adults
	0.05	Normal Children
	0.25	Children with cystic fibrosis
Cerebrospinal Fluid	0.00	Normal Children
	0.01	Children with viral meningitis
	0.13	Children with bacterial meningitis
Synovial Fluid	0.014	Normal
	0.338	Inflammatory arthritis
Blood Serum	0.003	Normal
	2.5	Acute bacterial infection
Vaginal Fluid	0.1	Before menstruation
	2.0	Just after menstruation

Source: E. D. Weinberg, 2001

assigned to blood serum, lymph, and cerebrospinal fluid (CSF), lactoferrin is responsible for maintaining an environment devoid of "free" iron in body secretions that are commonly exposed to microorganisms. These include milk, tears, tubotympanum mucus, nasal exudate, bronchial mucus, saliva, gastrointestinal fluids, cervicovaginal mucus, and seminal fluid. Note that the only body fluid not protected by either transferrin or lactoferrin is urine. The large size of the two siderophilins (78kDa) would prevent healthy kidneys from excreting them into urine. To protect us against urinary tract infections, we depend on the flushing action of the urine.

In the chart listing examples of the quantities of lactoferrin in human body fluids, note that the concentration of lactoferrin markedly increases at sites of bacterial infections. The defense protein is a major component of granules contained in circulating white blood cells called neutrophils. The latter accumulate in infected areas and release the granules with subsequent liberation of Lf. Inherited inability to produce sufficient granules and neutrophilic lactoferrin is associated with recurrent infection and, in untreated persons, death.

A second protein called lysozyme (LZ) generally accompanies lactoferrin. The two defense proteins function as a team. Lactoferrin prevents bacterial growth and survival by trapping iron while lysozyme destroys the walls of the bacterial cells. The large concentration of lactoferrin in tears, together with lysozyme, efficiently protects ocular tissues from most bacterial pathogens.

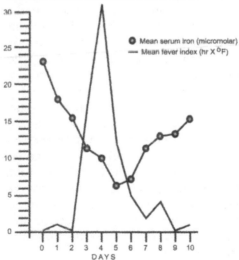

HYPOFERREMIC RESPONSE TO INFECTION
Four human volunteers were exposed to Francisella tularensis on day zero. They developed typical clinical illness as indicated by fever on days 3-8. Note how the serum iron level drops when the fever rises, then returns to normal as the fever abates.

● Mean serum iron (micromolar)
— Mean fever index (hr $\times {}^{0}$F)

DAYS

Source: E. D. Weinberg, 1984

165

Hypoferremic Infection

These two natural (nonimmune) proteins permit much lesser reliance on secretory antibody for antibacterial defense. Accordingly, possible scarring of delicate ocular tissues as a result of antigen-antibody reactions is minimized.

Upon host invasion, the reserves are mobilized.

A dozen years before the discoveries by Schade and Caroline of iron withholding proteins, iron concentrations in blood serum had been observed to be lowered in patients with infections or cancers. A clinical pathologist, A. Locke, monitored iron levels in sera from a great variety of patients with different illnesses. He found that sera from persons undergoing inflammatory defense are hypoferremic. As patients recovered, normal levels of iron would promptly return. Other research workers subsequently demonstrated that this rapid profound shift in iron metabolism is independent of dietary iron and is regulated by hormone-like chemicals called cytokines. As cited in chapter 3, a cytokine called interleukin-6 signals hepatocytes to secrete hepcidin into the blood. Hepcidin depresses dietary iron assimilation and stimulates macrophages to hoard iron.

Serum iron levels begin to decline during the incubation phase of the infectious disease and quickly rise to normal as the patient improves. Moreover, the intestinal absorption of dietary iron, but not of other nutrients, is likewise markedly decreased early in the incubation phase. The similar correlation of depression of serum iron levels and of transferrin iron saturation is observed with increasing severity of cancer. The role of interleukin-6 and hecidin in this phase of iron withholding is described in greater detail in chapter 3.

Hypoferremia is a feature of a condition called anemia of chronic disease (ACD). This condition, when seen by some physicians, can be mistaken for iron-deficiency anemia and iron pills may be prescribed. In hypoferremia (anemia of chronic disease), though the serum iron, transferrin, total iron-binding capacity, and percentage of saturation of transferrin with iron are all lowered, the serum ferritin will be elevated. The elevated serum ferritin is a prime indicator that the iron withholding defense system is activated. This distinction differentiates ACD from iron-deficiency anemia.

166

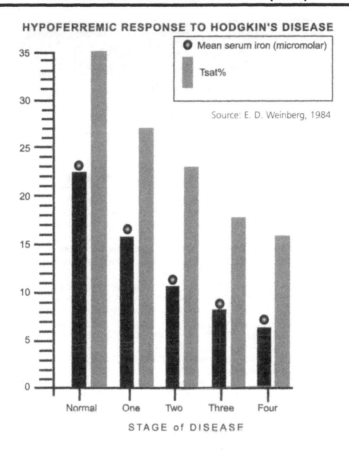

HYPOFERREMIC RESPONSE TO HODGKIN'S DISEASE

- ● Mean serum iron (micromolar)
- ▉ Tsat%

Source: E. D. Weinberg, 1984

STAGE of DISEASE

The various features of the iron withholding defense system can be grouped into two sets. In the constitutive set, the components are available and functioning fully at all times in health and in disease. In the set mobilized by cytokines, the features respond to microbial and neoplastic cell invasions; they are indispensable elements in the health-restoring inflammatory process.

In some invasions, the battle occurs within host cells. Siderophilins in body fluids are quite useful in lowering "free" iron in extracellular tissue spaces and fluids. But it is also necessary for such host cells as macrophages to be able to withhold iron from pathogens such as tuberculosis bacteria that are

167

The Iron Withholding Defense System

Constitutive Components

Siderophilins	■ Transferrin in serum, lymph, cerebrospinal fluid ■ Lactoferrin in secretions of lachrymal and mammary glands and of respiratory, gastrointestinal and genital tracts.

Ferritin within host cells

Processes Induced at Time of Invasion

- Suppression of assimilation of up to 80% of dietary iron*
- Suppression of iron efflux from macrophages that have digested dying red blood cells to result in up to 70% lowering of serum iron.
- Increased synthesis of ferritin to sequester withheld iron*
- Release of neutrophils from the bone marrow into circulation and then into site of infection*
- Release of lactoferrin from neutrophil granules followed by binding of iron in invaded sites.
- Macrophage scavenging of lactoferrin-iron in invaded sites
- Liver release of haptoglobin and hemopexin proteins into circulation (to bind and remove hemoglobin and hemin, respectively).
- Production of nitric oxide by macrophages to disrupt iron metabolism of invaders**
- Suppression of growth of microbial cells within macrophages by depressing expression of transferrin receptors and by enhancing formation of Nramp1 by the host cells**
- Stimulation of antibody-forming lymph cells to product antibodies against antigen used by invaders to acquire iron.

* Activated by interleukin-1 or -6 or by tumor necrosis factor-alpha
** Activated by interferon-gamma

Source: E. D. Weinberg, 1999

capable of growing within these host cells. A key cytokine that mobilizes alteration of macrophage iron metabolism is interferon-gamma. This compound induces a suppression of transferrin receptor expression that enables the invaded cells to starve the pathogen in its quest for iron.

Interferon-gamma also induces the infected macrophages to produce nitric oxide. This substance disrupts the ability of the

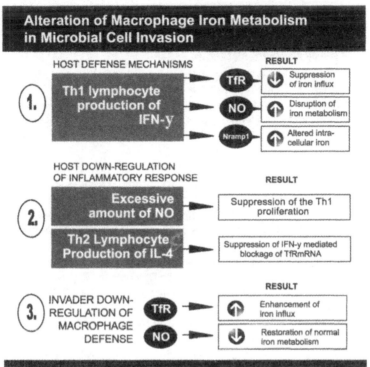

Source: E. D. Weinberg, 2000

pathogen to utilize iron properly. Additionally, interferon-gamma increases macrophage synthesis of NRAMP1, a protein that alters intracellular distribution of iron to further hamper the invader.

When the danger of invasion is over, the inflammatory response must be halted promptly. Two ways in which this can be accomplished are shown in the illustration above. Accumulation of nitric oxide inhibits proliferation of Th1 lymphocytes, and Th2 lymphocyte production of interleukin-4 causes the suppression of IFN-y-mediated blockage of transferrin receptor mediated RNA. Some microbial invaders can compel their host macrophages to increase the amount of acquired iron and to decrease formation of nitric oxide. Other mechanisms of interference with iron withholding defense are described in chapters that follow.

References:

Brandhagen, D. J., V. F. Fairbanks, and W. Baldus. "Recognition and Management of Hereditary Hemochromatosis." *American Academy of Family Physicians* 65 (2002): 853–66.

Ganz, T. "Hepcidin a Key Regulator of Iron Metabolism and Mediator of Anemia of Inflammation." *Blood* 102 (2003): 783–88.

Holmberg, C. G., and C. B. Laurell. "Investigations in Serum Copper: Nature of Serum Copper and Its Relation to the Iron-Binding Protein in Human Serum." *Acta Chemica Scandinavia* 1 (1947): 944–50.

Kochan, I. "The Role of Iron in Bacterial Infections with Special Consideration of Host-Tubercle Bacillus Interaction." *Current Topics in Microbiology and Immunology* 60 (1973): 1–30.

Locke, A., E. R. Main, and D. O. Rosbach. "The Copper and Non-Hemoglobinous Iron Contents of the Blood Serum in Disease." *Journal of Clinical Investigation* 11 (1932): 527–42.

Schade, A. L., and L. Caroline. "Raw Hen Egg White and the Role of Iron in Growth Inhibition of *Shigella Dysenteriae, Staphylococcus Aureus, Escherichia Coli,* and *Saccharomyces Cerevisiae*." *Science* 100 (1944): 14–15.

———. "An Iron-Binding Component in Human Blood Plasma." *Science* 104 (1946): 340–41.

Weinberg, E. D. "Iron and Susceptibility to Infectious Disease." *Science* 184 (1974): 952–56.

———. "Iron Withholding: A Defense against Infection and Neoplasia." *Physiology Reviews* 64 (1984): 65–101.

———. "The Development of Awareness of Iron-Withholding Defense." *Perspectives in Biology and Medicine* 36 (1993): 215–21.

———. "Iron Loading and Disease Surveillance." *Emerging Infectious Diseases* 5 (1999): 346–52.

———. "Modulation of Intramacrophage Iron Metabolism During Microbial Cell Invasion." *Microbes and Infections* 2 (2000): 85–89.

———. "Human Lactoferrin: A Novel Therapeutic with Broad Spectrum Potential." *Journal of Pharmacy and Pharmacology* 53 (2001): 1303–10.

15

Conditions That Antagonize the Iron Withholding Defense System

---

"It is important to distinguish between hypoferremia as a physiologic response and severe iron deficiency, a pathologic condition."

—*S. Kent and E. D. Weinberg*

The most obvious antagonist of the iron withholding defense system is iron. Unfortunately, to ensure that no one remains iron deficient, considerably excessive quantities of the metal are incorporated in processed foods, multivitamin supplements, and infant milk formulas. Overconsumption of red meats and alcohol intensifies the problem. On the horizon are super chelators and bioengineered foods designed to override our natural iron regulatory mechanisms.

Iron deficiency is claimed to be extensive, but indicators are ambiguous. Some health agencies consider a person anemic when hemoglobin values are 12.0–13.2 g/dL. Levels such as these are perfectly normal for many people. Hemoglobin values differ by age, race, and gender. East Asians, Hispanics, Japanese, and Native Americans have hemoglobin values similar to that of white Americans (Caucasians). African Americans normally have lower hemoglobin ranges than do Caucasians, and females of both black and white races have lower hemoglobin averages than the established adult ranges.

When groups of individuals are studied without compensating for these ethnic or gender differences, a higher incidence of iron-deficiency anemia will be found. Also, important to consider are individual differences. Large numbers of humans with hemoglobin values between 10 and 12 g/dL are included in such studies, yet these values permit this group to function normally and without symptoms of anemia.

According to iron-deficiency anemia experts, Drs. Cook, Skikne, Lynch, and Reusser of Kansas University Medical College, an estimated 3 percent of children age 6 months to 2 years of age, 2.6 percent of premenopausal and 1.9 percent of post-menopausal females, and about two-tenths of 1 percent of males in the United States are iron deficient. In this estimate, about 3 million rather than 5 million females are iron deficient as reported by the US Centers for Disease Control and Prevention. This discrepancy occurs only as a result of a difference in hemoglobin values used in the investigation of incidence. That is, the CDC used a slightly higher hemoglobin value range to define iron-deficiency anemia than was used by Drs. Cook, Skikne, Lynch, and Reusser.

Investigators Waalen, Felitti, and Beutler at Scripps Research Institute, California, measured the hemoglobin concentration values of 25,559 participants; 12,731 were male, 12,828 were female. In all parts of the study, hemoglobin concentrations were greater in males than in females. These investigators concluded that the difference between sexes is not due to iron deficiency.

Furthermore, though it is not prominent in the United States, developing countries with a high incidence of iron-deficiency anemia might be better served to investigate contamination of the water and food sources. Many inhabitants of these underdeveloped countries are infested with intestinal parasites, which cause blood loss. With blood loss there is iron loss. Endeavoring to eradicate the contaminants that cause bleeding might contribute to the reduction of iron-deficiency anemia better than eating genetically altered or iron-fortified foods.

To determine more realistically the incidence of iron-deficiency anemia, we need studies that take blood loss into consideration, separate the various groups of individuals by age, gender, and ethnicity, and use appropriate hemoglobin ranges.

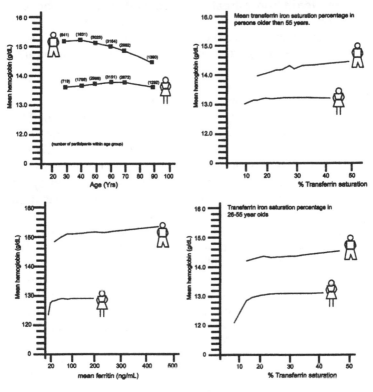

Source J Waalen et al.

Another group of individuals often mistakenly believed to be iron deficient are persons who are undergoing an inflammatory defense response (anemia of chronic disease [ACD]) to infection or cancer. As mentioned in earlier chapters, individuals with ACD have lowered hemoglobin and a low percentage of transferrin iron saturation. The reduced percentage is an important component of host defense. Supplemental iron is not appropriate for cases of anemia of chronic disease.

Unlike persons who truly are iron deficient, the serum transferrin receptor value of those with ACD remains normal. A normal value indicates that the person is not iron deficient. Additionally, though the hemoglobin, serum iron, transferrin, and transferrin-iron saturation percentage values will be lower than normal, serum ferritin will be elevated in response to the inflammation. Even during pregnancy, lowering of the transferrin-iron saturation percentage is consistent and compatible with fine health.

Are iron supplements appropriate for pregnant women?

In the United States, iron supplements are prescribed routinely for pregnant women as a customary part of prenatal care, even without evidence of iron deficiency or anemia. Between 25–65 mg of elemental iron generally are recommended to be taken daily. However, numerous clinical trials consistently have failed to demonstrate that supplemental iron improves maternal or fetal outcomes. Moreover, hematologic values are similar in women who take iron supplements and in women who do not, and there is no evidence that maternal iron values influence the hematologic profile of the newborn.

In a well-controlled study in England, 12 healthy volunteers who did not take iron supplements were monitored at 12, 24, and 36 weeks of gestation, and again at 18 months after delivery. The diet of the women contained 13 mg/day of iron. For iron balance in the trimester 1, only about 1 mg/day is necessary to be absorbed. The table below shows the dramatic changes in absorption of iron from the normal diet during gestation. In the second trimester, absorption is 5 times higher than in trimester I or in nonpregnancy and 9 times higher in trimester III.

Iron Absorbed in Pregnancy			
WEEKS OF GESTATION			18 Months after delivery
12	24	36	
0.94*	4.7*	8.6*	1.5*

*Mean milligrams of iron absorbed daily from a balanced diet containing 13 milligrams of iron.

Source J F R. Barrett et al.

In the second trimester, the extra iron is required for expansion of the red blood cell mass. Further iron must be absorbed in trimester III for the developing fetus and placenta. The increased absorption in the latter 6 months of pregnancy is a well programmed, consistent process rather than an emergency response to a nonexistent anemia. For most women, a balanced diet contains an adequate amount of iron for the entire period of gestation.

Accordingly, supplemental iron is not needed by nonanemic pregnant women for successful gestations. Although without beneficial value, might iron supplementation be a possible source of harm? Four categories of potential danger have been documented.

First, iron supplements are a potential cause of unintentional pediatric ingestion fatalities. In an 8-year summary of US poison control centers, iron accounted for 30 percent of all fatalities.

Most of the deaths occurred in the 1- to 2-year age group, often in homes of pregnant women. As little as 1000–2000 mg of iron can cause death. Thus if the toddler believed that the maternal tablets (of about 50 mg) were candy and ingested 20 of them, a death could occur.

A second potential danger of iron supplementation is the suppression of absorption of zinc during pregnancy by excessive intestinal iron. As little as 38 mg iron/day for a few weeks can reduce zinc absorption. More problems may arise were the amount of ingested zinc to be increased, inasmuch as this metal may interfere with absorption of a third essential nutrient, copper.

A third possible hazard has been reported in a study in Finland of 2688 pregnant women. The group was split at random into two sets: 1336 routinely took approximately 100 mg elemental iron daily. The other set of 1352 women took no supplemental iron except for those persons whose hemoglobin declined below 10 gm/dL and then only until their hemoglobin rose to 11 gm/dL. Of the children from the iron-supplemented mothers, 32 were hospitalized for convulsions. Of the children from the noniron set, only 17 were hospitalized for convulsions. The chance that this difference could have occurred randomly is less than 1 in 20. The authors noted that these results suggest that fetal exposure to high maternal iron increases the risk of seizures in the first year of life. They recommended that additional studies be done to further evaluate this possible hazard.

In a US study, ferritin levels in cord serum were recorded at the time of delivery of 278 children. Five years later, psychomotor development of the children was tested. Those in the highest quartile (fourth) of ferritin values had a 3.3 fold increased risk of a subnormal development score, as compared with children in the two middle quartiles. However, the authors reminded us that elevated ferritin could indicate a maternal infection as well as excessive iron.

The fourth possible risk of increasing the iron burden of pregnant women concerns the development of preeclampsia. In women with this dangerous complication of pregnancy, the iron saturation percentage of transferrin consistently is about double that of healthy pregnant women. For instance, in a set of 17 women with preeclampsia and 19 women with uncomplicated pregnancy, the mean Tf iron saturation value in the former was 35 percent, in the latter 18 percent. Studies are not yet available that compare the incidence of preeclampsia in pregnant women on various levels of iron supplements with the incidence in those who avoid supplements and derive a natural quantity of iron from dietary sources. Nevertheless, obstetric research clinicians have concluded that "it would seem inadvisable, in the absence of evidence of iron deficiency, to give iron supplements to pregnant women at high risk for preeclampsia" (Griffith and Abrams, 2001).

Is iron-fortified milk formula appropriate for infants 0-6 months?

"Human milk-feeding seems to be adequate to prevent iron-deficiency anemia during the first 6 months of life, and possibly much longer" (Griffith and Abrams, 2001).

At delivery, normal full-term infants are brimming with iron deposits that will be essential for their rapid growth in the first half year of their postnatal life. Examples of their iron values are given in the following table. Numerous studies have shown that hematological values are similar in exclusively breast-fed infants, in those fed low iron from milk formula, and in those given high-iron milk formula.

Iron values of full-term infants					
Months of Age	0.5	1.0	2.0	4.0	6.0
Tsat%*	67	65	34	27	27
Serum Ferritin	NA	356	247	99	53

*Tsat%: Transferrin/iron saturation percentage   Source: B. Duncan et al.

The iron content of human milk is highest at delivery (~17 µM) and decreases during lactation to about 5 µM at 6 months. The concentration of iron is not affected by either maternal iron deficiency or maternal iron supplementation. As much as 50 percent of the milk iron is absorbed by the nursing infant, but this provides only about 0.2 mg/day. Thus during the first 6 months of postnatal life, full-term infants largely rely on prenatal iron deposits. By 6 months, iron-fortified weaning foods have begun to provide exogenous iron, about 4 mg/day.

Often, however, formula feeding of young infants is necessary. Although absorption of iron from formula might not be as efficient as from human milk, the quantity of the metal added to formula should be prophylactic rather than grossly excessive. In a study of healthy full-term infants who were not breast-fed, 164 were given formula with 116 µM iron; 158 were fed formula with 9 µM. Information provided by the infants' physicians, healthcare visitors, and parents demonstrated that the excess iron failed to promote better health. Hematological values, height, and weight were comparable in both sets. Fortunately, in this study, infectious disease complications did not arise. A similar study reported that infants fed formula with 28 µM iron "meets the requirement of healthy term infants up to 6 months of age and that higher concentrations are unnecessary and may pose some risks."

As cited in chapter 12, virulence of intestinal pathogens is markedly increased by high-iron formulas. In an outbreak among 200 formula-fed infants under 6 months, 75 became ill with salmonellosis. The sick infants were 3 times more likely to have received formula with an iron content greater than 179 µM. Moreover, as mentioned in chapter 12, avoidance of unnecessary postnatal iron loading would be expected to lower the incidence of infant botulism and of sudden infant death syndrome.

In preterm infants, prenatal transfer of maternal iron may be less than complete. Conflicting opinions exist about the precise amounts of additional iron, if any, that are required by preterm infants as well as the most appropriate time to give iron supplementation. In a recent study of two elevated levels of iron fortification of milk formula, higher rates of respiratory tract infections in preterm infants occurred with the higher iron level. Moreover, as compared with breast-feeding, use of milk formula in preterm infants has been associated with an elevated risk of necrotising enterocolitis.

Other severe neonatal diseases of preterm infants that may be related to early excessive iron loading by caregivers include the retinopathy (blindness) of prematurity, bronchopulmonary dysplasia, and subependymal and intraventricular hemorrhage. In a review on iron-induced oxidative radical injury in premature infants, Sullivan has noted that the low content of the children's serum transferrin may provide an insufficient antioxidant capacity to defend against these diseases. To provide protection from these catastrophic illnesses, he recommends injecting preterm infants with adult-donor plasma (to provide a high content of unsaturated transferrin) rather than whole blood (which has a high content of iron). Other therapeutic uses of unsaturated transferrin will be discussed in chapter 17.

Is mass medication of young children with injected or oral iron appropriate?

"Oral iron has been associated with increased rates of malaria and increased morbidity from other infections."

—S. L. Oppenheimer, 2001

In 1956, injected iron was reported to increase markedly the virulence of bubonic plague bacteria in rats. Many subsequent animal studies with a great variety of potentially pathogenic microorganisms have confirmed this dangerous effect of iron. The virulence-enhancing action of injected iron also has been reported in young children.

As cited in chapter 12, a sevenfold increase in septicemia and meningitis due to *Escherichia coli* and related bacteria occurred in Maori neonates within one week of injection of 10 mg/kg iron (as dextran). Sera of the infants promptly became hyperferremic. In laboratory tests, the iron-loaded sera supported extensive growth of bacterial strains of *E. coli* that generally are unable to multiply in blood that has normal amounts of iron. The rate of death in this ill-advised, tragic experiment is shown in the image below.

Iron injection and death from sepsis in Maori infants

Year	No. of Live Births	Iron injection	No. of Deaths
1963-4	697	NO	0
1965-9	1853	YES (some)	6
1970-2	1582	YES (most)	16
1973-4	1098	NO	0

Source: D. M. J. Berry and A. W. Reeve

In 1986, over 200 New Guinea infants at 2 months of age were injected with ~25 mg/kg iron (as dextran). At 6 and 12 months, the rate of malaria in the iron-injected group was twice that of the over 200 controls. The chance that this result might have occurred randomly was 1 in 100. Furthermore, in the first year of life in the iron-burdened group, the rate of pneumonia was 5.5 fold greater at 6 months and the rate of middle ear infections at various times was 2.3 fold greater than in the healthy noninjected controls. As with *E. coli*, the level of transferrin iron saturation percent in humans is critical in defense against *Streptococcus pneumoniae*. Saturation levels above normal permit multiplication of the pneumonia bacteria in the bloodstream with resulting increased rate of disease and death.

In a recent exhaustive review commissioned by the World Health Organization, Oppenheimer has summarized three decades of studies of infection in iron-supplemented children. He noted that oral iron in children of all ages in tropical countries in doses greater than 2 mg/kg/day has been associated with increased risk of clinical malaria and other infections, including pneumonia. None of the studies yielded a reduction in rates of infection. The author reminded us also that, since iron overload is common in patients with AIDS, mass iron supplementation in geographic areas of high AIDS density should be investigated urgently. Most importantly, Oppenheimer recommended that iron therapy, if necessary, should be oral rather than injected and based on laboratory evidence that the children are actually iron deficient.

Potential hazards of injected iron for older children and adults

Excessive quantities of injected iron are well recognized to be associated with an above-normal rate of infection and death. Iron dextran is a complex of ferric hydroxide with a carbohydrate polymer of high molecular weight (165 kilodaltons). The complex is designed to be engulfed by macrophages which split the iron from the polymer and bury it in intracellular ferritin. However, about 2–6 percent of the iron in the injected preparation is not complexed and hopefully must be captured by serum transferrin. Long-term persistence of this "labile" iron has been observed in 20 percent of recipient patients.

Persons on hemodialysis may receive various numbers of injections of iron dextran. In a study of 5833 US patients, rates of hospitalization and death were significantly increased in those who received more than 10 injections (100 mg iron/dose) in any 6-month period.

The iron in iron dextran is highly teratogenic (fetal injury and death) in pregnant mammals, including nonhuman primates. Thus it should not be used in pregnant women. Its use must be avoided also in persons with known or suspected infections.

Studies on the possible reactivation of latent malignant cells by iron dextran are not presently available.

As with iron dextran, the injection of whole blood provides a considerable excess of iron that must quickly be packaged into ferritin to avoid harm. Each unit of blood contains 200–250 mg of iron. A small portion of this large quantity of the metal is being continually released as hemoglobin from decaying red blood cells. A review of thirteen studies of incidence of postoperative infection with transfusions given at the time of surgery found that in twelve the number of transfusions was correlated positively with an increasing chance of subsequent infection. Indeed, in eight of the thirteen studies, the number of transfusions was the most significant predictor of possible development of infection.

In most, but not all, studies in animal models, an association between blood transfusions and development of bacterial infections also has been demonstrated. In humans, recurrence of cancers has been reported to be associated with the number of transfusions in fourteen of twenty-seven studies.

Although many, if not all, transfusions of whole blood might be appropriate in surgical patients to restore oxygen carrying capacity, the use of transfusions in medical patients may be more equivocal. A study of transfusion practice in 438 medical patients in a teaching hospital and in a community hospital demonstrated that the rate of nonjustifiable transfusions was as high as 35 percent. Patients' records were reviewed by five specialists. Eighteen percent of the transfusions were viewed as not justifiable by at least four of the five physicians. Another 17 percent of the transfusions were classified as equivocal because two or three of the reviewers judged them to be not justifiable.

Potential hazards of oral iron for older children and adults

Excessive quantities of oral iron are less hazardous than injected iron because of the fortunate barrier to absorption provided by our enterocytes. These intestinal lining cells prevent up to 90 percent of the ingested metal from gaining access to our bloodstream. They trap the iron, deposit it in their ferritin, then die and are excreted in the feces. However, a portion of the metal remains labile and stimulates free radical formation by bacteria that live in our large intestine. As mentioned earlier, free radicals are mutagenic and could induce colon cancer.

The feces of human volunteers who took 18 mg of iron (as ferrous sulfate) per day contained higher quantities of labile iron than in feces collected when the subjects were on their normal diet. The labile iron was associated with an increase in free radical generating capacity of the fecal samples.

In a subsequent study, rats were fed either 29 mg/kg or 102 mg/kg of iron for 6 months. Intestinal samples taken directly from the rats showed that the excess iron caused a significant increase in free radical generating capacity in the colon and increased lipid peroxidation in the cecum. The cecum in rats is anatomically equivalent to the proximal colon in humans, which is our most vulnerable site for development of colon cancer.

In a study in rats susceptible to inflammatory bowel disease (IBD), iron supplementation was found to increase microscopic signs of inflammation and oxidative stress. In humans with iron-overload disorders, IBD is a common complaint.

As cited in chapter 14, the intestinal barrier to iron assimilation is elevated considerably during microbial invasions. Decreased intestinal absorption of iron in response to infection has been observed in humans, rats, and chicks. Responsibility for retention of the additional iron in the intestine rests with the enterocytes. With increased content of iron, cultures of human enterocyte-like cells (Caco-2 cells) have been observed to become more susceptible to bacterial invasion. Thus it might be prudent for persons taking supplemental iron to aid their enterocytes by halting supplements during episodes of infection.

In healthy persons, about 10–20 percent of food iron is absorbed. The amount should balance the daily loss of 0.5–2.0 mg iron in perspiration, urine, and feces. Menstruating women need an extra milligram of iron/day to balance that lost in monthly bleeding. Dietary iron is available as heme and non-heme iron. In the United States, about 80 percent of the metal is in the latter form; in vegetarians, it would be close to 100 percent. Several factors can alter the absorbed amount of non-heme iron. For example, processed foods (flour, bread, cereals, peanut butter, potato chips, candy bars, popcorn, powdered soft drinks, etc.) have various kinds of added nonheme iron that differ considerably in absorption. A rough estimate is that human food processors add at least 10 percent (and possibly as much as 25 percent) to the burden of nonheme iron that must be withheld by our enterocytes.

Reducing agents such as ascorbic acid (vitamin C) change the valence of nonheme iron from the ferric to the ferrous state. The latter is more soluble and thus more readily absorbed in the duodenal portion of our small intestine. Other promoters of iron absorption are meat and alcohol, each of which enhances formation of stomach acid. The acid helps to maintain a low pH value in the duodenum, which favors the solubility of ferrous iron.

Fortunately, several factors aid our enterocytes in preventing excessive intestinal assimilation of nonheme iron. Most importantly, foods of vegetable origin often contain a powerful iron chelator called phytic acid. This compound traps nonheme iron and conveys it to fecal excretion. Regrettably, some plant foods are now being bioengineered to produce an enzyme (a phytase) which would destroy phytic acid. Important groups, such as the Iron Disorders Institute, are urging manufacturers and distributors to label these products clearly to warn potential consumers.

Potential hazards of inhaled iron for everyone

As mentioned in earlier chapters, inhaled iron can be quite dangerous in the respiratory tract as an initiator of cancer and as a nutrient for growth of cancer cells and microbial pathogens. Moreover, some of the lung macrophages that become iron loaded can migrate through blood vessels to cause an elevated risk of vascular damage. Vehicles for inhaled iron cited earlier include asbestos, tobacco smoke, and iron-contaminated air particulates.

A vehicle not previously mentioned is iron-contaminated water. Underwater swimmers and divers in rural ponds contaminated by iron smelters are at increased risk for inhaling *Naegleria fowleri*, normally a nonpathogenic water protozoan. The added iron permits the protozoan to survive in the human respiratory tract, migrate through the bloodstream, and cause a fatal meningitis in the central nervous system.

183

References:

Barrett, J. F. R., P. G. Whittaker, J. G. Williams, and T. Lind. "Absorption of Non-Haem Iron from Food during Normal Pregnancy." *British Pediatric Journal* 309 (1994): 79–82.

Barry, D. M. J., and A. W. Reeve. "Iron and Infection." *British Medical Journal* 296 (1988): 1736.

Duncan, B., R. B. Schifman, J. J. Corrigan Jr, and C. Schaefer. "Iron and the Exclusively Breast-Fed Infant from Birth to Six Months." *Journal of Pediatric Gastroenterological Nutrition* 4 (1985): 421–25.

Esposito, B. P., W. Breuer, I. Slotki, and Z. T. Cabantchic. "Labile Iron in Parenteral Iron Formulations and Its Potential for Generating Plasma Nontransferrin-bound Iron in Dialysis Patients." *European Clinical Investigation* 32 (2002): S42–49.

Feldman, H., J. Santanna, W. Guo, H. Furst, E. Franklin, M. Joffe, S. Marcus, and G. Faich. "Iron Administration and Clinical Outcome in Hemodialysis Patients." *Journal of American Society of Nephrologists* 13 (2002): 734–44.

Foster, S. L., S. H. Richardson, and M. L. Failla. "Elevated Iron Status Increases Bacterial Invasion and Survival and Alters Cytokine/Chemokine mRNA Expression in Caco-2 Human Intestinal Cells." *Journal of Nutrition* 131 (2001): 1452–58.

Friel, J. K., W. L. Andrews, K. Aziz, P. G. Kwa, G. Lepage, and M. R. L'Abbe. "A Randomized Trial of Two Levels of Iron Supplementation and Developmental Outcome in Low Birth Weight Infants." *Journal of Pediatrics* 139 (2001): 254–60.

Griffith, I. J., and S. A. Abrams. "Iron and Breastfeeding." *Pediatric Clinicians of North America* 48 (2001): 401–13.

Haddock, R. L., S. N. Cousens, and C. C. Guzman. "Infant Diet and Salmonellosis." *American Journal of Public Health* 81 (1991): 997–1000.

Hambidge, K. M., N. F. Krebs, L. Sibley, and J. English. "Acute Effects of Iron Therapy on Zinc Status during Pregnancy." *Obstetrics and Gynecology* 4 (1987): 593–96.

Hemminki, E., and J. Merilanen. "Long-Term Follow-up of Mothers and Their Infants in a Randomized Trial on Iron Prophylaxis during Pregnancy." *American Journal of Obstetrics and Gynecology* 173 (1995): 205–9.

Hemminki, E., K. Nemet, M. Horvath, M. Malin, D. Schuler, and S. Hollan. "Impact of Iron Fortification of Milk Formulas on

Infants' Growth and Health." *Nutrition Research* 15 (1995): 491–503.

Hernell, O., and B. Lonnerdal. "Iron Status of Infant Fed Low-Iron Formula: No Effect of Added Bovine Lactoferrin or Nucleotides." *American Journal of Clinical Nutrition* 76 (2002): 858–64.

Hubel, C. A., A. V. Kozlov, V. E. Kagan, R. W. Evans, S. T. Davidge, M. K. McLaughlin, and J. M. Roberts. "Decreased Transferrin and Increased Transferrin Saturation in Sera of Women with Preeclampsia: Implications for Oxidative Stress." *American Journal of Obstetrics and Gynecology* 175 (1996): 692–700.

Jackson, S., and T. W. Burrows. "The Virulence Enhancing Effect of Iron on Nonpigmented Mutants of *Pasteuerella Pestis.*" *British Journal of Experimental Pathology* 37 (1956): 577–83.

Kent, S., and E. D. Weinberg. "Hypoferremia Adaptation to Disease?" *New England Journal of Medicine* 320 (1989): 672.

Lambert, C. C., and R. L. Hunter. "Low Levels of Unsaturated Transferrin as a Predictor of Survival in Pneumococcal Pneumonia." *Annals of Clinical Laboratory Sciences* 20 (1990): 140–46.

Litovitz, T., and A. Manoguerra. "Comparison of Pediatric Poisoning Hazards: An Analysis of 3.8 Million Exposure Incidents." *Pediatrics* 89 (1992): 999–1006.

Lund, E. K., S. G. Wharf, S. J. Fairweather-Tait, and I. T. Johnson. "Oral Ferrous Sulfate Supplements Increase the Free Radical-Generating Capacity of Feces from Healthy Volunteers." *American Journal of Clinical Nutrition* 69 (1999): 250–55.

Lund, E. K., S. J. Fairweather-Tait, S. G. Wharf, and I. T. Johnson. "Chronic Exposure to High Levels of Dietary Iron Fortification Increases Lipid Peroxidation in the Mucosa of the Rat Large Intestine." *Journal of Nutrition* 131 (2001): 2928–31.

Newsome, A. L., and W. E. Wilhelm. "Inhibition of Naegleria Fowleri by Microbial Iron-Chelating Agents: Ecological Implications." *Applications of Environmental Microbiology* 45 (1983): 665–68.

Oldenburg, B., J. C. Koningsberger, G. P. Van Berge Henegouwen, B. S. Van Asbeck, and J. J. Rarx. "Iron and Inflammatory Bowel Disease." *Alimentary Pharmacological Therapy* 15 (2001): 429–38.

Oppenheimer, S. I. "Iron and Its Relation to Immunity and Infectious Disease." *Journal of Nutrition* 131 (2001): S616–35.

Oppenheimer, S. I., F. D. Gibson, S. B. Macfarlane, J. B. Moody, C. Harrison, A. Spencer, and O. Bunari. "Iron Supplementation Increases Prevalence and Effects of Malaria: Report on Clinical

Studies in Papua New Guinea." *Transcripts of Royal Society of Tropical Medicine and Hygiene* 80 (1986): 603–12.

Rayman, M. P., J. Barlis, R. W. Evans, C. W. G. Redman, and L. J. King. "Abnormal Iron Parameters in the Pregnancy Syndrome Preeclampsia." *American Journal of Obstetrics and Gynecology* 187 (2002): 412–18.

Saarinen, U. M., and M. A. Siimes. "Developmental Changes in Serum Iron, Total Iron-Binding Capacity, and Transferrin Saturation in Infancy." *Journal of Pediatrics* 91 (1977): 875–77.

Saxena, S., J. M. Weiner, A. Rabinowitz, J. Fridey, I. A. Shulman, and R. Carmel. "Transfusion Practice in Medical Patients." *Archives of Internal Medicine* 153 (1993): 2575–80.

Schein Pharmaceuticals, Inc. "Iron Dextran Injection, USP." In *Physician's Desk Reference*, 2478–80. 51st ed. Montvale, NJ: Medical Economics Co., 1997.

Sullivan, J. L. "Iron, Plasma Antioxidants, and the Oxygen Radical Disease of Prematurity." *American Journal of Diseases in Children* 12 (1988): 1341–44.

Tamura, T., R. L. Goldenberg, J. Hou, K. E. Johnston, S. P. Cliver, S. L. Ramey, and K. G. Nelson. "Cord Serum Ferritin Concentrations and Mental and Psychomotor Development of Children at Five Years of Age." *Journal of Pediatrics* 140 (2002): 165–70.

Tartter, P. I. "Does Blood Transfusion Predispose to Cancer Recurrence?" *American Journal of Clinical Oncology* 12 (1989): 169–71.

Triutzi, D. J., N. Blumberg, and J. M. Heal. "Association of Transfusion with Postoperative Bacterial Infection." *Critical Reviews of Clinical Laboratory Science* 28 (1990): 95–107.

Tuthill, D. P., M. Cosgrove, F. Dunstan, M. L. Stuart, J. C. K. Wells, and D. P. Davies. "Randomized Double-Blind Controlled Trial on the Effects on Iron Status in the First Year Between a No-Added-Iron and Standard Infant Formula Received for Three Months." *Acta Paediatrica* 91 (2002): 119–24.

Waalen, J., V. Felitti, and E. Beutler. "Haemoglobin and Ferritin Concentration in Men and Women: Cross Sectional Study." *British Medical Journal* 325 (2002): 137.

Weinberg, E. D. "Iron Withholding: A Defense Against Infection and Neoplasi." *Physiological Reviews* 64 (1984): 65–102.

———. "Cellular Iron Metabolism in Health and Disease." *Drug Metabolism Reviews* 22 (1990): 531-79.

————. "Iron-Enriched Rice: The Case for Labeling." *Journal of Medicine: Food* 3 (2000): 189-91.

Woolf, S. H. "US Preventive Surveillance-Task Force: Routine Iron Supplementation during Pregnancy." *Journal of American Medical Association* 270 (1993): 2846–54.

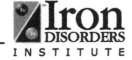
PART III

Practical Guide to Diagnosis, Treatment, and Prevention

16
Diagnosis

"Most physicians diagnose only a few cases of hereditary hemochromatosis in their practice because they do not routinely test for iron overload."

—*David J. Brandhagen et al.*

Primary (inherited) and secondary (acquired) conditions of iron overload both have similar consequences, which make it essential to determine the cause of iron overload for a complete diagnosis and commencement of therapy. Iron overload is confirmed with a combination of clinical and laboratory findings often prompted by abnormal routine blood work or the patient's complaint of symptoms.

Though the symptoms of iron overload are not specific, chronic fatigue is among the first complaints of patients with iron overload, whether the cause is primary or secondary. Besides chronic fatigue, individuals with iron overload due to hereditary type I hemochromatosis are often seen with arthralgia and impotence initially, with liver disease, diabetes and heart trouble later on. By comparison, patients with thalassemia major display heart trouble and hypogonadism initially, and liver disease and diabetes thereafter.

Symptoms, findings, or diseases associated with iron overload include arthritis, diabetes mellitus (especially type II), heart trouble or arrhythmia, liver disease, and mildly evaluated liver enzymes—especially ALT. Also associated with iron overload are amenorrhea, anterior pituitary failure, impotence and loss of

Clinical Features of Patients with Hemochromatosis

Symptoms
  Asymptomatic
    Abnormal serum iron studies on routine
      screening chemistry panel
    Evaluation of abnormal liver tests
    Identified by family screening
    Identified by population screening
  Non-specific, systemic symptoms
    Weakness, fatigue, lethargy, apathy, weight loss

  Specific Organ-related Symptoms
    Abdominal pain secondary to hepatomegaly
    Arthralgias
    Diabetes
    Amenorrhea
    Loss of libido, impotence
    Congestive heart failure, arrhythmias
Signs
  Asymptomatic
    Hepatomegaly
  Symptomatic
    Liver
      Hepatomegaly
      Cutaneous stigmata of chronic liver disease
      Splenomegaly
      Portal hypertension (ascites, encephalopathy)
    Joints
      Arthritis
      Joint swelling
    Heart
      Dilated cardiomyopathy
      Congestive heart failure
    Skin
      Increased pigmentation
    Endocrine
      Testicular atrophy
      Hypogonadism
      Hypothyroidism

Source. S. A Harrison and B R Bacon

libido, inappropriate increase in skin pigmentation, depression, hypothyroidism, infertility, viral hepatitis, liver cancer, NASH, and porphyria cutanea tarda (PCT).

In conditions where iron overload and anemia occur simultaneously, as in thalassemia major, or for individuals who are transfusion dependent, life expectancy is generally shortened. Iron-induced cardiac disease remains the main cause of death in patients with thalassemia major, despite conventional chelation therapy.

Most patients with classic type I hereditary hemochromatosis who are diagnosed prior to severe organ disease such as diabetes mellitus or cirrhosis will have a normal life expectancy.

Tests that can determine iron overload

Tissue iron overload can be determined in most conditions using fasting serum iron, total iron binding capacity (TIBC), and serum ferritin. Some investigators use UIBC (unbound iron-binding capacity). Though not widely used in the United States, UIBC is an excellent alternative to the TIBC. UIBC is less costly and has fewer false positives than TIBC.

Tests: to determine iron overload

Fasting serum iron   Serum iron/TIBC
Total iron binding capacity   X 100%= Tsat% (Normal 25-35%)

Serum ferritin: See ranges in ferritin chart

Liver biopsy with quantitative iron stain (used in some cases, especially those with normal TS% with elevated serum ferritin)

Hepatic Iron Content (HIC): 4500 mcg (80 mcmol) per gram of dry weight or 3-4+ iron stain

Tsat%= transferrin-iron saturation percentage

Source: Iron Disorders Institute, 2004

The percentage of transferrin saturation is calculated by dividing serum iron by TIBC and multiplying by 100 percent. Normal range for transferrin iron saturation percentage is 25–35 percent. If the patient has an elevated transferrin iron saturation percentage greater than 45 percent with an accompanying elevated serum ferritin, iron overload is present and phlebotomy can commence. If UIBC is used to calculate the percentage of saturation, the calculation is serum iron divided by [serum iron + UIBC] x 100 percent.

If initial test to determine transferrin iron saturation percentage has not been performed fasting and the finding is greater than 55 percent, the test should be repeated fasting. Fasting involves nothing by mouth after midnight or prior to blood work. Also, a patient should discontinue any vitamin supplements that contain great amounts of vitamin C, A, or iron, which can affect the result of the test. Further, patients should cut back on sugary fruit juices, and be sufficiently hydrated prior to blood work.

Important Ferritin Reference Ranges	ferritin	Adult Males	Adult Females
	Normal Range	up to 300ng/mL	up to 200ng/mL
	In treatment*	below 100ng/mL	below 100ng/mL
	Ideal maintenance	25-75ng/mL	25-75ng/mL
Adolescents, Juveniles, Infants & Newborns of normal height and weight for their age and gender			
Male ages 10-19 23-70ng/mL		Infants 7-12 months 60-80ng/mL	
Female ages 10-19 6-40ng/mL		Newborn 1-6 months 6-410ng/mL	
Children ages 6-9 10-55ng/mL		Newborn 1-30 days 6-400ng/mL	
Children ages 1-5 6-24ng/mL			

*undergoing therapeutic phlebotomy

Source: Iron Disorders Institute, 2004.

	TIBC	Serum Iron	Ferritin
Newborn	130-275 mg/dL	100-250 mcg/dL	
Age 1-30 days			6-400 ng/mL
Age 1-6 months			6-410 ng/mL
Infant (age 7-12 months)	220-400 mg/dL	40-100 mcg/dL	60-80 ng/mL
Child (1-5 years of age)	220-400 mg/dL	50-120 mcg/dL	6-24 ng/mL

Source: Iron Disorders Institute, 2004

Reference Ranges

hemoglobin	Adult Males	Adult Females
Normal Range	14.0-18.0g/dL	12.0-16.0g/dL
Adolescents, Juveniles, Infants & Newborns of normal height and weight for their age and gender		
Age 6-18 years 10.0-15.5g/dL	Age 2-6 mos 10.0-17.0g/dL	
Age 1-6 years 9.5-14.0g/dL	Age 0-2 weeks 12.0-20.0g/dL	
Age 6 mos-1 year 9.5-14.0g/dL	Newborn 14.0-24.0g/dL	

Source: Iron Disorders Institute, 2004

LAB TEST RESULTS	Hemoglobin	Hematocrit	Ferritin	Transferrin Iron Saturation Percentage
Iron Overload	NORMAL 12-17 g/dL	NORMAL 36-42%	Elevated	Greater than 45%
Iron-Deficiency Anemia	Less than 10 g/dL	Less than 30%	Less than 15 ng/mL	Less than 15%

Source: Iron Disorders Institute, 2004

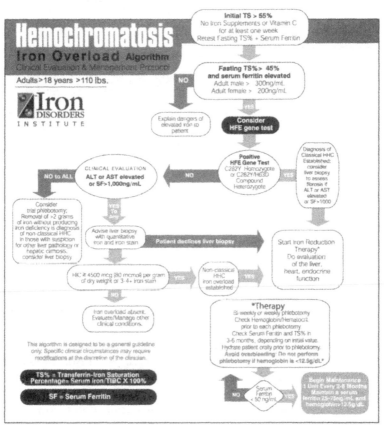

Source: Iron Disorders Institute, 2004

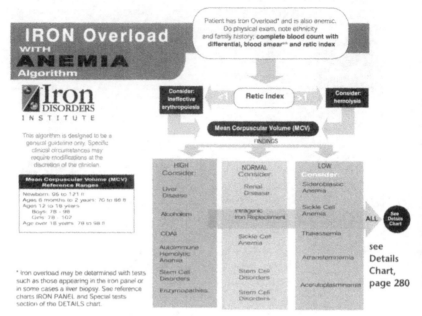

IRON Overload
WITH
ANEMIA
Algorithm

Iron
DISORDERS
INSTITUTE

This algorithm is designed to be a
general guideline only. Specific
clinical circumstances may
require modifications at the
discretion of the clinician.

Patient has Iron Overload* and is also anemic.
Do physical exam, note ethnicity
and family history; **complete blood count with
differential, blood smear** ** and retic index**

Consider:
ineffective
erythropoiesis

Retic Index

Consider:
hemolysis

Mean Corpuscular Volume (MCV)
FINDINGS

Mean Corpuscular Volume (MCV)
Reference Ranges

Newborn: 95 to 121 fl
Ages 6 months to 2 years: 70 to 86 fl
Ages 12 to 18 years
 Boys: 78 - 98
 Girls: 78 - 102
Age over 18 years: 78 to 98 fl

HIGH Consider:	NORMAL Consider:	LOW Consider:
Liver Disease	Renal Disease	Sideroblastic Anemia
Alcoholism	Iatrogenic Iron Replacement	Sickle Cell Anemia
CDAII	Sickle Cell Anemia	Thalessemia
Autoimmune Hemolytic Anemia		Atransferrinemia
Stem Cell Disorders	Stem Cell Disorders	Aceruloplasminemia
Enzymopathies	Stem Cell Disorders	

ALL **See Details Chart**

see
Details
Chart,
page 280

* Iron overload may be determined with tests
such as those appearing in the iron panel or
in some cases a liver biopsy. See reference
charts IRON PANEL and Special tests
section of the DETAILS chart.

**For excellent images, visit The American Society of Hematology web site:
www. hematology.org. Click on "education" then on "image bank." For PDF version of copies
of chapters from *The Iron Disorders Institute Guide to Anemia*, e-mail your request to:
publications@irondisorders.org, or visit the Physician's Section: http://www.irondisorders.org.

Elevated serum iron can be an indicator that iron overload is
present, but serum iron alone is not a reliable way to determine
excessive tissue iron. Serum iron is influenced by many factors,
such as time of day, and for this reason must be done while fasting for accuracy. Fasting does not affect serum ferritin, but ferritin is an acute-phase reactant and can be elevated if inflammation is present. Inflammation can occur as a result of taking
certain medications, such as hormone replacement therapy,
and in the presence of chronic disease and infection.

Both the fasting transferrin iron saturation percentage and
serum ferritin will be elevated in persons with classic hemochromatosis (type I) if tissue iron is excessive. However, in about
30–50 percent of patients with acute viral hepatitis and alcoholic liver disease, both serum ferritin and transferrin iron saturation percentage can be elevated.

Individuals with non-alcoholic fatty liver disease (NAFLD), also called non-alcoholic steatohepatitis (NASH), can have an elevated serum ferritin with a normal or only slightly elevated transferrin iron saturation percentage. Along with iron overload, NASH patients will exhibit hyperinsulinemia induced by insulin resistance, two factors significantly associated with NAFLD in obese patients.

High serum ferritin can occur in the absence of elevated iron or of inflammation. For example, patients who have hyperferritinemia-cataract syndrome are not iron loaded and should not be phlebotomized. Hyperferritinemia-cataract syndrome is an inherited condition of early onset cataracts. Though the serum ferritin is elevated, it is not due to tissue iron overload but some defect resulting in overproduction of ferritin. Many times these patients are inappropriately bled, with unpleasant results. Patients are usually young, male, have elevated serum ferritin, but normal serum iron and complain of eye pain when subjected to bright lights. An ophthalmologist can confirm diagnosis.

A physical examination to ascertain hepatomegaly or splenomegaly is important, albeit somewhat subjective. If either organ is palpable a liver biopsy may be indicated, especially if liver enzymes are abnormal.

Liver enzymes

The levels of liver enzymes alone cannot provide a prognosis nor do they always correlate with the extent of liver damage. Patients with iron overload or cirrhosis can have normal or only slightly elevated alanine transaminase (ALT) or aspartate aminotransferase (AST). In hereditary hemochromatosis, ALT is elevated in only about 50 percent of the cases and then only moderately elevated (less than 2.5 times normal).

ALT helps to determine the presence of inflammation of the liver (hepatitis), which may indicate liver damage (cirrhosis, tumor, cancer). If the liver is injured, high levels of ALT are released into the blood. This enzyme can be elevated by certain drugs, such as acetaminophen, anti-seizure meds, cholesterol-lowering drugs, and anti-depressants. Heart attack, infections such as mononucleosis, and pancreatitis can also result in elevated ALT. Generally most elevated ALT levels are indicative of liver disease, which can be due to iron overload disease (hemochromatosis), copper overload (Wilson's disease), non-alcoholic steatohepatitis (NASH), alpha-1-antitrypsin deficiency, celiac sprue, or disease of the muscle. ALT is sometimes referred to as SGPT (serum glutamate pyruvate transaminase).

Aspartate aminotransferase (AST) is an enzyme found in the liver, heart, muscle, and bone. Used in conjunction with other tests, AST can help determine disease in any one of these organs. AST is most helpful in determining events such as a heart attack. When cells of the muscle (including the heart) or bone or liver are injured, these cells are destroyed (lysed). AST is released into the blood, causing an elevated level of the enzyme in serum. AST levels change; they are elevated within 8 hours of an injury such as heart attack but fall back to normal within days following the incident. In chronic disease, the AST remains constantly elevated. AST is also sometimes referred to as SGOT (serum glutamic oxaloacetic transaminase).

Alkaline phosphatase (ALP) is an enzyme found in the liver and bone. Injury to either organ will cause ALP to be released into the bloodstream. Elevated levels usually indicate an obstruction somewhere within the liver, such as gallstones. Elevated ALP can also be an indication of inflammation (heptatitis), bone disease, or liver cancer. Elevated ALP is normal in children, especially teenagers, who are undergoing rapid growth and physical changes, which includes bone growth. In these cases, a pediatrician will want to measure the GGT level, which will be normal if the elevated ALP is due to bone growth.

Gamma glutamyl transferase (GGT) is found in the greatest quantities in the liver and biliary tract cells. GGT is also found to a lesser degree in kidney, spleen, heart, brain, intestine, and prostate gland. GGT can be elevated in a heart attack, renal failure, chronic obstructive pulmonary disease (COPD), diabetes, and alcoholism, but GGT is most effective in diagnosing an obstruction in the biliary tract.

When both ALP and GGT are elevated, it is generally due to liver disease. GGT is also very helpful in detecting chronic alcohol ingestion. The GGT will often be elevated in persons who

iron panel	IRON PANEL TESTS					
	Serum Iron	Serum Ferritin	Transferrin Iron Saturation Percentage	Total Iron Binding Capacity (TIBC)	Transferrin	Serum Transferrin Receptor
Hemochromatosis	↑	↑	↑	↓	↓	NORMAL TO LOW
Iron-Deficiency Anemia	↓	↓	↓	↑	↑	HIGH
Sideroblastic Anemia	↑	↑	↑	↓	↓	NORMAL TO HIGH
Thalassemia	↑	↑	↑	↓	↓	HIGH
Porphyria Cutanea Tarda	↑	↑	↑	↓	↓	NORMAL
Anemia of Chronic Disease (ACD)	↓	↑ OR NORMAL	↓	↓	↓	NORMAL
African siderosis	↑	↑	↑	↓	↓	NORMAL TO LOW

The Physician's Reference Chart is provided with the guidance of The Iron Disorders Institute Scientific Advisory Board and consultants to the board from the National Institutes of Health and the US Centers for Disease Control and Prevention. Larger versions of all charts are available upon request: publications@irondisorders.org

Iron Profile in Selected Conditions

Condition	IRON PANEL TESTS						
	Hemoglobin	Serum Iron	Serum Ferritin	Transferrin Iron Saturation Percentage	Total Iron Binding Capacity (TIBC)	Transferrin	Serum Transferrin Receptor
Hemoglobinapathies, Stem cell disorders, Chronic hymolysis Sickle Cell Anemia G6PD Sideroblastic Anemia Thalassemia CDA II Autoimmune Hemolytic Anemia	↓	↑	↑	↑	↓	↓	NORMAL TO HIGH
Aceruloplasminemia	↓	↓	↑ OR NORMAL	↓	↓	↓	NORMAL
Atransferrinemia	NORMAL	↓	↑	↑	↓	↓	NORMAL TO LOW
Hemochromatosis	NORMAL	↑	↑	↑	↓	↓	NORMAL TO LOW
Anemia of Chronic Disease (ACD)	↓	↓	↑ OR NORMAL	↓	↓	↓	NORMAL

NOTE: Many of these conditions occur concomitantly with other illnesses confounding the findings.

Source: Iron Disorders Institute, 2004

199

have three or more alcoholic drinks per day. GGT can also be elevated in patients taking anti-convulsants. A normal GGT with elevated ALP is suggestive of bone activity, such as growth or deterioration. GGT can also be elevated following a heart attack.

Liver biopsy

Liver biopsy is no longer used to diagnose hereditary hemochromatosis, but it remains the Gold Standard for determining the extent of liver damage and hepatic iron load. In some conditions such as fatty liver diseases, where the serum ferritin is elevated but transferrin iron saturation percentage is normal or only modestly elevated, the liver biopsy might be used for complete diagnosis.

A possible hazard of liver biopsy of cirrhotic patients is the seeding of cancer cells at the subcutaneous site of the needle puncture. In a set of 150 patients, 4 (2.66 percent) developed tumor nodules within 2 years after the procedure.

LIVER IRON ASSESSMENT

Hepatic Iron Index (HII)= hepatic iron concentration (μmol/g dry weight) divided by the patient's age in years. HII values greater than 1.9 is diagnostic for hemochromatosis.
Hepatic Iron content (HIC) greater than 4500 mcg (80 mcmol) per gram of dry weight or 3-4+ iron stain substantiates abnormally elevated liver iron stores.
The liver biopsy remains the most widely accepted means of establishing the extent of liver damage such as cirrhosis or fibrosis. Also, it is recommended that for individuals with serum ferritin greater than 1,000ng/mL, liver biopsy be considered.

Source. K. V Kowdley, et al

A sample of the tissue obtained from liver biopsy is stained with Prussian Blue or Perl's stain. The sample is examined under a microscope where iron will appear as dark spots on the pathologist's slide. Without stain, iron cannot be seen. Staining the tissue sample confirms the presence of iron; drying, weighing the tissue sample, then analyzing it for iron content confirms the amount of iron contained in the organ biopsied. Hepatic iron >80 μmol/g or hepatic index >1.9 confirms hemochromatosis, or iron overload.

Cirrhosis is often a consequence of undetected iron overload. Conventionally, cirrhosis is confirmed with a liver biopsy, which is invasive and can be refused by a patient. Knowing whether a patient has cirrhosis is important to the prognosis. Patients with hemochromatosis are at twentyfold risk of liver cancer. When cirrhosis is present at the time of diagnosis of hemochromatosis, the risk of liver cancer can be as high as two-hundred-fold.

Alternatives to the liver biopsy include specialized MRI, computerized axial tomography (CAT) scan, or ultrasound. Or a physician might look at the liver using a laparoscope, an instrument inserted through the abdomen that relays pictures back to a computer screen. In most of these procedures an iron load can be detected and estimated to some degree, but damage such as cirrhosis cannot be determined.

Investigators found a high correlation between their index and liver iron content. They recorded 16 clinical and laboratory variables in 193 Canadian C282Y homozygous patients. Each patient had a liver biopsy to determine the presence or absence of cirrhosis. From these data, they devised an index for the non-invasive prediction of cirrhosis. They tested their index on participants of the study and found it to accurately predict cirrhosis in an average of 81 percent of patients. The index is derived from a combination of serum ferritin greater than or equal to 1,000 ng/mL, platelet levels of 200 x 10^9 /L or less, and AST levels above the upper limit of normal (10–40 IU/L). Physicians might consider this index prior to ordering a liver biopsy in their C282Y homozygous patients.

US investigators provide important guidelines for the necessity of liver biopsy. After studying 182 US patients with hemochromatosis, they concluded that patients with HHC whose serum ferritin levels are less than 1000 ng/mL are unlikely to have cirrhosis. Their findings strengthen earlier reports that HHC patients who are younger than 40, C282Y homozygous, with no hepatomegaly and with serum ferritin <1,000 ng/dL have less than a 1 percent chance of cirrhosis. Supported by the more recent findings, liver biopsy to screen for cirrhosis may be unnecessary in these patients, regardless of age or serum liver enzyme levels.

Alternatives to liver biopsy

Today physicians have several ways to confirm iron over-load, such as quantitative phlebotomy and specialized imaging such as MRI and SQUID.

Specialized magnetic resonance imaging (MRI) can detect the presence of iron in organs such as the liver, heart, lungs, pancreas, and brain. An MRI can even detect iron in small glands such as the pituitary but is an especially useful and non-invasive diagnostic tool for quantification of hepatic and car-diac iron concentration. Iron will appear as dark areas on the film. A trained radiologist will be able to distinguish the differ-ence between darkness caused by a tumor and darkness caused by iron.

Quantitative phlebotomy

In standard phlebotomy, about 1 pint or 450–500cc of blood is removed. This unit contains approximately 200–250 milligrams of iron. Quantitative phlebotomy is the technique where the total amount of iron ultimately removed is calculated to determine whether the total body iron load is increased. Four grams of iron is found in about 16–20 pints of blood. Individuals who have 4 grams or more of mobilizable iron by quantitative phlebotomy can be diagnosed as having iron over-load. Investigators Phatak and Barton studied the correlation between liver iron content and phlebotomy-mobilized iron; they determined that phlebotomy-mobilized iron is an accept-able way to diagnose hemochromatosis in a patient. Previously a conclusive diagnosis of hemochromatosis could not be made in this way. Genetic testing can be considered in these cases.

Experimental technology

Another very accurate method of measuring iron is through a radiologic study performed by a machine called SQUID (Superconducting Quantum Interference Device). Studies of patients with thalassemia demonstrate that SQUID tests offer measurements that tightly correlate with liver biopsy results. This

202

new technology is presently available at Columbia Presbyterian Medical Center, New York City, and Children's Hospital, Oakland, California.

Quantum Magnetics, Inc., a wholly owned subsidiary of InVision Technologies, Inc., is developing a POC device for iron-overload hereditary diseases such as hemochromatosis, thalassemia, and sickle cell anemia. The device is based on the company's magnetic sensor technology developed as a noninvasive procedure to determine iron levels in the body, primarily the liver.

Thermal imaging: Teletherm Infared of Tampa, Florida, has developed a high-resolution dynamic infrared (DIR) imaging system that was used with great success by the Department of Neurological Surgery, Mayo Clinic and Foundation, Rochester, Minnesota. These investigators found that DIR imaging exhibited the distinct thermal footprints of 14 of 16 brain tumors. Dynamic infrared imaging is emerging as an alternative to mammography. With studies to support its potential to qualify excess iron in the body, this technology might also become an alternative to the very expensive MRI to detect iron in the liver, heart, and brain.

Genetic testing

Genetic testing is helpful to determine if the potential for an iron-loading condition is present. More than 90 percent of those diagnosed with primary hemochromatosis who are of Northern European descent are homozygotes for the C282Y mutation of *HFE.* Genetic testing is also used for some conditions where iron overload and anemia occur together: some forms of sideroblastic anemia, thalassemia, CDAII, African siderosis (ferroportin 1 mutations), and juvenile hemochromatosis (hemojuvelin). In each of these conditions, genetic testing provides helpful information about the potential for disease and the potential for inheritance patterns of offspring of these individuals. Genetic testing alone is insufficient for a complete diagnosis because it offers no information about tissue iron levels, which is more critical to the prognosis.

Genetically testing a patient for the presence of C282Y and H63D mutations of *HFE* is a good noninvasive way to diagnose hereditary hemochromatosis early, before chronic disease occurs. Also, genetic testing is helpful for individuals planning a family, so that they can begin preventive measures early.

The best time to determine the possibility of hemochromatosis in youths is around age 18 for *HFE*-related hemochromatosis and after the age of 3 years for other inherited iron-loading disorders with early age onset. Parents should be cautioned that iron is essential for proper growth and development and should not be withheld or diminished while the child is in phases of rapid growth and development. Except in rare cases of neonatal hemochromatosis, which is almost always fatal, newborns and infants have a naturally elevated saturation percentage, in some cases 90 percent. They also have elevated serum ferritin.

Prior to performing genetic tests, a patient should be informed of the possible consequences. In studies of asymptomatic hemochromatosis patients, investigators found that "insurance denial and increased premium rates are reported commonly among individuals with hemochromatosis without end organ damage. However, the overall proportion of those with active insurance, the quality of life, and the psychological well-being of these subjects were similar to those of unaffected siblings."

The differential diagnosis and screening

Physicians can include the possibility of elevated tissue iron in their differential diagnosis. There are obvious benefits to the early diagnosis of iron overload because the consequences of iron overload can be severe, even fatal. Iron overload may underlie a great variety of diseases and health problems.

Opportunistic screening during routine health assessments such as college entrance exams, employment physicals, and routine physicals is recommended. In the case of classic hereditary hemochromatosis or African siderosis, an inexpensive serum iron with TIBC (total iron binding capacity) can help to identify an iron-loaded patient presymptomatically by a physician who is "screening" for excess iron. Physicians who correctly diagnose one patient with hemochromatosis iron overload have the opportunity to diagnose an entire family.

Elevated liver enzymes or elevated serum iron can prompt

a physician to suspect iron loading and confirm diagnosis with further testing. In a 1996 US Centers for Disease Control and Prevention 1996 HHC Patient Survey, 2861 patients responded. Over 45 percent of those who responded to the survey were diagnosed presymptomatically because of abnormal lab tests.

According to the Iron Disorders Institute Patient Services Department, elevated serum iron is among the most common reasons given for how the diagnosis of HHC was obtained. Prior to 1997, serum iron was included in routine blood panels such as the Executive Panel offered by LabCorp of America and its subsidiaries. However, physicians are no longer prompted to examine iron loads because of abnormal serum iron levels, unless they know to order them specifically.

In November 25, 1996, San Diego Regional Laboratory of Allied Clinical Laboratories, Inc. pled guilty to submitting a false claim to Medicare and to the California Medicaid Program for unnecessary blood tests and was fined $5 million as a result. Allied was then owned by LabCorp, which agreed to pay $182 million to the Department of Health and Human Services Medicare/Medicaid Program to resolve the allegations.

The matter of overcharging came to the attention of California law enforcement officials after a doctor noticed that the laboratory he was using routinely did tests that he did not ask for directly. Unfortunately, this led to the removal of serum iron and serum ferritin from the frequently used panel.

Thereafter, in an effort to reduce Medicare costs, the Health Care Finance Administration (HCFA) policy guidelines for reimbursement was changed—unbundling tests from such panels. HCFA presumed that people were being tested unnecessarily, and that money from these extra tests was creating a windfall for some laboratories. Thus no reimbursement would be made for such tests unless a physician ordered them specifically to confirm diagnosis. Serum iron and serum ferritin were among the casualties of this major change to reimbursement guidelines.

What was overlooked by HCFA policy decision-makers was that elevated serum iron had contributed to the correct diagnosis of possibly as many as one-third of the persons diagnosed with hemochromatosis during the years between 1990 and part of 1997. Some of these individuals had gone to their physician seeking a cause for symptoms; some went for routine physicals and were diagnosed presymptomatically because of abnormal blood work, especially elevated serum iron.

References:

Adams, P. C., A. E. Kertesz, C. E. McLaren, R. Barr, A. Bomford, and S. Chakrabarti. "Population Screening for Hemochromatosis: A Comparison of Unbound Iron-Binding Capacity, Transferrin Saturation, and C282Y Genotyping in 5,211 Voluntary Blood Donors." *Hepatology* 31 (2000): 1160–64.

Alustiza, J. M., J. Artetxe, A. Castiella, C. Agirre, J. I. Emparanza, P. Otazua, M. Garcia-Bengoechea, J. Barrio, F. Mujica, and J. A. Recondo. "MR Quantification of Hepatic Iron Concentration." *Radiology* 230 (2004): 479–84.

Bacon, B. R. "Hemochromatosis: Diagnosis and Management." *Gastroenterology* 120 (2001): 718–25.

Barton, J. C., and C. Q. Edwards, eds. *Genetics, Pathophysiology, Diagnosis and Treatment.* Cambridge: Cambridge University Press, 2000.

Beaton, M., D. Guyader, Y. Deugnier, R. Moirand, S. Chakrabarti, and P. Adams. "Noninvasive Prediction of Cirrhosis in C282Y-Linked Hemochromatosis." *Hepatology* 36 (2002): 673–78.

Bonkovsky, H. L., R. B. Rubin, E. E. Cable, A. Davidoff, T. H. Pels Rijcken, and D. D. Stark. "Hepatic Iron Concentration: Noninvasive Estimation by Means of MR Imaging Techniques." *Radiology* 212 (1999): 227–34.

Bonkovsky, H. L., and R. W. Lambrecht. "Iron-Induced Liver Injury." *Clinical Liver Diseases* 4 (2000): 409–29.

Brandhagen, D. J., V. F. Fairbanks, and W. Baldus. "Recognition and Management of Hereditary Hemochromatosis." *American Academy of Family Physicians* 65 (2002): 853–66.

Burke, M. D. "Liver Function: Test Selection and Interpretation of Results." *Clinical Laboratory Medicine* 22 (2002): 377–90.

Chapoutot, C., P. Perney, D. Fabre, P. Taourel, J. M. Bruel, D. Larrey, J. Domergue, A. J. Ciurana, and F. Blanc. "Needle-Tract Seeding after Ultrasound-Guided Puncture of Hepatocellular Carcinoma: A Study of 150 Patients." *Gastroenterology Clinical Biology* 23 (1999): 552–56.

Elmberg, M., R. Hultcrantz, A. Ekbom, L. Brandt, S. Olsson, R. Olsson, S. Lindgren, L. Loof, P. Stal, S. Wallerstedt, S. Almer, H. Sandberg-Gertzen, and J. Askling. "Cancer Risk in Patients with Hereditary Hemochromatosis and in Their First-Degree Relatives." *Gastroenterology* 125 (2003): 1733–41.

Fridlender, Z. G., and D. Rund. "Myocardial Infarction in a Patient with Beta-Thalassemia Major: First Report." *American Journal of Hematology* 75 (2004): 52–55.

Galhenage S. P., C. H. Viiala, and J. K. Olynyk. "Screening for Hemochromatosis: Patients with Liver Disease, Families, and Populations." *Current Gastroenterology Reports* 6 (2004): 44–51.

Garrison, Cheryl, ed. *The Iron Disorders Institute Guide to Hemochromatosis.* Nashville, TN: Cumberland House, 2001.

———. *The Iron Disorders Institute Guide to Anemia.* Nashville, TN: Cumberland House, 2003.

Harrison, S. A., and B. R. Bacon. "Hereditary Hemochromatosis: Update for 2003." *Journal of Hepatology* 38 (2003): 14–23.

Hsiao, T. J., J. C. Chen, and J. D. Wang. "Insulin Resistance and Ferritin as Major Determinants of Nonalcoholic Fatty Liver Disease in Apparently Healthy Obese Patients." *International Journal of Obesity Related Metabolic Disorders* 28 (2004): 167–72.

Kowdley, K. V., T. D. Trainer, J. R. Saltzman, M. Pedrosa, E. L. Krawitt, T. A. Knox, K. Susskind, D. Pratt, H. L. Bonkovsky, N. D. Grace, and M. M. Kaplan. "Utility of Hepatic Iron Index in American Patients with Hereditary Hemochromatosis: A Multicenter Study." *Gastroenterology* 113 (1997): 1270–77.

Lieber, C. S. "Biochemical and Molecular Basis of Alcohol-Induced Injury to Liver and Other Tissues." *New England Journal of Medicine* 319 (1988): 1639–50.

McDonnell, S. M., B. L. Preston, S. A. Jewell, J. C. Barton, C. Q. Edwards, P. C. Adams, and R. Yip. "Survey of 2,851 Patients with Hemochromatosis Symptoms and Response to Treatment." *American Journal of Medicine* 106 (1999): 619–24.

Morrison, E. D., D. J. Brandhagen, P. D. Phatak, J. C. Barton, E. L. Krawitt, H. B. El-Serag, S. C. Gordon, M. V. Galan, B. Y. Tung, G. N. Ioannou, and K. V. Kowdley. "Serum Ferritin Level Predicts Advanced Hepatic Fibrosis among U.S. Patients with Phenotypic Hemochromatosis." *Annals of Internal Medicine* 138 (2003): 627–33.

Park, J. D., N. J. Cherrington, and C. D. Klaassen. "Intestinal Absorption of Cadmium Is Associated with Divalent Metal

Transporter 1 in Rats." *Toxicology Science* 68 (2002): 288–94.

Pennell, D. J. "Cardiovascular Magnetic Resonance: Twenty-First Century Solutions in Cardiology." *Clinical Medicine* 3 (2003): 273–78.

Phatak P. D., and J. C. Barton. "Phlebotomy-Mobilized Iron as a Surrogate for Liver Iron Content in Hemochromatosis Patients." *Hematology* 8 (2003): 429–32.

Piga, A., C. Gaglioti, E. Fogliacco, and F. Tricta. "Comparative Effects of Deferiprone and Deferoxamine on Survival and Cardiac Disease in Patients with Thalassemia Major: A Retrospective Analysis." *Haematologica* 88 (2003): 489–96.

Raiola, G., M. C. Galati, V. De Sanctis, M. Caruso Nicoletti, C. Pintor, M. De Simone, V. M. Arcuri, and S. Anastasi. "Growth and Puberty in Thalassemia Major." *Journal of Pediatric Endocrinology Metabolism* suppl. 2 (2003): 259–66.

Shaheen, N. J., L. B. Lawrence, B. R. Bacon, J. C. Barton, N. H. Barton, J. Galanko, C. F. Martin, C. K. Burnett, and R. S. Sandler. "Insurance, Employment, and Psychosocial Consequences of a Diagnosis of Hereditary Hemochromatosis in Subjects without End Organ Damage." *American Journal of Gastroenterology* 98 (2003): 1175–80.

Simsek, S., P. W. B. Nanayakkara, J. M. F. Keek, L. M. Fber, K. F. Bruin, and G. Pals. "Two Dutch Families with Hereditary Hyperferritinaemia-Cataract Syndrome and Heterozygosity for an *HFE* Related Haemochromatosis Gene Mutation." *Netherlands Journal of Medicine* 61 (2003): 291–95.

Westwood, M. A., L. J. Anderson, D. N. Firmin, P. D. Gatehouse, C. H. Lorenz, B. Wonke, and D. J. Pennell. "Interscanner Reproducibility of Cardiovascular Magnetic Resonance T2* Measurements of Tissue Iron in Thalassemia." *Journal of Magnetic Resonance Imaging* 18, (2003): 616–20.

Witte, D. L., W. H. Crosby, C. Q. Edwards, V. F. Fairbanks, and F. A. Mitros. "Hereditary Hemochromatosis." *Clinica Chimica Acta* 245 (1996): 139–200.

17
Treatment

"It must be remembered that the goal of treatment is not to make patients iron deficient and/or anemic, but rather to deplete excess iron stores and to achieve serum iron values in the low normal range."

—S. A. Harrison and B. R. Bacon

Depending upon hemoglobin status, de-ironing is achieved primarily in one of two ways: therapeutic phlebotomy or the pharmacological removal of iron by chelation. Chelation is generally reserved for reducing iron levels in patients with anemia due to repeated blood transfusion or ineffective erythropoiesis. The latter is more prone to be associated with de novo iron overload. Both methods of de-ironing are addressed in this chapter, beginning with iron overload without anemia.

For patients with hemoglobin values of 12.5 g/dL or greater, therapeutic phlebotomy is the most efficient means of reducing excessive iron levels. Standard therapeutic phlebotomy is the removal of 1 unit of blood, approximately 500cc from a vein in the arm. The unit of blood removed contains approximately 200–250 mg of iron. Standard phlebotomy is relatively straightforward, safe, and can be done in any facility that does therapeutic blood removal.

Besides the standard phlebotomy, other methods of blood removal for the nonanemic patient include minimal or half-unit removal, double red cell apheresis, use of a chest port or the removal of blood from the femoral vein. These methods are reserved for unique cases where the standard phlebotomy is difficult or the patient has very high iron levels and where removing greater amounts of iron is needed.

Serum ferritin, hemoglobin value, and transferrin iron saturation percentage are all three key to the frequency and method of blood removal employed. Measuring serum ferritin alone is inadequate, because serum ferritin is an acute phase reactant and it can be elevated greatly in conditions not related to iron overload, such as hyperferritinemia-cataract syndrome (HFC). HFC is a hyper production of proteins that results in early onset cataracts. Bleeding these individuals can cause a rapid drop in hemoglobin, which could result in a heart attack. The hemoglobin of an iron-overload patient will rebound after every treatment. As red blood cells are removed, the bone marrow is stimulated to produce new red blood cells, which triggers release of iron from ferritin.

Several other factors influence de-ironing therapy: a person's age, weight, gender, general health, reloading pattern, the volume and frequency of blood removed, fluid intake, diet, and behavior such as tobacco and alcohol use, which can contribute to dehydration, medication, compliance with therapy, presence of anemia, or concomitant disease such as viral hepatitis, cancer.

Age

When phlebotomy is warranted for a juvenile or an elderly or frail individual, often these patients are not able to tolerate the large needle or removal of a full unit of blood. They can have fragile or difficult-to-find veins. The elderly can often be dehydrated and in poor health. Their hearts are especially vulnerable to arrhythmia. One approach for these patients is minimal therapeutic extraction or removal of 250–300cc using a butterfly needle and vacuum bag twice during a week, depending upon the iron load.

Generally when iron overload is seen in juveniles, if not due to juvenile hemochromatosis, the cause of iron overload is likely due to repeated blood transfusion, which is often used to treat patients with thalassemia major, and some sickle cell anemia patients. A pediatric hematologist or gastroenterologist should be consulted in cases of juvenile iron loading. Iron panel test

210

results for children, especially those younger than three, can be misleading. With the exception of neonatal hemochromatosis, which is quite rare, newborns and infants have a naturally elevated serum ferritin and transferrin iron saturation percentage. Refer to the diagnosis chapter or the reference section of this book for the serum ferritin and transferrin iron saturation reference ranges for infants and toddlers.

Weight

Individuals who weigh less than 110 pounds do not have the body mass to support standard extraction. For these individuals minimal therapeutic extraction can be considered.

Gender

Males and females typically have a different body mass and females can menstruate. With menstrual blood loss there is iron loss. During the menstrual cycle a woman's natural iron regulatory system takes care to increase absorption of iron from her diet. Her normal absorption rate of 0.5–1 milligram is stepped up to 1.5–2 milligrams per day—the female body's natural response to blood loss.

The average period lasts anywhere from 2–5 days. Blood loss during this time is estimated to be as little as 60–250 milliliters or about 2 tablespoons for a light period, to as much as 1 cup for a heavy period. A unit of blood, which is 450–500cc, extracted by phlebotomy is about 1 pint or 2 cups in volume and contains about 200–250 milligrams of iron.

During childbirth or a heavy period, blood loss can be as much as 1 cup, about one-half pint of blood, which contains about 100–125 milligrams of iron.

General health

When other conditions are present such as diabetes mellitus; liver disease such as cirrhosis, alcoholic steatohepatitis and non-alcoholic steatohepatitis; infection, neurological disorders, anemia, chronic hemolysis, heart trouble, arthritis, depression, or cancer, a combined therapeutic approach is needed to address iron overload and the concomitant condition. Less frequent phlebotomy or partial phlebotomy augmented by iron

211

chelation therapy might be considered. Some extremely ill or complicated patients might require hospitalization.

Diet and behavior

Tobacco and alcohol use can dehydrate a patient, concentrating hemoglobin, which can increase the time it takes to remove a unit of blood. If one consumes red meat frequently, reloading of iron can be more rapid, because red meat contains the most highly bioavailable type of dietary iron: heme. Other substances, which are outlined in greater detail in the next chapter, influence iron absorption. Key are the enhancers: alcohol, vitamin C, meat, and sugar; and the inhibitors: tea, coffee, and supplemental calcium.

Cooking in glass or ceramic cookware is recommended for someone who is in the initial de-ironing phase of treatment. Prolonged cooking in cast iron pots or skillets should be avoided during this time. Afterward, these pots can be used on a limited basis, but the patient should be aware that iron filings can break off cast iron pots and grills and contaminate food.

Patients with iron overload should avoid consumption of raw shellfish and should take care when walking barefoot on the beach or swimming in oceans. *Vibrio vulnificus* is a bacterium that can cause death due to sepsis in an iron-loaded person.

Fluid

Patients undergoing routine phlebotomy become dehydrated and may need fluid replacement. Dehydration can also occur due to inadequate daily fluid intake, excessive alcohol consumption, or smoking.

Prior to treatment

Labwork to determine hemoglobin/hematocrit must be done prior to phlebotomy. In the uncomplicated patient (does not have anemia), pretreatment hemoglobin should be 12.5 g/dL or higher before phlebotomy is done. Patients should be advised that supplemental vitamin C (ascorbate) in excess of 200 mg daily and frequent consumption of soft drinks or sugary juices may affect some test results such as blood glucose (HbA1C) and transferrin iron saturation percentage. Patients should refrain from use of these substances and should be properly hydrated prior to receiving treatment.

Patients should report difficulties prior to phlebotomy such as unusual fatigue, experiences with rolling or difficult-to-find veins, as well as any concerns that might be related to their condition and quality of therapy. Restless legs syndrome (RLS) is often a symptom reported by patients who have been overbled. RLS is an uncontrollable urge to move limbs, especially the legs. The condition causes sleep disturbances, which results in fatigue. In studies of patients with RLS, investigators found that RLS is most frequently found in patients whose serum ferritin is less than 50 ng/mL. In another study of blood donors, RLS was reported by patients with serum ferritin values less than 20 ng/mL, regardless of normal hemoglobin value.

Phlebotomy treatment schedule

Once a treatment frequency schedule has been established, it is up to the patient to be compliant with therapy. A patient can be properly diagnosed and not comply with therapy, frequently skipping or allowing too much time to lapse between phlebotomy treatments. This can result in reaccumulation of iron and might necessitate another round of more aggressive phlebotomies. Some reasons for noncompliance that have been reported to Iron Disorders Institute Patient Services include discomfort or painful experience with therapy, usually due to problems inserting the needle, fear of needles, symptoms such as weakness or fatigue, schedules, or financial reasons.

Rebounding hemoglobin/hematocrit

Following phlebotomy, hemoglobin/hematocrit will rebound or remain within normal range for patients who have iron overload. As blood is extracted, bone marrow is stimulated to make new red blood cells. Red blood cell production is best challenged when hemoglobin levels are at 12.5–13.0 g/dL; therefore, to avoid overbleeding a patient, pretreatment hemoglobin should be 12.5 g/dL or greater.

Treatment Options

Treatment for iron overload in those who do not have concurrent anemia is therapeutic phlebotomy. Most patients are candidates for standard phlebotomy. **Patients should have a pretreatment hemoglobin of 12.5g/dL.** Quantities removed by phlebotomy can vary from minimal extraction of 250cc up to large volume extraction of 600cc. Extraction continues until ferritin reaches 25ng/mL on one occasion but hemoglobin does not drop below normal range for age, weight or gender.

| | TYPE OF PHLEBOTOMY | | |
	STANDARD	MINIMAL VOLUME	LARGE VOLUME
Patient Profile	most patients	for youths, persons who are frail, small in stature or weight, or who have coexistent illness such as heart problems*	unique cases such as adults with extremely high iron levels and other medical complications
Procedure	extracted from vein in the arm using 16-gauge needle (similar to routine blood donation)	extracted from vein in the arm using 20- to 22-gauge butterfly needle with vacuum bag	chest port surgically implanted near collar bone area
Duration of Procedure	15-20 minutes	15-20 minutes	15-20 minutes
Approx. Volume Blood Removed	450-500 cc of blood	250-300 cc of blood	600 cc of blood
Approx. Iron Removed	approx. 250 mg of iron	approx. 125 mg of iron	approx. 300 mg of iron
Frequency of Treatment	one or two times weekly	one or two times monthly	one or two times weekly
Important Notes	increasing the frequency to twice a week should be considered to facilitate more rapid iron depletion	frequency may be increased depending on patient tolerance *patient may have small, inaccessible, scarred or rolling veins *patient may be unable to tolerate standard volume of blood removal	serious procedure not to be considered a routine option

AVOID OVER-BLEEDING

Forced-sustained anemia

A now outdated and no longer recommended method of de-ironing involved bleeding an iron-overload patient until the hemoglobin remained at 10.0 g/dL for a period of 2–3 weeks, and the serum ferritin was lowered to less than 10 ng/mL.

The practice of forced sustained anemia was thought to be the only way to remove hemosiderin, an inert byproduct of iron. However, more recent findings provide that when ferritin reaches 10 ng/mL there is no detectable hemosiderin in the liver. Also, forcing hemoglobin to remain below normal for a prolonged period of time may, in fact, result in other health problems later on.

The greatest advances in therapy for hemochromatosis patients with iron overload come from the National Institutes of Health Hemochromatosis Protocol. More than 100 hemochromatosis patients are enrolled in the unique program. Initially, the purpose of the study was to determine a protocol for HHC blood use. Since 2001, investigation has been expanded to

- Define efficacy of mean corpuscular volume (MCV) as a guide to phlebotomy therapy during induction and maintenance phases of treatment in HHC.
- Compare utility and cost of MCV as a replacement for transferrin saturation and ferritin as monitoring tools during phlebotomy.
- Create standardized system (SOP) for use of HHC donor blood for transfusion.

In the study, 130 patients with iron overload were referred for phlebotomy therapy (9 patients between 1987 and 1997; and 122 between 1998 and 2002). Diagnosis was established with genetic testing, a transferrin saturation >45 percent and an elevated serum ferritin as well as a liver biopsy. Patients without the common mutations of *HFE* (C282Y or H63D) were admitted to the study if their serum ferritin was >1500 ng/mL, with elevated liver enzymes.

Results and conclusions of the protocol

"During induction therapy, the MCV increased transiently because of reticulocytosis, and then stabilized for a prolonged period before decreasing more sharply, which reflected iron-limited erythropoiesis. Iron depletion was achieved after a median of 38 phlebotomies and removal of 9.0 g of iron. Maintenance phlebotomy was targeted to maintain the MCV at 5–10 percent below prephlebotomy values and the Hb at >13 g per dL. Transferrin saturation fluctuated considerably during treatment, but remained below 35 percent during MCV-guided maintenance therapy. In this study, ferritin values were not useful guides to the pace of phlebotomy. The median maintenance therapy phlebotomy interval was 7.5 weeks (range, 6–16), which corresponded to an average daily iron removal of 35–67 microg per kg. Most patients showed evidence of iron reaccumulation at phlebotomy intervals of 8 weeks or more."

Conclusions
- •Forced-sustained anemia is not necessary to de-iron a patient.
- •MCV is an inexpensive means of determining when a patient has been successfully de-ironed. When used in conjunction with Hgb, it is a clinically useful guide to the pace of phlebotomy therapy for hemochromatosis.
- •Double red cell apheresis is safe and practical for some patients.

For physicians who wish to use MCV-guided phlebotomy, the targeted endpoint of MCV is 3 percent below baseline (normal range: 82–98fL), at which time the ferritin level is less than 30 ng/mL and the transferrin saturation is less than 30 percent.

Serum ferritin and inflammatory conditions

In the uncomplicated patient, serum ferritin drops about 30 ng/mL with each standard unit of blood removed. Because serum ferritin is an acute phase reactant, special consideration must be given to serum ferritin values of patients with inflammatory conditions that might affect serum ferritin levels, such as arthritis, kidney disease, liver disease, autoimmune, or infection. Response to drugs used to treat some inflammatory conditions, such as interferon for viral hepatitis, is improved after the iron load is reduced.

Frequency of extractions

Terms such as aggressive phlebotomy, minimal or partial extraction, or maintenance phlebotomy are used to define the frequency and quantity of blood removed. For adult patients with iron overload but without anemia or who are not transfusion dependent, the critical level of serum ferritin is 1000 ng/mL. In patients whose serum ferritin is below 1000 ng/mL with an accompanying transferrin iron saturation percentage greater than 55 percent, aggressive extraction is important. Aggressive extraction is the removal of 2 or more standard units per week.

Adults with moderately high ferritin but at levels which are below 1,000 ng/mL and an accompanying transferrin iron saturation percentage greater than 55 percent might also begin with aggressive phlebotomy for the initial period of therapy but slow to weekly extractions once the serum ferritin is in the 450–650 ng/mL range. Thereafter, phlebotomies can be reduced to every 2 weeks or once a month, depending upon the patient. If de-ironing is not successful in this phase, weekly extractions may be resumed.

Tolerance

Most people will tolerate phlebotomy without many side effects. Fatigue is the common problem reported. Of 353 venesected patients, 43 percent had problems with needle puncture, 63 percent experienced immediate fatigue, 28 percent found the treatment tedious. There are techniques that can be employed to reduce problems. Refer your patients to the Iron Disorders Institute (IDI) web site or contact IDI for a free booklet about phlebotomy.

Patients should be encouraged to keep good records during the entire treatment process. Patients often believe that they will remember details, but many do not. A careful diary of events can provide clues later that may not seem relevant at the time. Notations about response to treatment can be significant in modifying treatment.

De-ironing is complete when ferritin reaches 25 ng/mL on one occasion (while pretreatment hemoglobin remains at 12.5 g/dL or greater). Thereafter to avoid anemia-related symptoms, such as restless legs syndrome, serum ferritin should remain in a range of 25–75 ng/mL with an accompanying transferrin saturation percentage <40 percent.

Once de-ironed, some patients will continue to have an elevated transferrin iron saturation percentage (Tsat) in spite of a normal serum ferritin and hemoglobin. If the pretreatment hemoglobin is 12.5 g/dL or greater, this patient can continue to donate blood. If however, the hemoglobin is below 12.5 g/dL but the Tsat is elevated, other causes can be considered before blood donation.

The patient may be dehydrated or deficient in nutrients such as B₆, B₁₂, or folate. They may also need antioxants such as selenium, vitamin E, and vitamin C. Often hemochromatosis patients will avoid vitamin C entirely because it enhances the absorption of iron. See diet and nutrition recommendations in the selected reference charts section in the back of the book.

Maintenance

Once a patent is de-ironed, they may require only four to eight phlebotomies a year. Again, the frequency of mainte-nance phlebotomy will be based on the same factors men-tioned earlier. Providing that a patient is compliant with routine blood donation, more than moderate consumption of alcohol and eating red meat frequently are probably the two greatest influences of iron reaccumulation.

Prognosis

Most patients with hemochromatosis will have a normal life expectancy. Outcome for the patient will vary depending upon when the condition was detected and treated. Also, much depends upon whether or not the patient was bled too aggres-sively, resulting in overbleeding and its complications.

Apheresis and double red cell apheresis (DRCA)

Red blood cell and plasma (RBCP) apheresis and double red cell apheresis (DRCA) can be used as an option to routine phle-botomy for some patients. These alternatives might be more costly to perform, but patients who have scheduling problems or who have to drive long distances for treatment might find this type of treatment helpful.

According to Dr. James Smith, Oklahoma Blood Institute, "The advantage to apheresis over standard phlebotomy is that a standard unit of blood contains about 40 percent red blood cells. A unit removed by apheresis contains nearly 80 percent RBC." If one does the math, it becomes apparent that one apheresis treat-

Results of Therapeutic Phlebotomy in Patients with Hemochromatosis

Complication of Iron Overload	Expected Treatment Outcome
None	Prevention of iron overload and normal life expectancy
Weakness, fatigue, lethargy	Resolution or marked improvement
Elevated liver enzymes	Resolution or marked improvement
Hepatomegaly	Resolution often occurs
Hepatic cirrhosis	No change
Increased risk for primary liver cancer	No change if at time of detection patient has cirrhosis
Right upper quadrant pain	Resolution or marked improvement Right upper quadrant pain in HHC patients is usually due to hepatic I/O URQP can also be due to gallbladder disease, portal vein thrombosis, hepatic lesions or primary liver cancer
Arthropathy	Improvement in arthralgias sometimes occurs; change in joint deformity is rare; progression is sometimes seen
Hypogonadotrophic hypogonadism	Resolution is rare
Diabetes mellitus	Occasional improvement; often temporary
Hypo/hyperthyroidism	Resolution is rare
Cardiomyopathy	Resolution sometimes occurs
Hyperpigmentation	Resolution usually occurs
Hyperferritinemia	Resolution
Excess absorption and storage of nonferrous metals	Little or no change: Cobalt, manganese, zinc, and lead
Infection with *Vibrio vulnificus* or other bacteria	Little or no change

Source: adapted with permission: Annals of Internal Medicine 129 (1998): 935.

ment removes approximately double the iron, or an impressive 500 mg per treatment, as compared with 250 mg. Though apheresis is more efficient than phlebotomy for iron removal, it is expensive and may not be affordable to many people.

Dr. Mary Townsend, Medical Director, Coffee Memorial Blood Center, agrees that apheresis can be considered by individuals with iron overload. Dr. Townsend points out that apheresis can be helpful for patients who live in rural areas and must travel long distances for treatment. These individuals can get the equivalent of two phlebotomies with one apheresis treatment.

A prescription for this type of procedure might read: "Two unit apheresis every two weeks until serum ferritin is lowered to 20 ng/mL or less as long as hematocrit remains greater than 35 percent and hgb remains within range of 14–18 g/dL."

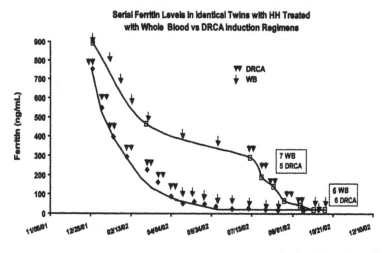

Source: C. D Bolan et al.

Apheresis is available in any blood center; however, it is not routinely offered as a treatment option for those with iron overload. The Warren Magnuson Clinical Center, the Oklahoma Blood Institute, and Reading Pennsylvania Hospital therapeutic laboratory are three centers known to be using apheresis specifically for the purposes of de-ironing. Requirements for apheresis are the same as for a regular blood donor. The person must be at least 17 years of age, weigh more than 110 pounds, and not have anemia.

Chest port

Patients with exceptionally high amounts of iron, usually confirmed by liver biopsy, might benefit from an implant or chest port. Chest port or central venous catheters are tubes threaded through the vein in the upper chest under the collarbone. Two types are commonly used: internal, which is surgically implanted under the skin, or external, where the entry site portion is visible outside the skin.

A phlebotomist who performs therapeutic phlebotomy is also qualified to remove blood through a port. Hemoglobin/-hematocrit levels are measured prior to extraction just as with other types of blood extraction. Blood is extracted from the port through a tube leading into a vacuum bag or bottle. This type of bag/bottle is needed to suction the blood through the needle into a tube and into a blood bag. Vacuum bags or bottles hold the same amount of blood, one unit or 450–500cc of blood, the same as a standard blood bag.

A saline solution is used to clean the port, followed by a heparin flush. Heparin is a blood thinner and used to prevent clotting, one of the problems of this device. Another problem with ports is that they can work their way out of the body and have to be replanted.

Butterfly needle

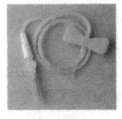

A smaller gauge needle makes insertion into the vein easier. Wings are pinched together to allow the phlebotomist a secure grip.

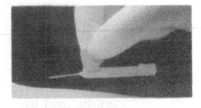

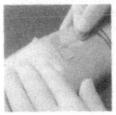

The needle is inserted into a vein in the arm and a connecting tube is attached to a blood bag.

Photographs courtesy of Becton Dickinson

Ports are not considered routine method for therapeutic phlebotomy. These devices are generally used to give medication in cases where a patient requires large amounts of medicine that must be given often, such as in AIDS and cancer patients. However, this device can work well for some patients where iron levels are extremely high, especially when access to veins is impaired or difficult.

Chest ports require surgical implantation. Most patients with iron overload are not candidates for this treatment option.

Minimal extraction

Individuals who are frail, elderly, small (less than 110 pounds), or whose veins are scarred and not accessible might benefit from a smaller needle such as the butterfly needle. This type of needle is usually a 20–22 gauge as compared with a 16- to 18-gauge needle used for standard phlebotomy. Because the needle is smaller, removal of a standard unit of blood will take longer. Some individuals, such as those with heart conditions, especially arrhythmia, might not need a full unit removed, in which case minimal extraction or half-unit (250cc) can be considered.

Recombinant human erythropoietin (rHuEPO)

The use of Epoietin (EPO) is suitable for some patients with iron overload, especially if they have anemia. Iron-overload patients with cardiomyopathy or cardiac arrythmias are possible candidates for EPO. Generally, EPO is not used for patients who can tolerate phlebotomy, but this drug has been tried experimentally on hemochromatotics with some degree of success. In one study of ten asymptomatic patients with serum ferritin >400 ng/mL, and transferrin saturation greater than 50 percent, and elevated liver enzymes, erythrocytapheresis (EA) with recombinant human erythropoietin (rHuEPO) and folic acid was performed on ten patients with hemochromatosis who were not anemic. The results were that red cell indices (red blood cell count), serum ferritin, and other iron metabolism parameters (serum iron, transferrin, and transferrin saturation), liver enzymes, and other laboratory data were considerably improved.

EPO is expensive and not approved for use with hemochromatosis. Benefits of EPO for persons with iron overload should be limited to those who cannot tolerate routine phlebotomy and who have ineffective erythropoiesis, such as a patient with sideroblastic anemia, CDAII, red cell enzymopathies, autoimmune hemolytic anemia, myelodysplastic syndromes, or kidney disease.

Iron chelation

Iron chelation therapy is used for patients with concomitant iron overload and anemia. Iron overload complicated by anemia can occur in sideroblastic anemia, thalassemia, sickle cell anemia, congenital dyserythropoietic anemia (CDAII), red cell enzymopathies, myelodysplastic syndromes, atransferrinemia, and aceruloplasminemia. Iron chelation has been used with success on patients with viral infections, atherosclerosis, and some types of cancer. The primary role of iron chelation is to prevent organ damage and premature death. Statistically 50 percent of patients with thalassemia major die of heart attack before the age of 35, primarily due to heart failure caused by myocardial iron overload.

Iron chelation is the removal of iron pharmacologically by chemicals formulated to bind specifically to iron so that it can be excreted in urine or feces. This type of chelation should not be confused with EDTA (ethylene-diamine-tetra-acetic acid) chelation. EDTA, a method used by some alternative medicine practitioners, is a broad-spectrum chelator, meaning that it binds with and removes a wide number of metals, including iron, but it is not specific. In contrast, desferrioxamine (Desferal) and deferiprone, a new oral chelator awaiting FDA approval, are highly specific for iron.

Candidates for iron chelation therapy are those who have iron overload with anemia. Often these are patients who require repeated blood transfusions, such as those with sickle cell anemia, thalassemia major, and some forms of cancers.

Desferal is not absorbed in the intestinal tract; therefore, this drug must be administered intravenously, which is done in an infusion center or hospital or subcutaneously, using a portable battery-operated infusion pump. Generally, the pump is worn at night, where slow infusion of the iron chelating agent is administered subcutaneously over a period of about 8 hours, 5–7 nights a week. Patients are given a step-by-step demonstration of how to sterilize the skin, insert the needle, and operate the pump.

Before Desferal is administered by either method, a test dose is given to be certain that there are no immediate reactions to the drug. Desferal is administered slowly at first, beginning with 1.0 gram, 3–4 times per week with monitoring of iron excretion in a cumulative 24-hour urine sample. If effective, the dose can then be adjusted upward, 1 gram at a time, up to 4 times per week, until the patient reaches a tolerable level. The dose should not exceed 50 milligrams/kg weight, or about 3 grams per day. Periodic examination of the patient is necessary until positive response to treatment is confirmed.

Patients might be given an additional 2 grams of Desferal intravenously for each unit of blood transfused. Desferal is administered separately from blood transfusions.

Pumps used for chelation therapy

A variety of pumps are available, including the CADD Micro, the Graseby pump, the new portable Crono ambulatory infusion pump, and the Eclipse C-Series Continuous Infusion System.

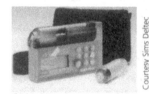

Courtesy Sims Deltec

CADD Micro

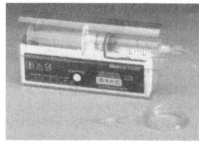

Courtesy Marcal Medical, Inc.

Graseby pump

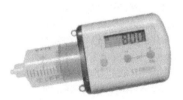

Crono ambulatory infusion pump
Courtesy Intrapump, Inc.

Product information is available in the resource section in the back of the book.

Side effects

The urine can become orange colored, which is a harmless side effect. Immediate symptoms of adverse reaction to Desferal chelation therapy might include: visual disturbances, blurred vision, rash or hives, itching, vomiting, diarrhea, stomach or leg cramps, fever, rapid heartbeat, hypotension (low blood pressure), dizziness, anaphylactic shock, and pain or swelling at site of intravenous entry. Long-term problems might include kidney or liver damage, loss of hearing, or cataracts.

Patients should report such symptoms immediately to their physician who can adjust dosage. Further, physicians should examine the patient's visual status with slit-lamp examination (means of examining the eye) and hearing status with audiometry or hearing test on a yearly basis. Liver enzymes (ALT, AST, GGT, and ALP), a kidney function test such as BUN, serum ferritin and transferrin iron saturation percentage should also be measured annually by the attending physician.

Also there are a number of needles available. Straight needles, butterfly, or thumbtack (also called button), or devices such as the MiniMed Sof-serter. The Sof-serter is a bit different from the other needles in that a spring-activated device inserts a tiny plastic catheter under the skin for infusion; the needle is removed after insertion.

Each patient is different and physicians can talk about the features and benefits of the various pumps and needles, such as size, portability, ease in operation, etc.

Tip

Mild topical anesthetic creams, such as Emla or Topicaine, will somewhat numb the skin so that the patient does not feel the needle stick. These creams are used by many hemochromatosis and pediatric patients who report good results.

Limitations of Desferal

Nursing mothers will need to talk with their physicians. It is not known how much of the drug gets into breast milk; thus, a mother who is receiving Desferal treatment might consider low iron–soy formula substitutes.

When to begin iron chelation therapy

Initiating chelation therapy depends upon several factors: the patient's overall health, hematologic values, especially hemoglobin, hematocrit, and the tissue iron levels. Tissue iron is determined by measuring serum ferritin, and fasting serum iron and TIBC (total iron-binding capacity). These results help the physician to monitor iron buildup and to address the excess iron as soon as possible. Addressing the excess promptly with chelation therapy is important. Free or unbound iron triggers the production of oxygen-free radicals and peroxidative tissue injury, especially to the heart, anterior pituitary, and liver. Some physicians will begin chelation therapy when serum ferritin is between 1,000–1,500 ng/mL. Serum ferritin should not be allowed to go above 2,500 ng/mL before beginning chelation.

Animal studies provide substantial evidence that iron overload can result in oxidative damage to lipids in vivo, once the concentration of iron exceeds a threshold level.

Experimental therapies

Iron chelators are being developed as possible adjuncts in management of infection, neurological disorders, cancer, and other conditions in which iron participates in the disease progression. Oral iron chelators, use of lactoferrin, hepcidin, and novel devices produced in the future may contribute to better compliance and offer an alternative to some iron overload patients, especially those who cannot tolerate Desferal (DF).

Oral chelators

One clinically available iron chelator, deferiprone (DP), developed in the 1980s, is administered orally 3 times/day. Complications are minimal except for an inhibition of white blood cell formation that occurs in about 1 percent of patients. Occurrence of this side effect must be determined promptly. Therefore, patients have blood count determinations every 2 weeks. If the side effect occurs, the patient must shift to Desferal. The cost of production of DP has been estimated to be only one-thirtieth that of DF. In India, DP is sold for 8 times less than DF. Sadly, in Europe, DP is sold for the same amount as DF; in the United States, sale of DP is prohibited.

Presently, compliance in use of DF has been improved in some patients by lowering the injections to 2 days/wk and adding DP to the weekly regimen. Moreover, there is some evidence that although removal of liver iron is helped by DF, greater removal of cardiac iron is achieved by DP. For example, in a 6-year study of 75 patients on DF, 20 percent developed cardiac disease and 3 died. In contrast, of 54 patients on DP, only 4 percent developed disease and none died.

At this time, an alternate oral iron chelator, Exjade® deferasirox (ICL670) Novartis Pharmaceuticals, is being tested in thalassemic adults. In a recent 2-week study, side effects were minimal and iron excretion was adequate. However, the authors noted that it will be necessary to completely evaluate possible complications as well as efficacy in long-term studies. Furthermore, no prediction has yet been made as to whether deferasirox might be more affordable than that of Desferal (Novartis) or deferiprone (Ferriprox Apotex, Canada) sold in Europe.

Other chelators

Biomedical Frontier's (BMF) starch-based synthetic chelator is used intravenously similar to Desferal, but BMF's product requires only a single dose that takes about an hour to administer to achieve similar results as 1 week of Desferal therapy, which requires 5–6 nightly infusions, lasting 8–12 hours per infusion. The BMF product must be administered with medical supervision, but a once-a-week trip to an infusion center may be an appealing alternative to the portable pump.

Non–iron-loaded patients often have specific disease processes that might be exacerbated by local deposits of the metal and for which iron chelation might be useful as an adjunct to classic forms of therapy. For example, a series of patients with coronary artery disease had a mean serum ferritin of 127 ng/mL as compared with healthy controls whose mean serum ferritin was 76 ng/mL. Arterial blood flow in the patients was improved by injection of DF. The chelator had no effect on blood flow in the controls. In rabbits in which high cholesterol was induced by diet, atherosclerosis was suppressed by deferiprone (DP). It may be recalled that elevated cholesterol is hazardous in the presence of elevated iron.

Characteristics of Leading Iron Chelators

Characteristics	deferoxamine (DF)	deferiprone (DP)	deferasirox (ICL670)
Source of drug	bacterial siderophore	synthetic compound	synthetic compound
Molecular size	561	139	383
Ratio chelator:iron	1:1	3:1	2:1
Removal of iron from: transferrin, lactoferrin ferritin, hemosiderin small molecules	NO YES YES	YES YES YES	Not Known
Metal binding in humans	Fe, Al, Cu, Zn	Fe, Al, Cu, Zn	Highly specific for Fe
Effective dose in humans	40-60 mg/kg body wt	50-100 mg/kg body wt	20 mg/kg body wt
Route of administration	subcutaneous/injected	oral	oral
Excretion in humans	urine, feces	urine	feces
Can be used by some pathogens to obtain iron	YES	NO	Not Known
Side effects at high doses	Auditory and visual disturbances	Arthralgia; agranulocytosis	Skin rash
Geographic availability:	World-wide	Europe, Asia India	In clinical trials

Source: E. D. Weinberg, 2003

Several studies have reported that growth of cultures of neoplastic and microbial cells is suppressed by either DF or DP. For instance, each of the chelators inhibited growth and induced death of human cervical carcinoma cell lines. Unfortunately, for unknown reasons, both DF and DP enhanced growth of human sarcoma cells that had been implanted in mice.

Compared with normal mammalian cells, bloodstream forms of trypanosomes (the protozoa that cause sleeping sickness) are 10 times more sensitive to iron depletion by DF. Strong antitrypanosome activity also is possessed by DP. Several clinical studies with patients infected with a protozoan that causes severe malaria, *Plasmodium falciparum*, have shown that DF in some situations can be a useful adjunct to established anti-malarial drugs. Both DF and DP suppressed multiplication of a fungal pathogen, *Pneumocystis carinii*, at concentrations that can be achieved in patient therapy.

A variety of low molecular weight compounds have been synthesized by chemists and are being studied as potential iron chelating drugs. Among these are HBED, desferrithiocin, alpha-

228

ketohydroxypyridines (in addition to DP), and pyridoxal isoni-cotinoyl hydrazones. Several compounds in these series have strong activity in culture systems and a few of the chelators have shown potency and safety in animal models. None are presently available for clinical use in humans.

A synthetic antioxidant, idebenone, has been reported to protect heart muscle cells against oxidative stress. It has been recommended for use in patients who have cardiac enlargement associated with a neurodegenerative disease, Friedreich's ataxia.

As cited in chapter 6, iron chelating drugs are being devel-oped for therapeutic use in neurodegenerative diseases. A novel compound, VK-28, can cross the blood-brain barrier. Upon injec-tion in rats, the iron chelator has been observed to protect the animals against developing Parkinson-type lesions. Two other iron chelators, DZR and MITOX, have been found to suppress multiple sclerosis-type lesions in rats. Mitox has already been approved for use in relapsing-remitting forms of MS in the United States and Germany.

Gallium is a metal that is so similar chemically to iron that it is bound by transferrin and carried by the protein by mistake into multiplying cells. As gallium accumulates inside cancer cells, it intereferes with their normal use of iron. Accordingly, gallium salts have been used to suppress growth of cells of lym-phomas and bladder cancer.

In order for transferrin to release its iron to endosomes inside cells, the pH value must be lowered. Chloroquine, a drug that has long been used to treat malaria, prevents the pH from being lowered. Thus the drug suppresses the ability of the malarial protozoan to obtain iron. Similarly, chloroquine pre-vents macrophages from loading iron, and in this way it can inhibit growth of those bacterial pathogens that infect and grow inside macrophages. The anti-inflammatory activity of chloroquine likewise is associated with its ability to prevent excessive iron accumulation in inflamed cells.

Iron deprivation of microbial pathogens also can be achieved by development of specific vaccines that contain iron acquisition antigens derived from the germs. The microbes are grown in culture media that contain very little iron. This forces the pathogens to markedly increase formation of their surface antigens that are necessary to bind and take in the metal. Humans and animals vaccinated with such preparations therefore are stimulated to form antibodies to the specific antigens. The antibodies will prevent subsequent invaders of the same kind from obtaining body iron for growth. It is noteworthy that persons who recover from such specific bacterial infections as meningococcal meningitis promptly begin forming antibodies to the iron acquisition antigens of the pathogen and thereby are resistant to reinfection for many years.

Natural chelators

In addition to low-molecular-mass chelators, two natural product iron–binding proteins are being developed for clinical use: transferrin and lactoferrin. The first would be employed in patients whose iron saturation of transferrin has temporarily been elevated, as in bone marrow recipients who are being conditioned with a week of cytotoxic chemotherapy. Moreover, both transferrin and lactoferrin suppress bacterial biofilm formation by binding iron. Lactoferrin is also being used or considered in a variety of sites as illustrated in the chart on the opposite page.

The transferrin (Tf) product is being evaluated for possible use in several medical conditions in which iron saturation of Tf is elevated as well as in patients who produce below normal levels of the protein. For example, Tf iron saturation often rises dramatically in patients who are undergoing cytotoxic chemotherapy prior to receiving bone marrow stem cells. The cytotoxic procedure temporarily halts red blood cell formation and also damages liver cells, thus releasing iron deposits. Iron saturation consistently approaches 100 percent in such patients.

Another potential medical use for the Tf product would be for anemic patients who undergo maintenance dialysis while being treated with erythropoietin plus intravenous iron supplements. Athough these treatments are appropriate for kidney-deficient patients with severe anemia, the therapy sometimes results in elevated Tf iron saturation, which increases risk of infection.

The transferrin product also might be useful in patients with cancers in whom their own Tf is below normal. For instance, in a set of 22 patients with nonsmall cell lung cancer, serum Tf

Possible Applications of Bovine or Recombinant Human Lactoferrin

Site	Suppression by lactoferrin of:
Available Now or in the Near Future	
Processed foods such as meat	Bacterial & Fungal Growth (to extend shelf life) life expectancy
Fish farms	Bacterial & fungal infection of fish
Animal feed for young poultry and mammals	Low-grade bacterial infections (to replace antibiotics now used for growth acceleration).
Infant milk formula	Bacterial pathogens in infant intestine
Oral cavity	Bacteria that live in biofilms and that cause tooth decay or periodontal disease; also, yeast infections
Throat	Streptococcal growth on tonsillar tissue; also, yeast infection
Small intestine (oral ingestion)	Bacterial pathogens and inflammation
Skin	Allergic inflammation
Possibly Available in the Future	
Eyes (eyedrops)	Bacterial & fungal infections
Joints (injection)	Bacterial pathogens and inflammation
Vagina (suppository)	Bacterial & fungal pathogen (but not protozoa)
Blood (intravenous injection)	Bacterial & fungal pathogen (but not *Neisseria*)
Colon (oral preparation encapsulated to prevent intestinal digestion)	Cancer cells

was 28–50 percent below normal, whereas serum albumen remained unaltered.

The Tf product might become useful also as an adjunct to antibiotics in patients with infections. As with lactoferrin, however, caution must be exercised to avoid using the product in patients who might be infected with pathogens that can extract iron from the protein.

The body site of the disease process that requires de-ironing would indicate whether to employ transferrin or lactoferrin. In sites in which the pH value might be lower than that of the bloodstream (e.g., inflamed areas), lactoferrin would be selected. The pH value (7.35) of the blood and lymph would be compatible with de-ironing activity of transferrin in these fluids.

Because cancer cells often are much more actively multiplying than are most normal cells, the former produce more Tf receptors and thus attract higher amounts of Tf. The protein can be chemically attached to anti-cancer drugs so as to act as a targeted carrier of the drugs to sites of cancer cells. In an earlier section of this chapter, the availability of human recombinant lactoferrin was noted. Development of this product now can be anticipated for use in a wide range of medical conditions that are worsened by elevated iron.

Another possible pharmaceutical used to treat iron overload might include hepcidin, a recently discovered hormone that regulates iron. Hepcidin is produced by the liver and is depressed in patients with iron overload. It might be useful as a pharmaceutical in the prevention of iron loading in persons with hereditary hemochromatosis.

Hydroxyurea (HU)

Hydroxyurea belongs to the group of medicines called antimetabolites and is fairly inexpensive compared to deferioxamine (Desferal). HU is used to treat some kinds of cancer and to prevent painful episodes associated with sickle cell anemia. HU is found to enhance fetal hemoglobin (Hb) production, which is significant for patients with beta-thalassemia.

Investigators report success with HU in both sickle cell and beta-thalassemia intermedia patients. Hydroxyurea therapy was initiated in study participants to increase the efficacy of erythropoiesis, thereby reducing the required transfusion volume and finally leading to a reduction of transfusional iron overload. An increase in total hemoglobin level was repeatedly reported during HU treatment in these patients. The effects in patients with beta-thalassemia major remain controversial. In one study, the marked elevation of total hemoglobin levels with HU permitted regular transfusions to be stopped in 7 children with transfusion-dependent beta-thalassemia. It was concluded that HU can eliminate transfusional needs in children with beta-thalassemia major, which could be particularly useful in countries such as Algeria, where supplies of blood or chelating agents are limited.

According to researchers at the National Heart, Lung, and Blood Institute (NHLBI) of the National Institutes of Health (NIH), when used to treat sickle cell anemia, hydroxyurea appears to increase the flexibility of sickled cells. In a NIH supported study, sickle cell anemia patients who took the drug hydroxyurea over a 9-year period experienced a 40 percent reduction in deaths, according to the first study to evaluate whether the treatment prolongs life.

Over 2½ years, the drug resulted in an almost 50 percent reduction in the number of painful crises and episodes of chest syndrome. Patients on hydroxyurea also required about 50 percent fewer transfusions and hospitalizations. The Food and Drug Administration (FDA) approved hydroxyurea in 1995 for the treatment of sickle cell anemia.

Pediatricians at Oakland Children's Hospital report that patients receiving HU might benefit from supplemental L-arginine. This amino acid is metabolized to nitric oxide (NO), which is a vasodilator. While arginine alone does not increase serum NO production in sickle cell disease (SCD) patients at steady state, it does when given together with HU. Hence, co-administration of arginine with HU may augment the NO response in SCD and improve utilization of arginine in patients at steady state. Others report that the effects of magnesium supplementation in patients with sickle cell anemia receiving hydroxyurea might be beneficial.

Bone marrow transplantation

Bone marrow transplantation has resulted in a cure for some patients with thalassemia major and sickle cell anemia. Italian investigators studied the reversibility of cirrhosis in six patients who were cured of thalassemia with bone marrow transplantation. When they compared liver biopsies of these patients done prior to and following transplantation, the reversal of cirrhosis in these patients was confirmed. Bone marrow transplantation procedure is complicated as exact marrow matches are needed for the procedure. Also there are risks and posttransplantation consequences such as infection due to the immunosuppressive medications used and possible rejection.

Moreover, after successful bone marrow transplantation, the

excess iron in the patient must still be removed by chelation or phlebotomy if hemoglobin values are sufficient.

Novel devices

Hemodialysis with a specialized device called the Hemopurifier™, manufactured by Aethlon Medical, may offer an alternative for patients who cannot tolerate standard infused Desferal treatment. The Hemopurifier device is used to remove iron from the body, but the process takes place outside the body, so that the drug Desferal never enters the patient's bloodstream. Side effects most commonly associated with iron chelation therapy are avoided. The Hemopurifier device is still being tested in clinical trials.

Supplementation and health food store claims

Health food store claims of oral products that remove heavy metals are simply false. Iron can only be removed efficiently from the body through blood loss, as with phlebotomy or by using specific iron chelating agents. Iron chelators approved for use in humans include deferoxamine (also spelled deferioxamine and often called DF), sold as brand name Desferal, and deferiprone (DP) or L1, sold as an oral iron chelator brand name Ferriprox.

Claims that inositol phosphate (IP6) will remove iron from the body are completely false. Though IP6 is an excellent inhibitor of nonheme iron absorption, it has not been proven capable of removing iron from ferritin.

When iron is removed by phlebotomy or chelation therapy, other nutrients may also be removed. A daily multivitamin without iron is highly recommended for these patients.

B-complex including folic acid helps to build red blood cells. Antioxidants such as vitamin E and selenium reduce the risk of free radical production. Also, patients undergoing phlebotomy can have increased levels of heavy metals such as cadmium, aluminum, gallium, and lead; they may also experience shifts in the levels of zinc. A good time to check for the presence of these heavy metals is when the patient is de-ironed. Other nutrients might be removed, and the patient may also experience shifts in levels.

Fresh fruits provide fluids, antioxidants, and fiber, and patients should be encouraged to consume these in spite of the vitamin C content. The concern about vitamin C with regard to iron overload is that supplemental C is often taken in excessively high amounts. When vitamin C consumption is derived from food sources it is usually in amounts of 100–200 mg, a safe amount for people with hemochromatosis. However, if a patient has diet restrictions for extremely high iron or diabetes, fruit may be limited to the less sugary variety, such as apples and berries.

References:
Akesson, A., P. Stal, and M. Vahter. "Phlebotomy Increases Cadmium Uptake in Hemochromatosis." *Environmental Health Perspectives* 108 (2000): 289–91.

Allen, R. P., and C. J. Earley. "Restless Legs Syndrome: A Review of Clinical and Pathophysiologic Features." *Journal of Clinical Neurophysiology* 18 (2001): 128–47.

Altura, R. A., W. C. Wang, L. Wynn, B. M. Altura, and B. T. Altura. "Hydroxyurea Therapy Associated with Declining Serum Levels of Magnesium in Children with Sickle Cell Anemia." *Journal of Pediatrics* 140 (2002): 565–69.

Bacon, B. R. "Hemochromatosis: Diagnosis and Management." *Gastroenterology* 120 (2001): 718–25.

Barton, J. C., and C. Q. Edwards, eds. *Genetics, Pathophysiology, Diagnosis and Treatment.* Cambridge: Cambridge University Press, 2000.

Ben-Shacher, D., N. Kahana, V. Kampel, A. Warshawsky, and M. B. H. Youdim. "Neuroprotective by a Novel Brain Permeable Iron Chelator, V-28, against 6-Hydroxydopamine Lesion in Rats." *Neuropharmacology* 46 (2004): 254–63.

Bergeron, R. J., J. Wiegand, and G. M. Brittenham. "HBED Ligand: Preclinical Studies of a Potential Alternative to Deferoxamine for Treatment of Chronic Iron Overload and Acute Iron Poisoning." *Blood* 99 (2002): 3019–26.

Bolan, C. D., C. Conry-Cantilena, G. Mason, T. A. Rouault, and S. F. Leitman. "MCV as a Guide to Phlebotomy Therapy for Hemochromatosis." *Transfusion* 41 (2001): 819–27.

Bonkovsky, H. L., R. W. Lambrecht, and Y. Shan. "Iron as a Co-morbid Factor in Nonhemochromatotic Liver Disease." *Alcohol* 30 (2003): 137–44.

Bradai, M., M. T. Abad, S. Pissard, F. Lamraoui, L. Skopinski, and M. de Montaiembert. "Hydroxyurea Can Eliminate Transfusion Requirements in Children with Severe ß-Thalassemia." *Blood* 102 (2003): 1529–30.

Brandhagen, D. J., V. F. Fairbanks, and W. Baldus. "Recognition and Management of Hereditary Hemochromatosis." *American Academy of Family Physicians* 65 (2002): 853–66.

Breidbach, T., S. Scory, R. L. Krauth-Siegel, and D. Steverding. "Growth Inhibition of Bloodstream Forms of Trypanosoma Brucei by the Iron Chelator Deferoxamine." *International Journal of Parasitology* 32 (2002): 473–79.

Britton, R. S., K. L. Leicester, and B. R. Bacon. "Iron Toxicity and Chelation Therapy." *International Journal of Hematology* 76 (2002): 219–28.

Cario, H., M. Wegener, K. M. Debatin, and E. Kohne. "Treatment with Hydroxyurea in Thalassemia Intermedia with Paravertebral Pseudotumors of Extramedullary Hematopoiesis." *Annals of Hematology* 81 (2002): 478–82.

Chapoutot, C., P. Perney, D. Fabre, P. Taourel, J. M. Bruel, D. Larrey, J. Domergue, A. J. Ciurana, and F. Blanc. "Needle-tract Seeding after Ultrasound-guided Puncture of Hepatocellular Carcinoma: A Study of 150 Patients." *Gastroenterology Clinical Biology* 23 (1999): 552–56.

Chitambar, C. R., and J. P. Wereley. "Expression of the Hemochromatosis (*HFE*) Gene Modulates the Cellular Uptake of Gallium." *Journal of Nuclear Medicine* 44 (2003): 943–46.

Cohen, A. R., P. Galanello, A. Piga, V. DeSanctis, and F. Tricta. "Safety and Effectiveness of Long Term Therapy with the Oral Iron Chelator Deferiprone." *Blood* 102 (2003): 1583-1587.

de Valk, B., and J. J. M. Marx. "Iron, Atherosclerosis, and Ischemic Heart Disease." *Archives of Internal Medicine* 159 (1999): 1542–48.

Duffy, S., E. S. Biegelson, M. Holbrook, J. D. Russell, N. Gokee, J. F. Keany Jr., and J. A. Vita. "Iron Chelation Improves Endothelial Function in Patients with Coronary Artery Disease." *Circulation* 103 (2001): 2799–2804.

Elmberg, M., R. Hultcrantz, A. Ekbom, L. Brandt, S. Olsson, R. Olsson, S. Lindgren, L. Loof, P. Stal, S. Wallerstedt, S. Almer,

H. Sandberg-Gertzen, and J. Askling. "Cancer Risk in Patients with Hereditary Hemochromatosis and in Their First-degree Relatives." *Gastroenterology* 125 (2003): 1733–41.

Facchini, F. S., N. W. Hua, and R. A. Stoohs. "Effect of Iron Depletion in Carbohydrate-intolerant Patients with Clinical Evidence of Nonalcoholic Fatty Liver Disease." *Gastroenterology* 122 (2002): 931–39.

Fleming, D. J., K. L. Tucker, P. F. Jacques, G. E. Dallal, P. W. Wilson, and R. J. Wood. "Dietary Factors Associated with the Risk of High Iron Stores in the Elderly Framingham Heart Study Cohort." *American Journal of Clinical Nutrition* 76 (2002): 1375–84.

Fridlender, Z. G., and D. Rund. "Myocardial Infarction in a Patient with Beta-thalassemia Major: First Report." *American Journal of Hematology* 75: (2004): 52–55.

Galhenage, S. P., C. H. Viiala, and J. K. Olynyk. "Screening for Hemochromatosis: Patients with Liver Disease, Families, and Populations." *Current Gastroenterology Reports* 6 (2004): 44–51.

Ganz, T. "Hepcidin, a Key Regulator of Iron Metabolism and Mediator of Anemia of Inflammation." *Blood* 102 (2003): 783–88.

Garrison, C., ed. *The Iron Disorders Institute Guide to Hemochromatosis.* Nashville, TN: Cumberland House, 2001.

———. *The Iron Disorders Institute Guide to Anemia.* Nashville, TN: Cumberland House, 2003.

Hausse, A. O., Y. Aggoun, D. Bonnet, D. Sidi, A. Munnich, A. Rotig, and P. Rustin. "Idebenone and Reduced Cardiac Hypertrophy in Friedreich's Ataxia." *Heart* 87 (2002): 346–49.

Harrison, S. A., and B. R. Bacon. "Hereditary Hemochromatosis: Update for 2003." *Journal of Hepatology* 38 (2003): 14–23.

Hoffbrand, A. V., A. Cohen, and C. Hershko. "Role of Deferiprone Therapy for Transfusional Iron Overload." *Blood* 102 (2003): 117–24.

Hsiao, T. J., J. C. Chen, and J. D. Wang. "Insulin Resistance and Ferritin as Major Determinants of Nonalcoholic Fatty Liver Disease in Apparently Healthy Obese Patients." *International Journal of Obesity Related Metabolism Disorders* 28 (2004): 167–72.

Jones, M. M., P. K. Singh, J. E. Lane, R. R. Rodrigues, A. Nesset, C. C. Suarez, B. J. Bogitsh, C. E. Carter. "Inhibition of Trypanosoma Cruzi Epimastigotes in Vitro by Iron Chelating Agents." *Arzneim-Forsch/Drug Research* 46 (1996): 1158–62.

Kassab-Chekir, A., S. Laradi, S. Ferchichi, A. Haj Khelil, M. Feki,

F. Amri, H. Selmi, M. Bejaoui, and A. Miled. "Oxidant, Antioxidant Status and Metabolic Data in Patients with Beta-thalassemia." *Clinica Chimica Acta* 338 (2003): 79–86.

Kicic, A., A. C. G. Chua, and E. Baker. "Desferrithiocin Is a More Potent Antineoplastic Agent Than Desferrioxamine." *British Journal of Pharmacology* 135 (2002): 1393–1402.

Kontoghiorghes, G. J., K. Neocleous, and A. Kolnagou. "Benefits and Risk of Deferiprone in Iron Overload in Thalassemia and Other Conditions." *Drug Safety* 26 (2003): 1557–92.

Lang, F., K. S. Lang, T. Wieder, S. Myssina, C. Birka, P. A. Lang, S. Kaiser, D. Kempe, C. Duranton, and S. M. Huber. "Cation Channels, Cell Volume and the Death of an Erythrocyte." *Pflugers Archives* 447 (2003): 121–25.

Leitman, S. F., J. N. Browning, Y. Y. Yau, G. Mason, H. G. Klein, C. Conry-Cantilena, and C. D. Bolan. "Hemochromatosis Subjects as Allogeneic Blood Donors: A Prospective Study." *Transfusion* 43 (2003): 1538–44.

Lessyer, R., R. I. Ward, R. R. Crichton, and J. R. Boelaert. "Effect of Chloroquine Administration on Iron Loading in the Liver and Reticuloendothelial System and on Oxidative Responses by Alveolar Macrophages." *Biochemical Pharmacology* 57 (1999): 907–11.

Li, H. Y., and Z. M. Qian. "Transferrin/Transferrin Receptor-Mediated Drug Delivery." *Medicinal Research Reviews* 22 (2002): 225–50.

Lieber, C. S. "Biochemical and Molecular Basis of Alcohol-induced Injury to Liver and Other Tissues." *New England Journal of Medicine* (1988) 319: 1639–50.

Malecki, E. A., and J. R. Connor. "The Case for Iron Chelation and/or Antioxidant Therapy in Alzheimer's Disease." *Drug Development Research* 56 (2002): 526–30.

Matthews, A. J., G. M. Vercellotti, H. J. Menchaca, P. H. S. Bloch, V. N. I. Michalek, P. H. Marker, J. Murar, and H. Buchwald. "Iron and Atherosclerosis: Inhibition by the Iron Chelator Deferiprone." *Journal of Surgical Research* 73 (1997): 35–40.

McDonnell, S. M., B. L. Preston, S. A. Jewell, J. C. Barton, C. Q. Edwards, P. C. Adams, and R. A. Yip. "Survey of 2,851 Patients with Hemochromatosis Symptoms and Response to Treatment." *American Journal of Medicine* 106 (1999): 619–24.

Morris, C. R., E. P. Vichinsky, J. van Warmerdam, L. Machado, D. Kepka-Lenhart, S. M. Morris Jr, and F. A. Kuypers.

"Hydroxyurea and Arginine Therapy: Impact on Nitric Oxide Production in Sickle Cell Disease." *Journal of Pediatric Hematology & Oncology* 25 (2003): 629–34.

Morrison, E. D., D. J. Brandhagen, P. D. Phatak, J. C. Barton, E. L. Krawitt, H. B. El-Serag, S. C. Gordon, M. V. Galan, B. Y. Tung, G. N. Ioannou, and K. V. Kowdley. "Serum Ferritin Level Predicts Advanced Hepatic Fibrosis among U.S. Patients with Phenotypic Hemochromatosis." *Annals of Internal Medicine* 138 (2003): 627–33.

Muretto, P., E. Angelucci, and G. Lucarelli. "Reversibility of Cirrhosis in Patients Cured of Thalassemia by Bone Marrow Transplantation." *Annals of Internal Medicine* 136 (2002): 667–72.

Niederau, C. "Hereditary Hemochromatosis." *Internist* 44 (2003): 191–205.

Nisbet-Brown, E., N. F. Olivieri, P. J. Giardina, R. W. Grandy, E. J. Heufeld, R. Sechaud, A. J. Krebs-Brown, J. R. Anderson, D. Albert, K. C. Sizer, and D. G. Nathan. "Effectiveness and Safety of ICL670 in Iron-loaded Patients with Thalassemia: A Randomized, Double-blind, Placebo-controlled, Dose-escalation Trial." *The Lancet* 361 (2003): 1597–1602.

Nittis, T., and J. D. Gitlin. "The Copper Iron Connection: Hereditary Aceruloplasminemia." *Seminars in Hematology* 39 (2002): 282–89.

Pennell, D. J. "Cardiovascular Magnetic Resonance: Twenty-first Century Solutions in Cardiology." *Clinical Medicine* 3 (2003): 273–78.

Phatak, P. D., and J. C. Barton. "Phlebotomy-mobilized Iron as a Surrogate for Liver Iron Content in Hemochromatosis Patients." *Hematology* 8 (2003): 429–32.

Pietrangelo, A. "EASL International Consensus: Conference on Haemochromatosis." *Journal of Hepatology* 33 (2000): 485–504.

Piga, A., C. Gaglioti, E. Fogliacco, and F. Tricta. "Comparative Effects of Deferiprone and Deferoxamine on Survival and Cardiac Disease in Patients with Thalassemia Major." *Haematologia* 88 (2003): 489–96.

Raiola, G., M. C. Galati, V. De Sanctis, M. Caruso Nicoletti, C. Pintor, M. De Simone, V. M. Arcuri, and S. Anastasi. "Growth and Puberty in Thalassemia Major." *Journal of Pediatric Endocrinology Metabolism* 16, suppl. 2 (2003): 259–66.

Richardson, D. R. "Potential of Iron Chelators as Effective Antiproliferative Agents." *Canadian Journal of Physiology & Pharmacology* 75 (1997): 1164–80.

Sattar, N., D. C. Scott, D. McMillan, D. Talwar, S. J. O'Reilly, J. G. S. Fell. "Acute Phase Reactants and Plasma Trace Element Concentrations in Non-small Cell Lung Cancer Patients and Controls." *Nutrition & Cancer* 28 (1997): 308–12.

Shedlofsky, S. I. "Does Iron Reduction Improve Sustained Viral Responses to Interferon Monotherapy in Hepatitis C Patients?" *American Journal of Gastroenterology* 97 (2002): 1093–95.

Silber, M. H., and J. W. Richardson. "Multiple Blood Donations Associated with Iron Deficiency in Patients with Restless Legs Syndrome." *Mayo Clinic Procedures* 78 (2003): 52–54.

Simonart, T., J. R. Boelaert, R. Mosselmans, G. Andrei, J. C. Noel, E. De Clercq, and R. Snoeck. "Anti-proliferative and Apoptotic Effects of Iron Chelators on Human Cervical Carcinoma Cells." *Gynecology Oncology* 85 (2002): 95–102.

Simsek, S., P. W. B. Nanayakkara, J. M. F. Keek, L. M. Fber, K. F. Bruin, and G. Pals. "Two Dutch Families with Hereditary Hyperferritinaemia-cataract Syndrome and Heterozygosity for an *HFE* Related Haemochromatosis Gene Mutation." *Netherlands Journal of Medicine* 61 (2003): 291–95.

Skikne, B. S., N. Ahluwalia, B. Fergusson, A. Chomko, and J. D. Cook. "Effects of Erythropoietin Therapy on Iron Absorption in Chronic Renal Failure." *Journal of Laboratory Clinical Medicine* 135 (2000): 452–58.

Sullivan, J. L. "Blood Donation May Be Good for the Donor." *Vox Sang* 61 (1991): 161–64.

Vichinsky, E. "Current Issues with Blood Transfusions in Sickle Cell Disease." *Seminars in Hematology* 38 (2001): 14–22.

Weilbach, F. X., A. Chan, K. V. Yoyka, and R. Gold. "The Cardioprotector Dexrazoxane Augments Therapeutic Efficacy of Mitoxantrone in Experimental Autoimmune Encephalomyelitis." *Clinical Experimental Immunology* 135 (2004): 49–55.

Weinberg, E. D. "Development of Clinical Methods of Iron Deprivation for Suppression of Neoplastic and Infectious Diseases." *Cancer Investigations* 17 (1999): 507–13.

———. "Therapeutic Potential of Human Transferrin and Lactoferrin." *American Society of Microbiology News* 68 (2002): 65–69.

———. "Iron Chelation in Chemotherapy." *Advances in Applied Microbiology* 52 (2003): 187–208.

Weinberg, G. A. "Iron Chelators as Therapeutic Agents Against

Pneumocystis." *Antimicrob Agents Chemotherapy* 38 (1994): 997–1003.

Westwood, M. A., L. J. Anderson, D. N. Firmin, P. D. Gatehouse, C. H. Lorenz, B. Wonke, and D. J. Pennell. "Interscanner Reproducibility of Cardiovascular Magnetic Resonance T2* Measurements of Tissue Iron in Thalassemia." *Journal of Magnetic Resonance Imaging* 18 (2003): 616–20.

Witte, D., W. Crosby, C. Edwards, V. Fairbanks, and F. Mitros. "Hereditary Hemochromatosis." *Clinica Chimica Acta* 245 (1996): 139–200.

18

Prevention of Excess Body Iron

"Iron overload is not benign. Often undiagnosed, it has been associated with a slew of chronic disorders. These include heart disease, diabetes, arthritis, and liver failure."

—G. D. Vogin and J. S. MacNeil

It is estimated that one-third of our population has some type of iron disorder—anemia, iron overload, or iron overload with anemia. Some of these disorders are complicated and more difficult to manage. But in the majority of these conditions, excessive tissue iron can be managed and even prevented when the same consideration is given to the potential of iron excesses as iron deficiencies.

A considerable variety of methods for prevention and reduction of the iron hazard now are available. The most obvious methods are those concerned with prevention of iron loading via the routes into our bodies of ingestion, injection (including blood transfusion), and inhalation. In each category of iron acquisition, ingestion, injection, and inhalation, the diminution of iron is achieved by various strategies.

Ingestion: dietary iron

When working properly, humans have a natural iron regulatory mechanism that assures adequate amounts of iron are absorbed from the diet. This mechanism has been observed in menstruating or pregnant females who absorb up to 50 percent more iron during the days of menstruation than when not menstruating. We can override this mechanism by consuming excessive amounts of heme primarily contained in red meat and excessive amounts of sugar, fats, iron-fortified foods, alcohol, and vitamin C. These foods and substances enhance the absorption of iron because they increase the bioavailability of the metal. Other foods or substances such as phytate, polyphenols (tannins in coffee and tea), calcium, eggs, and soy protein reduce the bioavailability of iron. According to Dr. Janet Hunt, Agricultural Research Team, Grand Forks Human Nutrition Research Center, "Iron absorption from food can vary up to tenfold depending on the bioavailability of iron."

". . . intakes of highly bioavailable forms of iron (supplemental iron and red meat) and of fruit, a dietary source of an enhancer of nonheme-iron absorption (vitamin C), promote high iron stores, whereas foods containing phytate (whole grains) decrease these stores. Individual dietary patterns may be important modulators of high iron stores."

—D. J. Fleming et al.

Humans consume heme and nonheme iron

Heme iron: Derived from organic sources such as the blood proteins hemoglobin and myoglobin contained in meat, this type of iron is in a form more easily absorbed by the body.

Nonheme iron: The majority of dietary iron is inorganic or nonheme iron. This type of iron is derived from grains, nuts, fruits, vegetables, fortificants, or contaminant iron from sources such as water, soil, and cooking utensils.

Absorption of heme and nonheme or plant-based iron can be increased or decreased depending upon substances or foods eaten. Heme iron, especially in red meat, is easily absorbed because it is in a form that is highly bioavailable to the body. Investigators of the Framingham Heart Study found that persons who consumed more than four servings of red meat per week had a threefold increase in iron stores than those who consumed four or fewer servings of red meat per week.

Red meats have a greater proportion of heme iron than do light meats. The proportion of heme varies from 50–80 percent in cooked red meats and from 25–40 percent in cooked light

IRON	per 3.2 oz serving MEAT		
	total iron MILLIGRAMS	heme iron percentage of total iron	heme iron MILLIGRAMS
VENISON	4.5	51	2.3
LAMB	3.1	55	1.7
BEEF			
RUMP STEAK	2.9	52	1.5
SIRLOIN STEAK	2.5	52	1.3
ROUND STEAK	3.2	50	1.6
TOP ROUND	2.5	48	1.2
GROUND	2.5	40	1.0
BRISKET	2.0	25	0.5
VEAL	1.9	40*	0.7*
PORK	1.3	23	0.3
PROCESSED MEATS			
SAUSAGE (VEAL)	0.7	40*	0.2*
BOILED HAM	0.7	40*	0.2*
LIVER PATE	5.0	16	0.8
CHICKEN	0.6	40*	0.2*
FISH			
COD	0.2	0.0	0.0
MACKEREL	0.7	0.0	0.0
SALMON	0.6	17	0.1
MUSSELS	4.6	48	2.2
LOBSTER	1.6	40*	0.6*
SHRIMP	2.6	40*	1.0*

* resources vary

Source. Iron Disorders Institute, 2004

meats (chicken, pork, or turkey). In addition to heme, meat also contains animal fats, which improve the absorption of non-heme iron. It has been calculated that 1 gram of meat (about 20 percent protein) has an enhancing effect on nonheme iron absorption equivalent to that of 1 milligram of ascorbic acid. A Latin American–type meal (maize, rice, and black beans) with a low iron bioavailability had the same improved bioavailability when either 75 grams of meat or 50 milligrams of ascorbic acid were added.

Both heme and nonheme iron absorption can be impaired by calcium, but the amount or form of calcium (dietary or supplemental) is still debated. Some investigators report that small amounts of calcium contained in a slice of cheese, for example, will not significantly impair heme absorption. Others provide that initally supplemental calcium will inhibit iron absorption, but over time, the body will adjust and increase absorption of iron to compensate. Another group of investigators found that when calcium is consumed in combination with bread, it will diminish iron bioavailabity. It is known that a single 3000-mg dose of calcium significantly impairs absorption of iron.

Vitamin C

Vitamin C (ascorbic acid) increases the intestinal absorption of nonheme iron. Cases of iron overload due to excessive and chronic ingestion of vitamin C have been reported. Vitamin C is an excellent antioxidant, but it can also work as a prooxidant. Pharmalogical doses of iron associated with high vitamin C intakes can result in uncontrolled lipid peroxidation. Patients with iron-loading conditions should not avoid vitamin C; they can modify the way in which they obtain this nutrient. The amounts of the vitamin contained in fresh fruits and vegetables, for example, are consistent with good health. When consumed along with an inhibiting substance, such as tannin in tea for example, studies suggest that greater than or equal to 50 mg ascorbic acid would be required to overcome the inhibitory effects on iron absorption of any meal containing greater than 100 mg tannic acid. However, if vitamin C supplements are to be employed, single doses should be 200 mg or less and the total kept under 500 mg/day and taken separately from meals.

Sugar

Researchers investigated the absorption rates of seven different beverages that contained sugar and were fortified with iron. They found that sugar improved the absorption of iron by as much as

4 times in some cases. Since this study, others have determined that the risk of high iron stores in the subjects who consumed more than 21 servings of fruit or fruit juice/wk was threefold higher than the subjects who consumed 14 servings/wk.

Alcohol

Twenty to 30 percent of chronic alcoholics have increased iron absorption. Alcohol can elevate intestinal iron absorption, possibly by increasing stomach acid secretion. Alcohol in moderation can be consumed safely provided that the person is in good iron balance. Those patients with liver abnormalities or other evidence of iron loading should cease all alcohol consumption.

A standard drink is defined as 13.5 grams of alcohol: 12 oz beer, 5 oz wine, or 1.5 oz distilled spirits. Moderate consumption is defined as two drinks per day for an adult male; one drink per day for females or those older than 65, regardless of gender. Options to consider might be nonalcoholic or low-alcohol content beer and wine. Though red wine is reported to be healthy for the heart, it is likely the polyphenol content in red wine that is providing the greater benefit. Except for the sedating quality of alcohol, a handful of red grapes will provide equal, if not greater, health benefit.

Beta-carotene: In studies of vitamin A, beta-carotene, and iron absorption, vitamin A did not significantly increase iron uptake under the experimental conditions employed. However, beta-carotene (6 micromol/L) significantly increased iron uptake compared to no beta-carotene addition. Moreover, in the presence of phytates or tannic acid, beta-carotene generally overcame the inhibitory effects of both compounds, depending on their concentrations.

Fortification

Fortification of processed foods with iron began in 1941; folic acid was added more recently. Many scientists, physicians, and the general public have assumed, without evidence, that fortification is harmless. But in recent years much evidence has accumulated that indicates that fortification can potentially cause more harm than good, especially in well-nourished countries.

247

Moreover, a team at the US Food and Drug Administration headed by Dr. Paul Whittaker assayed the actual levels of iron and folic acid in 29 breakfast cereals. They found that the actual level of iron in a realistic single serving was as much as 380 percent higher than the label declaration. Folate levels similarly were inflated.

The authors noted that because iron is a significant risk factor for heart disease and several types of cancer, it would be helpful to have available additional cereals without iron fortification. They noted also that high levels of folic acid can mask a deficiency of vitamin B_{12}, a serious matter, especially among the aging or vegetarian population.

Indeed for individuals with undiagnosed genetic hemochromatosis, the fortification may be exacerbating iron levels and contributing to the potential for chronic disease. Iron deficiency still remains a serious health matter, especially in third world countries. Therefore it seems reasonable for companies to continue to fortify foods with iron intended for distribution in third world countries.

Even in light of what is known about the potential for iron overload, food manufacturers continue the formulation of super additive iron compounds such as EDTA+Fe and Ferrochel™ to address iron deficiency. These super compounds exceed absorption capabilities of the commonly used fortificant ferrous sulfate.

Ferrochel is an iron bis-glycine chelate. Two molecules of glycine ("bis" meaning two), a nonessential amino acid, are combined with one atom of iron. Albion Laboratories, Salt Lake City, Utah, owns the patent rights to produce this type of chelate, which is much more effective at delivering a highly bioavailable form of iron than ferrous sulfate.

EDTA+Fe is a chelate of iron and EDTA (ethylenediamine-tetra-acetic acid). It, too, performed well in the same absorption studies. Both EDTA and bis-glycine chelated iron were absorbed at the rate of 2–3 times that of ferrous sulfate. When combined with phytase, the enzyme that breaks down phytates in fiber, Ferrochel and EDTA increased the bioavailability of iron even more.

Genetic modification of foods

Earlier, we noted that heme iron is more readily absorbed into the bloodstream than nonheme iron. In the past few years, successful attempts have been made to increase the absorbency of nonheme iron by genetically altering such plant staples as rice.

Genetically modified rice that compels the plant to incorporate in its seeds a two- to threefold increased iron content was described by two research groups in 1999. In the first report, compared with the normal iron content of rice seeds of 11 micrograms iron/gram, the transgenic seeds accumulate up to 38 micrograms iron per gram. In the second investigation, the content of iron was doubled in the modified rice seeds. Most alarmingly, a gene for a heat-resistant phytase enzyme also was introduced. The phytase destroys phytic acid, a plant iron-trapping compound that functions to prevent humans and animals from overabsorbing nonheme iron. In addition, a gene for a cysteine-rich protein was inserted in the rice; this protein enhances iron absorption!

The investigators in the two research groups noted that iron deficiency can be a serious problem when vegetable-based diets are the primary food source. They sincerely believe that iron-enriched rice could provide improved nutrition to many persons, especially in developing countries. Sadly, they expressed no concern that their genetically modified products could be a serious health hazard to large numbers of humans who have thalassemia, African siderosis, hemochromatosis, or other conditions of iron overload.

Companies who produce such products should consider labelling the packages in large print in appropriate languages: *Use of this product may be dangerous to persons with iron-loading conditions.*

Oral iron supplements

For persons with normal iron metabolism the body attempts to suppress the amount of iron gotten from oral supplements. Researchers at the USDA Grand Forks Human Nutrition Research Center conducted a study of the effects of iron supplements on the body's control of iron absorption. In a randomized, placebo-controlled trial, heme and nonheme iron absorption by healthy men and women were measured from a test meal containing a hamburger, potatoes, and milkshake. These absorption measurements were made before and after a period of 12 weeks when the 57 participants were given 50 mg of supplemental iron or placebo daily while they consumed their usual diets.

Serum ferritin and fecal ferritin were measured during supplementation and for a period of 6 months after supplementation was discontinued. Volunteers who took iron supplements— even those with initial ferritin less than 21 ng/mL—adapted to absorb less nonheme iron, but not less heme iron from meat.

Daily iron supplements caused these volunteers to absorb 36 percent less nonheme iron and 25 percent less total iron from food, and to have higher iron stores than those in the placebo group. The higher ferritin persisted for six months post supplementation, except in individuals who had low iron stores at the beginning of the study. Since iron stores were greater after iron supplementation, this study demonstrated that adaptation in absorption did not completely prevent accumulation of excessive iron.

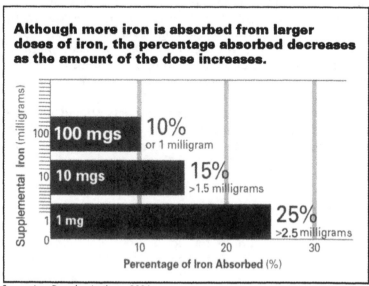

Although more iron is absorbed from larger doses of iron, the percentage absorbed decreases as the amount of the dose increases.

Source. Iron Disorders Institute, 2004

The adaptation to reduce iron absorption even in volunteers with low iron stores may indicate a localized control system to prevent excessive iron exposure of intestinal cells. The study is consistent with two systems at work, one that regulates how much iron we must absorb for normal function, and the iron withholding defense system, which protects us from nurturing harmful pathogens with excesses of iron we don't presently need.

Yet in a recent US survey of 411 men and 605 women between 67 and 96 years of age who took supplemental iron, 23 percent had highly elevated iron deposits (serum Ft >300 ng/mL in men and >200 ng/mL in women). An additional 44 percent of men (serum Ft 100–300 ng/mL) and 29 percent of women (serum Ft 100-200 ng/mL) were mildly iron elevated. The authors noted that "the use of unprescribed iron supplements in free-living elderly white Americans is probably unnecessary and could be detrimental given the reported association between elevated iron stores and the risk of some chronic diseases."

In a study of iron-supplemented infants compared to non-supplemented, the infants who received the supplemental iron had significantly lower plasma retinol concentrations and a significantly higher prevalence of vitamin A deficiency, as defined by a plasma retinol concentration <0.70 micromol/L, than did the nonsupplemented infants. In contrast, the modified relative dose response of the iron-supplemented infants indicated greater liver stores of vitamin A.

In yet another study, pregnant females given modest amounts of supplemental iron experienced zinc deficiencies. These and other findings call into question the practice of routinely recommending supplemental iron for pregnant women.

Pregnancy and iron needs*

In a British study of 12 pregnant women, iron absorbed from a normal diet was increased fivefold at 24 weeks of gestation and ninefold at 36 weeks, as compared with the amount absorbed at the seventh week during the pregnancy.

For many decades, a large number of pregnant women have been advised to routinely take iron supplements, some-

*From The Iron Disorders Institute Guide to Anemia, reprinted with permission

times as frequently as 3 times daily, even without laboratory evidence of subnormal hemoglobin values. The routine procedure, even though it may be unnecessary, often is considered to be harmless and to have some unknown benefit. However, in 1993 a US Prevention Service Task Force of the Office of Disease Prevention and Health Promotion, US Public Health Service, carefully reviewed 50 published studies about iron supplementation. The task force concluded that controlled trials have failed to demonstrate that iron supplementation or changes in hematologic indexes actually improve clinical outcome for the mother or newborn. Additionally, the review found "no evidence that giving iron during pregnancy will reduce the incidence of childhood anemia or abnormal cognitive development."

There is agreement, however, that pregnant women who have subnormal hematologic values of 11.0 g/dL or less and are iron deficient should take supplemental iron. The American Academy of Family Physicians and the Institutes of Medicine recommend that pregnant females have serum ferritin measured along with hemoglobin values to assure that moderately low normal hemoglobin values are in fact due to iron deficiency and not due to an undetected illness. Iron supplementation during this time is best monitored by a physician and discontinued once anemia is corrected.

A few studies have examined the possibility that high as well as low hemoglobin values might be detrimental to the mother or fetus. In Wales, a study of 54,000 pregnancies found that prenatal mortality, low birthweight, and preterm birth were more common in women with hemoglobin values either less than 10.4 g/dL or greater than 13.2 g/dL than in women who had hemoglobin within the range of 10.5–13.1 g/dL. Similarly, in the United States, a study of 22,000 pregnancies found that incidence of perinatal mortality was as much as twofold higher in women with hemoglobin values of 8 g/dL, and up to fivefold higher in women with hemoglobin values of 14 g/dL, than women with hemoglobin ranges of 9–13 g/dL. In the same study, incidence of low birthweight and neonatal prematurity were greater in women whose hemoglobin were less than 8 g/dL or higher than 14 g/dL.

In a *Journal of the American Medical Association* article entitled "Maternal Hemoglobin Concentration During Pregnancy and Risk of Stillbirth," Dr. Olof Stephansson and his colleagues report that stillbirths nearly doubled in women whose hemoglobin values were 14.5 g/dL or higher. The report went on to state that anemia, or hemoglobin values less than 11.0 g/dL, was not significantly associated with risk of stillbirth. It should be noted that hemoglobin will be elevated in women who are dehydrated or who smoke.

Iron is a known prooxidant. Females with increased transferrin saturation and decreased unsaturated iron-binding capacity are at increased risk for preeclampsia due to oxidative stress, which decreases serum antioxidant that would normally protect against redox-active iron.

Supplemental iron for expectant mothers with normal iron metabolism does not significantly affect hemoglobin values for her or for the fetus. In these women, iron that the body does not absorb will be excreted. What is absorbed and not used will be placed in ferritin.

To assure iron balance, females, even those who are pregnant or nursing, whose hemoglobin and ferritin levels are within normal range are not candidates for iron supplements.

Lactating and nursing females

A well-established belief is that another time of high iron demand for females is during lactation. Though lactating females can be iron deficient, the cause is probably due to blood loss as a result of childbirth, and not necessarily because they need extra iron to nourish a newborn. Another reason for iron deficiency during lactation is that during the third trimester the mother sends a large quantity of iron to her developing offspring. If her diet is iron-poor at this time, she will experience iron-deficiency anemia. Lactating mothers indeed require extra calories and adequate fluids to enable them to produce milk, but it is not necessarily true that they need supplemental iron. Nor is it true that supplemental iron taken by the mother will have an effect on her milk. Studies of breast milk of females with hemochromatosis or other iron overload diseases indicate that the excess iron stored in the tissues did not have an effect

253

on the iron levels in the breast milk, suggesting that there is a complex iron regulatory system to assure that the proper balance of iron gets into human milk.

Unless a new mother's hemoglobin values are below 11.0 g/dL, an iron-rich diet which includes lean red meat, fresh fruits and vegetables, which are rich in vitamin C and beta-carotene, will likely provide sufficient amounts of iron for her and her newborn. For women who cannot afford meat, such as those who live in developing countries or come from low-income families, iron-fortified foods and supplemental iron may be essential. Conversely, healthy females who can afford meat and who consume adequate amounts, along with other iron-rich foods, should not experience iron-deficiency anemia. A health care provider can monitor hemoglobin values and diet to assure that the right balance of iron is maintained.

Accidental iron poisoning

A known danger of routine supplemental iron is that of pediatric iron poisoning, usually in toddlers 1–2 years of age. Ingestion of as little as 15 30-mg iron tablets may be lethal. Iron supplements were the single most frequent cause of pediatric unintentional ingestion fatalities, accounting for 30.2 percent of such fatalities reported over an 8-year period. As of 2000, iron overdose remains a significant public health threat to young children. The frequency of pediatric iron overdose injuries increased in 1986 and has not declined. Safety cap or unit-dose packaging of iron supplements should be used when iron supplementation is established as appropriate for an expectant mother. Parents should take any child they suspect has ingested more than a single dose of iron pills to the emergency room immediately.

Iron doping

Ingrained in our culture is the notion that iron cures fatigue and enhances endurance. To assure sufficient stamina and energy, some athletes will take iron supplements, thinking that the added iron will be beneficial to performance.

Ferritin determinations in 1998 on 249 French elite road cyclists revealed that 83 had levels between 306 and 1671 ng/mL; the median was 504 ng/mL. Their transferrin iron saturation percentage ranged from 20–76 percent with a median of 39 percent. Eighty-nine percent of the cyclists had taken iron supplements. The greater the amount of supplements, the higher were the body iron burdens. The authors stated that the possibility that this strong association might have occurred by chance was less than 1 in 500. Not surprisingly, they noted also that the elevated iron values persisted after the cyclists ceased to take the iron supplements. It has been known for many decades that humans cannot excrete body iron deposits.

The authors of the cyclist study emphasized that "even when mild, iron excess may expose to long-term complications and should be removed at least at the time when professional cyclists retire. To prevent iatrogenic (i.e., induced by health professionals) iron overload, supplementation with iron must be done according to serum ferritin follow-up."

Many investigations in animal models have confirmed the potential danger of excessive dietary iron. A recent study exemplifies these types of enquiries. Chronic ulcerative colitis in mice and its subsequent carcinogenesis was significantly increased by elevated dietary iron. In 16 animals fed high iron, colorectal tumor incidence occurred in 88 percent. In 16 fed adequate iron for good health, tumor incidence was 19 percent.

Excessive oral iron can contribute to colorectal cancer. When iron is ingested in large doses, the amounts not absorbed by the body are excreted in feces. This iron sits, however, for a period of time in the colon, providing ample nourishment for harmful pathogens, including cancer cells.

"It is likely that as many people are being injured by iron supplementation as are receiving medical benefit from it. Those individuals who are particularly at risk are the top 5 percent of US vitamin users who may be taking up to five times the daily allowance for iron . . . iron doping of healthy individuals to improve performance may well have dire health consequences not less severe than anabolic steroids."

—R. L. Nelson

Lowering the bioavailability of iron

Besides reducing the amount of food items that enhance the bioavailability of iron, one can consume foods and substances that inhibit the absorption of iron.

Certain foods or food products inhibit the absorption of dietary iron. The most easily inhibited form is nonheme iron. Among the most prominent, effective products are phytate, tannins in tea and coffee, oxalates, and various polyphenols and calcium. Eggs also inhibit the absorption of nonheme iron. The component in eggs that impairs absorption of iron is not known, though its inhibiting factor has been established in several separate studies. One boiled egg can reduce absorption of iron in a meal by as much as 28 percent. Previously, it was believed that nothing could impair the absorption of heme iron. Investigators in Europe and the United States have reported that calcium, especially when taken in the form of supplements, can inhibit heme as well as nonheme iron.

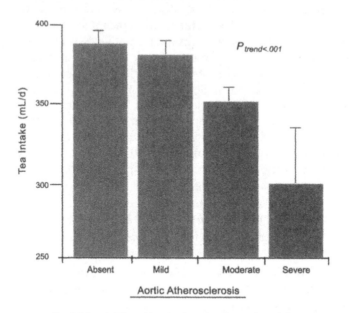

Tea intake at different levels of aortic atherosclerosis in a general population of 3,454 older men and women. The tea intake measurements of 250-400 (mL/d) are equivalent to about 2-3 cups per day.

Source: J M Geleijnse et al
Adapted with permission

256

Tannins are natural iron-trapping products contained in green and black teas. These phenolic compounds have a strong affinity for nonheme iron and thus are especially useful in preventing absorption of iron that has been indiscriminately added to processed foods. An example of the powerful protection against disease provided by iron chelators in teas is the report of 3454 women and men above 55 years of age who were free of cardiovascular disease and then were observed for 3 years for possible development of calcified plaques in abdominal aortas. Those subjects who drank 1–2 cups per day had only half as much chance of developing atherosclerosis as did non–tea drinkers. Consumption of 4 cups per day lowered the risk to one-third as great as those who drank no tea.

Osteoporosis is another example of a chronic disease exacerbated by iron loading. Thus, not surprisingly, habitual consumption of tea has been found to have significant beneficial effects on bone mineral density of the total body, lumbar spine, and hips.

Hemochromatotic patients have been observed to lower dietary iron absorption by about one-third by drinking tea. Likewise, patients with thalassemia markedly reduce their nonheme iron absorption by consuming tea.

DIMINUTION OF INGESTED IRON

Decrease consumption of red meats (heme iron)

Avoidance of iron-adulterated processed foods

Elimination of self-directed consumption of iron supplements

Avoidance of foods that are genetically modified to incorporate more iron

Decreased consumption of alcohol

Decreased consumption of sugar

Decreased consumption of vitamin C

Increased consumption of plant foods high in phytic acid

Increased use of phenolic compounds such as tannin

Use of natural chelators such as lactoferrin in human milk

Source: Iron Disorders Institute, 2004

Phytates are excellent natural chelators of iron. Foods such as bran, corn, beans, and peas are high in phytate. As mentioned earlier, however, super chelated iron additives and genetically modified foods can override the inhibiting qualities of substances such as phytates. These super chelators and genetically modified food products must be avoided by all persons who have any type of iron loading or who tend to load even moderate amounts of iron.

Inositol phosphate-6 (IP6) (phytic acid) is an excellent iron chelator among plant natural products. IP6 is inositol hexaphosphate and so named because of six (hex) phosphates; there are also IP3, 4, and 5, but these forms do not impair iron absorption. In experiments, IP6 inhibited absorption of 40–65 percent of iron in the intestine. IP6 does not remove iron from ferritin and is therefore not an alternative to phlebotomy.

Increased use of natural chelators

Natural products with strong iron-binding ability have long been employed by plants and animals to protect against disease. For example, animals and humans produce a powerful iron-trapping compound called lactoferrin (Lf). It is present in secretions that are constantly exposed to potential pathogens: milk, tears, nasal exudate, saliva, bronchial mucous, gastrointestinal fluids, vaginal mucous, and seminal fluid. Also, lactoferrin is released from circulating white blood cells at body sites of microbial infections and other disease processes. In addition to its antimicrobial power, Lf has anti-viral, anti-cancer, and anti-inflammatory activity.

The very large amount of Lf in breast milk suppresses growth of iron-dependent pathogenic bacteria in the intestine of the nursling. Accordingly, the gut of the breast-fed human infant, in the absence of iron supplements, develops a natural mix of nonpathogenic bacteria that do not require iron. As mentioned in earlier chapters, numerous studies have confirmed the association of iron-dependent bacteria in the gut of infants fed milk formula (which lacks Lf) with an increased risk for infant botulism, salmonellosis, and sudden death.

Both bovine and human recombinant Lf have now become available for possible use in therapy of a variety of infectious

258

INCREASED USE OF NATURAL IRON CHELATORS
Use human milk, which is high in lactoferrin; low in iron
Use tea or coffee at mealtime
Use plant foods high in phytic acid

Source: Iron Disorders Institute, 2004

and inflammatory diseases. As a human natural product, human Lf should have minimal or no side effects. However, it should be used with caution in persons infected with *Helicobacter pylori*, a cause of gastritis and stomach ulcers. This bacterial pathogen can utilize the human lactoferrin-trapped iron for growth. Thus the bacterium might multiply to a greater extent in a person who ingests the Lf protein. In contrast, the pathogen cannot extract iron from bovine lactoferrin.

Diminution of injected iron

Parenteral (nonoral) introduction of iron into the body can be potentially hazardous because physiologic barriers are not in place to regulate absorption. Thus the intramuscular or intravenous injection of iron compounds or of red blood cells should be considered only if laboratory evidence unequivocally indicates erythrocyte deficiency.

DIMINUTION OF PARENTERAL IRON
Inject iron dextran only if unequivocally justified
Transfuse blood or erythrocytes if unequivocally justified
Substitute erythropoietin +minimal iron for blood transfusions when possible

Source: Iron Disorders Institute, 2004

Most importantly, a lifelong log that accurately documents the quantities of injected iron should be maintained for each patient. Note that a single unit of whole blood or of packed red blood cells contains 0.2 gram of iron. Similarly, a single injection of iron dextran contains 0.2 gram iron. As recorded in earlier chapters, deterioration of various organs has begun to become apparent in patients who have been burdened with 10 grams of iron.

Erythropoietin (EPO), a hormone produced by the kidneys, functions to stimulate formation of red blood cells in the bone marrow. In patients who have lost kidney function and who are on dialysis, blood transfusions formerly were required. Fortunately, human recombinant EPO now is available so that blood transfusions can be discontinued. The ability of EPO to stimulate production of red blood cells is dependent on availability of functional iron. Oral administration of iron generally is effective. Neither hemoglobin, hematocrit, nor ferritin values should be allowed to exceed normal limits. Injected iron is less safe than oral iron. For example, in a group of 618 dialysis patients with normal hematocrits, iron dextran was associated with an increased risk of death.

Diminution of Inhaled Iron

In preventing absorption of iron into the bloodstream, respiratory tract defense against the inhaled metal is not as effective as is intestinal tract defense against ingested iron. However, the alveolar (lung) macrophages do attempt to keep the lungs as free of nonprotein bound iron as possible. Also, transferrin in lung epithelial linings is active in trapping iron. Furthermore, during inflammatory episodes, lactoferrin is sent from the

DIMINUTION OF INHALED IRON

Use iron-free chrysotile in place of iron-loaded amosite, crocidolite, tremolite asbestos

Use mask to avoid inhalation of urban air particulates

Use mask and protective clothing when mining, cutting or grinding ferriferous substances

Eliminate use of tobacco, which contains high amounts of iron

Source: Iron Disorders Institute, 2004

blood to the diseased area to increase the scope of iron with-holding defense.

To ensure excellent respiratory tract health, all sources of inhaled iron should be excluded. Clearly, the most common source is tobacco smoke, whether actively or passively inhaled. In theory, were the tobacco plant to be genetically modified so that it contained lower amounts of iron in its leaves, the tobacco product might become quite safe to smoke.

The second most common source of inhaled iron is urban air particulate matter. Other sources are less common but no less hazardous. Recommended to wear masks and protective cloth-ing are iron miners; steel foundry and furnace operators; metal grinders, glazers, and buffers; steel machinists and turners; and asbestos workers. Contaminated clothing should be laundered professionally rather than at home. Persons who scrape iron-loaded tremolite asbestos from surface rocks to use as white-wash for interior and exterior house walls should be warned of the very high possibility that they and members of their fami-lies might develop lung cancers.

Routine blood donation

Reduction of body iron by regular depletion of red blood cells with routine blood donation is another way to reduce the risk of disease. In a study in Italy of 332 blood donors compared with 399 non–blood donors, giving blood was associated with longer life survival, especially between 50 and 70 years of age.

Whole blood contains approximately 0.5 mg iron/mL. Blood loss from normal menstruation of 30–60 mL/month results in excretion of 180–360 mg/yr. The risk of heart disease in women increases significantly after hysterectomy (with or without removal of ovaries) and after natural menopause. As long as women continue to menstruate, protection from heart disease persists, even among those who have high cholesterol. Healthy nonmenstruating women, as well as healthy men, can maintain low body iron burdens by donating blood 2–3 times a year.

Indeed, therapeutic blood-letting was standard medical practice from ancient times until the nineteenth century. It was used by peoples of ancient China and India, aboriginal people of North and South America, and Germanic tribes of Europe.

Blood-letting was described by Homer and Galen and practiced by European physicians for many centuries. Early American practitioners such as Dr. Benjamin Rush were noted for reliance on blood-letting. Its use throughout the world for several millennia suggests that therapeutic bleeding may be effective for a wide variety of diseases.

In patients with hemochromatosis, red blood cell formation is usually normal. Therefore, they generally can be safely de-ironed by a series of phlebotomies. Removal of 200–250 mg iron by each blood-letting is quickly replaced by mobilization of iron from tissue deposits. Folic acid supplements may be useful for catalyzing rapid formation of new red blood cells. Depletion of iron deposits typically requires weekly phlebotomies until the serum ferritin level of 25 ng/mL is attained. At each phlebotomy, the hemoglobin value should be ascertained; the level should be maintained at least at 12.5 g/dL.

REDUCTION OF BODY IRON BURDEN

Donate blood regularly

Avoid premature hysterectomy (if possible)

Ingest baby aspirin daily

Remain compliant with therapeutic phlebotomies for iron overload as in hemochromatosis

Do daily, vigorous exercise

Source: Iron Disorders Institute, 2004

Because iron loading is not stopped by depletion, periodic phlebotomies, often 3–6 per year, must be continued for life. Iron deposits in some body sites are more resistant to mobilization and require prolonged phlebotomy treatment for complete iron removal. With successful de-ironing, lethargy decreases, skin pigmentation clears, liver abnormalities (other than cirrhosis if present) improve, and cardiac symptoms are alleviated.

In the general population, the lowered disease rates achieved with daily ingestion of aspirin also are associated with de-ironing. Gastrointestinal microbleeding caused by the drug results in loss of iron comparable to that of menstrual blood loss. In a recent 3-year study of 1351 coronary disease patients who took a daily aspirin tablet compared with the same number of coronary disease patients who did not, 4 percent of the former and 8 percent of the latter died. That this difference might have occurred at random was stated by the authors to be less than 1 in 1000. Vigorous exercise also results in measurable blood loss through both perspiration and the gastrointestinal tract.

Prevention of saturation of iron withholding defense system by prompt chemotherapy of infections

In patients with AIDS, iron loading is often seen together with occurrence of opportunistic infectious diseases. Opportunistic pathogens include strains of such bacteria as *Hemophilus, Mycobacterium, Salmonella,* and *Streptococcus* and of such fungi and protozoa as *Candida, Cryptococcus, Leishmania,* and *Pneumocystis.* Prompt antibiotic therapy of these opportunistic infections as well, of course, as concurrent anti-viral therapy of AIDS, should delay or suppress this particularly destructive aspect of iron withholding. Patients with AIDS also are advised to stop smoking and, if possible, to eliminate iron supplements and blood transfusions.

> Prevent the saturation of iron withholding defense system by prompt therapy of infections.

Pharmaceutical deprivation of iron: deferoxamine and deferiprone

Iron chelator drugs can, in theory, be useful in either or both of two categories of disease: (a) to continuously de-iron persons who tend to constantly load iron, and (b) to remove iron from specific disease processes in infection, cancer, arthritis, etc. An iron chelator that might be effective in treating infections or cancers need not also be useful or safe in therapy of iron overload. Such a drug would be used for relatively brief periods, whereas an iron chelator for persons who have chronic transfusional iron loading (thalassemia, sicklemia, etc.) would be employed through-out the lifetime of the patient.

Conversely, an iron chelator useful in transfusional iron load-ing might be toxic in a patient who is only slightly iron loaded or whose distribution of excessive iron is confined to a suscep-tible body site of infection, cancer, arthritis, etc.

Iron deprivation of microbial pathogens also can be achieved by development of specific vaccines that contain iron acquisition antigens derived from the germs. The microbes are grown in culture media that contain very little iron. This forces the pathogens to markedly increase formation of their surface antigens that are necessary to bind and take in the metal. Humans and animals vaccinated with such preparations there-fore are stimulated to form antibodies to the specific antigens. The antibodies will prevent subsequent invaders of the same kind from obtaining body iron for growth. It is noteworthy that persons who recover from such specific bacterial infections as meningococcal meningitis promptly begin forming antibodies to the iron acquisition antigens of the pathogen and thereby are resistant to reinfection for many years.

Decreased longevity

In a US representative cohort of 10,714 adults, 2.3 percent had a serum transferrin iron saturation value of more than 55 percent. During a 22-year study, the iron-loaded set had a sig-nificantly greater risk of all-cause mortality (RR 1.6 [95 percent CI 1.17–2.21]). Iron-burdened persons had decreased survival even after controlling for smoking, hypertension, and high cho-lesterol. The authors noted that the iron risk factor for mortality is too often unrecognized in a substantial proportion of adults.

In a 12-year follow-up study of 9229 adults, intakes of dietary iron and red meat were examined. Persons who had elevated transferrin saturation plus high dietary iron (>18 mg/day) had an increased all-cause mortality risk (RR 2.90 [95 percent CI 1.39–6.04]) compared with those with normal trans-ferrin iron saturation and low iron intake. Similarly, elevated transferrin iron saturation plus high red meat consumption (7 times/week) increased risk of death (RR 2.26 [95 percent CI 1.45–3.52]).

Persons with normal transferrin iron saturation values and high dietary iron or high red meat consumption did not show an increased risk in all-cause mortality. Furthermore, persons with elevated iron saturation but normal iron intake had a normal risk of death. The authors proposed that therapy of iron-loaded persons should focus on dietary restrictions instead of or in addition to phlebotomy.

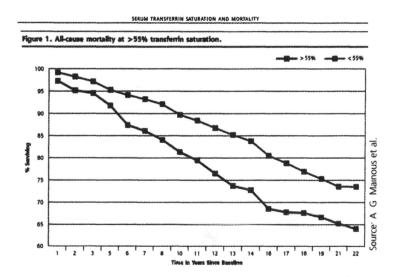

SERUM TRANSFERRIN SATURATION AND MORTALITY

Figure 1. All-cause mortality at >55% transferrin saturation.

These studies reemphasize the necessity of including transferrin saturation values in routine biochemical profiles of adults of all ages, and not least, of the critical need to lower elevated iron as early as possible. Just as persons are urged to use cholesterol-lowering drugs while their cardiovascular system remains intact, so must persons be urged to lower their iron burden while their overall health remains uncompromised.

References:
Barrett, J. F., P. G. Whittaker, J. G. Williams, and T. Lind. "Absorption of Non-Haem Iron from Food during Normal Pregnancy." *British Medical Journal* 309 (1994): 79–82.

Barton, J. C., S. M. McDonnell, P. C. Adams, P. Brissot, L. W. Powell, C. Q. Edwards, J. D. Cook, and K. V. Kowdley. "Management of Hemochromatosis." *Annals of Internal Medicine* 129 (1998): 932–39.

Beard, J., and B. Tobin. "Iron Status and Exercise." *American Journal of Clinical Nutrition* 72 (2001): S594–97.

Bendich, A. "Calcium Supplementation and Iron Status of Females." *Nutrition* 17 (2001): 46–51.

Besarab, A., W. K. Bolton, J. K. Browne, J. C. Egrie, A. R. Nissenson, D. M. Okamoto, S. I. Schwab, and D. A. Goodkin. "The Effects of Normal as Compared with Low Hematocrit Values in Patients with Cardiac Disease Who Are Receiving Hemodialysis and Epoetin." *New England Journal of Medicine* 339 (1998): 584–90.

Bolan, C. D., C. Conry-Cantilena, G. Mason, T. A. Rouault, and S. F. Leitman. "MCV as a Guide to Phlebotomy Therapy for Hemochromatosis." *Transfusion* 41 (2001): 819–27.

Casale, G., M. Bignamini, and P. de Nicola. "Does Blood Donation Prolong Life Expectance?" *Vox Sang* 45 (1983): 398–99.

Centers for Disease Control and Prevention. "CDC Criteria for Anemia in Children and Childbearing Aged Women." *Morbidity & Mortality Weekly Report* 38 (1989): 400–4.

Cook, J. D., and C. A. Finch. "Assessing Iron Status of a Population." *American Journal of Clinical Nutrition* 32 (1979): 2115–19.

Cook, J. D., and M. B. Reddy. "Ascorbic Acid Has a Pronounced Enhancing Effect on the Absorption of Dietary Nonheme Iron When Assessed by Feeding Single Meals to Fasting Subjects." *American Journal of Clinical Nutrition* 73 (2001): 93–98.

Davidsson, L., T. Walcyk, N. Zavaleta, and R. F. Hurrell. "Improving Iron Absorption from a Peruvian School Breakfast Meal by Adding Ascorbic Acid or Na (2)EDTA." *American Journal of Clinical Nutrition* 73 (2001): 283–87.

de Alarcon, P. A., M. E. Donovan, G. B. Forbes, S. A. Landaw, and J. A. Stockman. "Iron Absorption in the Thalassemia Syndromes and Its Inhibition by Tea." *New England Journal of Medicine* 300 (1979): 5–8.

de Valk, B., J. J. M. Marx. "Iron, Atherosclerosis, and Ischemic Heart Disease." *Archives of Internal Medicine* 159 (1999): 1542–48.

Deugnier, Y., O. Loreal, F. Carre, A. Duvallet, F. Zoulim, J. P. Vinel, J. C. Paris, D. Blaison, R. Moirand, B. Turlin, Y. Gandon, V. David, A. Megret, and M. Guinot. "Increased Body Iron in Elite Road Cyclists." *Medicine, Science, Sports & Exercise* 34 (2002): 876–80.

266

Duane, P., K. B. Raja, R. J. Simpson, and T. J. Peters. "Intestinal Iron Absorption in Chronic Alcoholism." *Alcohol and Alcoholism* 27 (1992): 539–44.

Fleming, J., P. F. Jacques, K. L. Tucker, J. M. Massaro, R. B. D'Agostino, P. W. F. Wilson, and R. I. Wood. "Status of the Free-Living, Elderly Framingham Heart Study Report: An Iron-replete Population with a High Prevalence of Elevated Iron Stores." *American Journal of Clinical Nutrition* 73 (2001): 638–46.

Fleming, D. J., K. L. Tucker, P. F. Jacques, G. E. Dallal, P. W. Wilson, and R. J. Wood. "Dietary Factors Associated with the Risk of High Iron Stores in the Elderly Framingham Heart Study Cohort." *American Journal of Clinical Nutrition* 76 (2002): 1375–84.

Garcia-Casal, M. N., I. Leets, and M. Layrisse. "Beta-Carotene and Inhibitors of Iron Absorption Modify Iron Uptake by Caco-2 Cell." *Journal of Nutrition* 130 (2000): 724–28.

Garn, S. M., M. T. Keating, and F. Falkner. "Hematological Status and Pregnancy Outcomes." *American Journal of Clinical Nutrition* 34 (1981): 115–17.

Garrison, C. *Cooking with Less Iron.* Nashville, TN: Cumberland House, 2002.

Garrison, C., ed. *Iron Disorders Institute Guide to Hemochromatosis.* Nashville, TN: Cumberland House, 2001.

Geleijnse, J. M., L. J. Launer, D. A. Van der Kuip, A. Hofman, and J. C. Witteman. "Inverse Association of Tea and Flavonoid Intakes with Incident Myocardial Infarction: The Rotterdam Study." *American Journal of Clinical Nutrition* 75 (2002): 880–86.

Geleijnse, J. T., L. J. Launer, A. Hofman, H. A. P. Pols, and J. C. M. Witteman. "Tea Flavonoids May Protect Against Atherosclerosis." *Archives of Internal Medicine* 159 (1999): 2170–74.

Gordeuk, V. R., G. D. McLaren, and W. Samowitz. "Etiologies, Consequences, and Treatment of Iron Overload." *Critical Reviews in Clinical Laboratory Sciences* 31 (1994): 89–133.

Goto, F., T. Yoshihara, N. Shigemoto, S. Toki, and F. Takaiwa. "Iron Fortification of Rice Seed by the Soybean Ferritin Gene." *Nature & Biotechnology* 17 (1999): 282–86.

Griffin, I., and S. Abrams. "Iron and Breastfeeding." *The Management of Breastfeeding* 48 (2001): 401–13.

Gum, P. A., M. Thamilarasan, J. Watanabe, E. H. Blackstone, M. S. Lauer. "Aspirin Use and All-cause Mortality among Patients Being Evaluated for Known or Suspected Coronary Artery Disease."

267

Journal of the American Medical Association 286 (2001): 1187–94.

Gura, T. "New Genes Boost Rice Nutrients." *Science* 285 (1999): 994–95.

Hallberg, L., and L. Hulthen. "Prediction of Dietary Iron Absorption: An Algorithm for Calculating Absorption and Bioavailability of Dietary Iron." *American Journal of Clinical Nutrition* 71 (2000): 1147–60.

Han, O., M. L. Failla, A. D. Hill, E. R. Morris, and J. C. Smith Jr. "Inositol Phosphates Inhibit Uptake and Transport of Iron and Zinc by a Human Intestinal Cell Line." *Journal of Nutrition* 124 (1994): 580–87.

Hemminki, E., and U. Rimpela. "A Randomized Comparison of Routine Versus Selective Iron Supplementation during Pregnancy." *Journal of the American College of Nutrition* 10 (1997): 344–51.

Hubel, C. A., A. V. Kozlov, V. E. Kagan, R. W. Evans, S. T. Davidge, M. K. McLaughlin, and J. M. Roberts. "Decreased Transferrin and Increased Transferrin Saturation in Sera of Women with Preeclampsia: Implications for Oxidative Stress." *American Journal of Obstetrics & Gynecology* 175 (1996): 692–700.

Kaltwasser, J. P., E. Werner, K. Schalk, C. Hansen, R. Gottschalk, C. Seidl. "Clinical Trial on the Effect of Regular Tea Drinking on Iron Accumulation in Genetic Haemochromatosis." *Gut* 43 (1998): 699–704.

Lachili, B., I. Hininger, H. Faure, J. Arnaud, M. J. Richard, A. Favier, and A. M. Roussel. "Increased Lipid Peroxidation in Pregnant Women after Iron and Vitamin C Supplementation." *Biology Trace Elements Research* 83 (2001): 103–10.

Layrisse, M., C. Martinez-Torres, M. Renzi, F. Velez, and M. Gonzalez. "Sugar as a Vehicle for Iron Fortification." *American Journal of Clinical Nutrition* 29 (1976): 8–18.

Layrisse, M., M. Garcia-Casal, L. Solano, M. Baron, F. Arguello, D. Llovera, J. Ramirez, I. Leets, and E. Tropper. "Iron Bioavailability in Humans from Breakfasts Enriched with Iron Bis-Glycine Chelate, Phytates and Polyphenols." *Human Nutrition and Metabolism* 9 (2000): 2195–99.

Litovitz, T., and A. Manoguerra. "Comparison of Pediatric Poisoning Hazards: An Analysis of 3.8 Million Exposure Accidents." *Pediatrics* 89 (1992): 999–1006.

Lonnerdal, B., and O. Hernell. "Iron, Zinc, Copper and Selenium Status of Breast-Fed Infants and Infants Fed Trace Element

Fortified Milk-Based Infant Formula." *Acta Pediatrica* 83 (1994): 367–73.

Mainous, A. G., J. M. Gill, and P. J. Carek. "Elevated Serum Transferrin Saturation and Mortality." *Annals of Family Medicine,* March/April 2004. http://www.annfammed.org.

Mainous, A. G., B. Wells, P. Carek, J. M. Gill, and M. E. Geesey. "The Mortality Risk of Elevated Serum Transferrin Saturation and Consumption of Dietary Iron." *Annals of Family Medicine,* March/April 2004, http://www.annfammed.org.

Mallory, M. A., C. Sthapanachai, and K. V. Kowdley. "Iron Overload Related to Excessive Vitamin C Intake." *Annals of Internal Medicine* 139 (2003): 532–33.

Meyers, D. G., D. Strickland, P. A. Maloley, J. J. Seburg, J. E. Wilson, and B. F. McManus. "Possible Association of a Reduction in Cardiovascular Events with Blood Donation." *Heart* 78 (1997): 188–93.

Morris, C. C. "Pediatric Iron Poisonings in the United States." *Southern Medical Journal* 93 (2000): 352–58.

Murphy, J. F., J. O'Riordan, R. G. Newcombe, E. C. Coles, and J. F. Pearson. "Relation of Haemoglobin Levels in First and Second Trimesters to Outcome of Pregnancy." *The Lancet* i (1986): 992–94.

Nelson, R. L. "Iron and Colorectal Cancer Risk: Human Studies." *Nutrition Reviews* 59 (2001): 140–48.

O'Brien, K. O., N. Zavaleta, J. Wen, and S. A. Abrams. "Prenatal Iron Supplements Impair Zinc Absorption In Pregnant Peruvian Women." *Journal of Nutrition* 130 (2000): 2251–55.

Oken, E., and C. Duggan. "Update on Micronutrients: Iron and Zinc." *Current Opinion in Pediatrics* 14 (2002): 350–33.

Pruchnicki, M. C., J. D. Coyle, S. Hoshaw-Woodard, and W. H. Bay. "Effect of Phosphate Binders on Supplemental Iron Absorption in Healthy Subjects." *Journal of Clinical Pharmacology* 42 (2002): 1171–76.

Richardson, D. R. "Potential of Iron Chelators as Effective Antiproliferative Agents." *Canadian Journals of Physiology Pharmacology* 75 (1997): 1164–80.

Roughead, Z. K., C. A. Zito, and J. R. Hunt. "Initial Uptake and Absorption of Nonheme Iron and Absorption of Heme Iron in Humans Are Unaffected by the Addition of Calcium as Cheese to a Meal with High Iron Bioavailability." *American Journal of Clinical*

Nutrition 76 (2002): 419–25.

Roughead, Z. K., and J. R. Hunt. "Adaptation in Iron Absorption: Iron Supplementation Reduces Nonheme-Iron But Not Heme-Iron Absorption from Food." *American Journal of Clinical Nutrition* 72 (2000): 982–89.

Salonen, J. T., T. P. Tuomainen, R. Salonen, T. A. Lakka, and K. Nyyssonen. "Donation of Blood Is Associated with Reduced Risk of Myocardial Infarction." *American Journal of Epidemiology* 148 (1998): 445–61.

Sandberg, A. S., M. Brune, N. G. Carlsson, L. Hallberg, E. Skoglund, and L. Rossander-Hulthén. "Inositol Phosphates with Different Numbers of Phosphate Groups Influence Iron Absorption in Humans." *American Journal of Clinical Nutrition* 70 (1999): 240–46.

Simonart, T., J. R. Boelaert, G. Andre, J. J. van den Oord, C. Degraef, P. Hermans, J. C. Noel, J. P. Van Vooren, M. Heenen, E. De Clerq, and R. Snoeck. "Desferrioxamine Enhances Aids-associated Kaposi's Sarcoma Tumor Development in a Xenograft Model." *International Journal of Cancer* 100 (2002): 140–43.

Simonart, T., J. R. Boelaert, R. Mosselmans, G. Andrei, J. C. Noel, E. De Clercq, and R. Snoeck. "Anti Proliferative and Apoptotic Effects of Iron Chelators on Human Cervical Carcinoma Cells." *Gynecology Oncology* 85 (2002): 95–102.

Stephansson, O., P. W. Dickman, A. Johansson, and S. Cnattingius. "Maternal Hemoglobin Concentration during Pregnancy and Risk of Stillbirth." *Journal of the American Medical Association* 284 (2000): 2611–17.

Sullivan, J. L. "Blood Donation May Be Good for the Donor." *Vox Sang* 61 (1991): 161–64.

———. "Iron Therapy and Cardiovascular Disease." *Kidney International* 55, suppl. 69 (1999): S135–37.

Tamura, T., R. L. Goldenberg, K. E. Johnston, S. P. Cliver, and C. A. Hickey. "Serum Ferritin: A Predictor of Early Spontaneous Preterm Delivery." *Obstetrics & Gynecology* 87 (1996): 360–65.

U.S. Preventive Services Task Force. "Routine Iron Supplementation during Pregnancy." *Journal of the American Medical Association* 270 (1993): 2846–54.

Vogin, G. D., and J. S. MacNeil. *Medscape Medical News*, December 10, 2002, http://www.medscape.com.

Weinberg, E. D. "The Development of Awareness of the Carcinogenic Hazard of Inhaled Iron." *Oncology Research* 11 (1999): 109–13.

————. "Development of Clinical Methods of Iron Deprivation for Suppression of Neoplastic and Infectious Diseases." *Cancer Investigation* 17 (1999): 507–13.

————. "Iron Therapy and Cancer." *Kidney International* 55, suppl. 69 (1999): S131–34.

————. "Iron-enriched Rice: The Case for Labeling." *Journal of Medcinal Food* 3 (2000): 189–91.

————. "Human Lactoferrin: A Novel Therapeutic with Broad Spectrum Potential." *Journal of Pharmacy and Pharmacology* 53 (2001): 1303–10.

Weinberg, G. A, J. R. Boelaert, and E. D. Weinberg. "Iron and HIV Infection." In *Micronutrients and HIV Infection.* Edited by H. Friis, 135–58. Boca Raton, FL: CRC Press, 2002.

Weinberg, R., S. R. Ell, and E. D. Weinberg. "Blood-letting, Iron Homeostasis and Human Health." *Medical Hypothesis* 21 (1986): 441–43.

Weiss, G. "Iron and Immunity: A Double-edged Sword." *European Clinical Investigators* 32 (2002): 70–78.

Wesselius, L. J., M. E. Nelson, and B. S. Skikne. "Increased Release of Ferritin and Iron by Iron-loaded Alveolar Macrophages in Cigarette Smokers." *American Journal of Respiratory Critical Care Medicine* 150 (1994): 690–95.

Whittaker P., P. R. Tufaro, and J. I. Rader. "Iron and Folate in Fortified Cereals." *Journal of the American College of Nutrition* 20 (2001): 247–54.

Wieringa, F. T., M. A. Dijkhuizen, C. E. West, D. I. Thurnham, Muhilal, and J. W. Van der Meer. "Redistribution of Vitamin A after Iron Supplementation in Indonesian Infants." *American Journal Clinical Nutrition* 77 (2003): 651–57.

Wu, C. H., Y. C. Yang, W. J. Yan, F. H. Lu, J. S. Wu, and C. J. Chang. "Epidemiological Evidence on Increased Bone Mineral Density in Habitual Tea Drinkers." *Archives of Internal Medicine* 162 (2002): 1001–6.

Zijp, I. M., O. Korver, and L. B. Tijburg. "Effect of Tea and Other Dietary Factors on Iron Absorption." *Critical Reviews in Food Science Nutrition* 40 (2000): 371–98.

271

Selected Reference Charts at a Glance

Tests: to determine iron overload

Fasting serum iron
Total iron binding capacity → Serum iron/TIBC X 100%= Tsat% (Normal 25-35%)

Serum ferritin: See ranges in ferritin chart

Liver biopsy with quantitative iron stain (used in some cases, especially those with normal TS% with elevated serum ferritin)

Hepatic Iron Content (HIC): 4500 mcg (80 mcmol) per gram of dry weight or 3-4+ iron stain

Tsat%= transferrin-iron saturation percentage   Source: Iron Disorders Institute, 2004.

Important Ferritin Reference Ranges		Adult Males	Adult Females
	Normal Range	up to 300ng/mL	up to 200ng/mL
	In treatment*	below 100ng/mL	below 100ng/mL
	Ideal maintenance	25-75ng/mL	25-75ng/mL
Adolescents, Juveniles, Infants & Newborns of normal height and weight for their age and gender			
	Male ages 10-19 23-70ng/mL	Infants 7-12 months 60-80ng/mL	
	Female ages 10-19 6-40ng/mL	Newborn 1-6 months 6-410ng/mL	
	Children ages 6-9 10-55ng/mL	Newborn 1-30 days 6-400ng/mL	
	Children ages 1-5 6-24ng/mL		

*undergoing therapeutic phlebotomy   Source: Iron Disorders Institute, 2004.

	TIBC	Serum Iron	Ferritin
Newborn	130-275 mg/dL	100-250 mcg/dL	
Age 1-30 days			6-400 ng/mL
Age 1-6 months			6-410 ng/mL
Infant (age 7-12 months)	220-400 mg/dL	40-100 mcg/dL	60-80 ng/mL
Child (1-5 years of age)	220-400 mg/dL	50-120 mcg/dL	6-24 ng/mL

Source: Iron Disorders Institute, 2004.

Reference Ranges

hemoglobin	Adult Males	Adult Females
Normal Range	14.0-18.0g/dL	12.0-16.0g/dL
Adolescents, Juveniles, Infants & Newborns of normal height and weight for their age and gender		
Age 6-18 years 10.0-15.5g/dL	Age 2-6 mos 10.0-17.0g/dL	
Age 1-6 years 9.5-14.0g/dL	Age 0-2 weeks 12.0-20.0g/dL	
Age 6 mos-1 year 9.5-14.0g/dL	Newborn 14.0-24.0g/dL	

Source: Iron Disorders Institute, 2004.

LAB TEST RESULTS	Hemoglobin	Hematocrit	Ferritin	Transferrin Iron Saturation Percentage
Iron Overload	NORMAL 12-17 g/dL	NORMAL 36-42%	Elevated	Greater than 45%
Iron-Deficiency Anemia	Less than 10 g/dL	Less than 30%	Less than 15 ng/mL	Less than 15%

Source: Iron Disorders Institute, 2004.

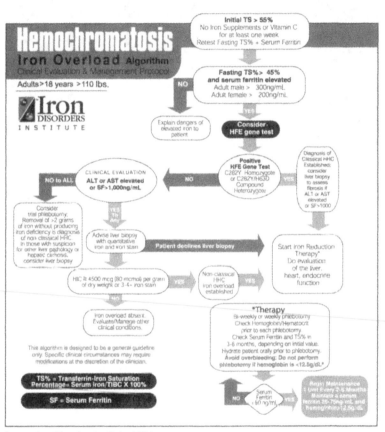

Source: Iron Disorders Institute, 2004.

iron panel	IRON PANEL TESTS					
	Serum Iron	Serum Ferritin	Transferrin Iron Saturation Percentage	Total Iron Binding Capacity (TIBC)	Transferrin	Serum Transferrin Receptor
Hemochromatosis	⬆	⬆	⬆	⬇	⬇	NORMAL TO LOW
Iron-Deficiency Anemia	⬇	⬇	⬇	⬆	⬆	HIGH
Sideroblastic Anemia	⬆	⬆	⬆	⬇	⬇	NORMAL TO HIGH
Thalassemia	⬆	⬆	⬆	⬇	⬇	HIGH
Porphyria Cutanea Tarda	⬆	⬆	⬆	⬇	⬇	NORMAL
Anemia of Chronic Disease (ACD)	⬇	⬆ OR NORMAL	⬇	⬇	⬇	NORMAL
African siderosis	⬆	⬆	⬆	⬇	⬇	NORMAL TO LOW

The Physician's Reference Chart is provided with the guidance of The Iron Disorders Institute Scientific Advisory Board and consultants to the board from the National Institutes of Health and the US Centers for Disease Control and Prevention. Larger versions of all charts are available upon request: publications@irondisorders.org.

Treatment Options

Treatment for iron overload in those who do not have concurrent anemia is therapeutic phlebotomy. Most patients are candidates for standard phlebotomy. **Patients should have a pretreatment hemoglobin of 12.5g/dL.** Quantities removed by phlebotomy can vary from minimal extraction of 250cc up to large volume extraction of 600cc. Extraction continues until ferritin reaches 25ng/mL on one occasion but hemoglobin does not drop below normal range for age, weight or gender.

	TYPE OF PHLEBOTOMY		
	STANDARD	MINIMAL VOLUME	LARGE VOLUME
Patient Profile	most patients	for youths, persons who are frail, small in stature or weight, or who have coexistent illness such as heart problems*	unique cases such as adults with extremely high iron levels and other medical complications
Procedure	extracted from vein in the arm using 16-gauge needle (similar to routine blood donation)	extracted from vein in the arm using 20- to 22-gauge butterfly needle with vacuum bag	chest port surgically implanted near collar bone area
Duration of Procedure	15-20 minutes	15-20 minutes	15-20 minutes
Approx. Volume Blood Removed	450-500 cc of blood	250-300 cc of blood	600 cc of blood
Approx. Iron Removed	approx. 250 mg of iron	approx. 125 mg of iron	approx. 300 mg of iron
Frequency of Treatment	one or two times weekly	one or two times monthly	one or two times weekly
Important Notes	increasing the frequency to twice a week should be considered to facilitate more rapid iron depletion	frequency may be increased depending on patient tolerance *patient may have small, inaccessible, scarred or rolling veins *patient may be unable to tolerate standard volume of blood removal	serious procedure not to be considered a routine option

AVOID OVER-BLEEDING

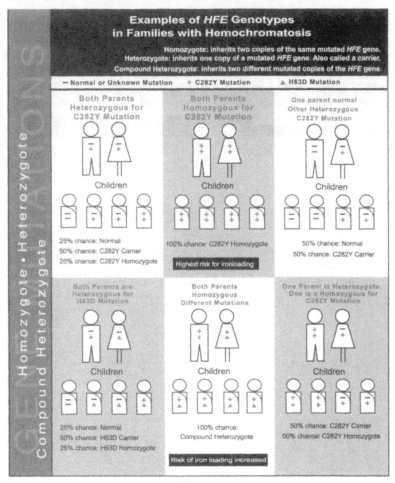

Examples of *HFE* Genotypes in Families with Hemochromatosis

Homozygote: inherits two copies of the same mutated *HFE* gene.
Heterozygote: inherits one copy of a mutated *HFE* gene. Also called a carrier.
Compound Heterozygote: inherits two different mutated copies of the *HFE* gene.

— Normal or Unknown Mutation   + C282Y Mutation   ▲ H63D Mutation

Both Parents Heterozygous for C282Y Mutation
Children
25% chance: Normal
50% chance: C282Y Carrier
25% chance: C282Y Homozygote

Both Parents Homozygous for C282Y Mutation
Children
100% chance: C282Y Homozygote
Highest risk for ironloading

One parent normal Other Heterozygous C282Y Mutation
Children
50% chance: Normal
50% chance: C282Y Carrier

Both Parents are Heterozygous for H63D Mutation
Children
25% chance: Normal
50% chance: H63D Carrier
25% chance: H63D Homozygote

Both Parents Homozygous Different Mutations
Children
100% chance:
Compound Heterozygote
Risk of iron loading increased

One Parent is Heterozygote. One is a Homozygous for C282Y Mutation
Children
50% chance: C282Y Carrier
50% chance: C282Y Homozygote

IMPORTANT NOTES

· Everyone inherits two copies of *HFE*
· Only the mutated copies C282Y and H63D are represented in this chart
  because these are the most significant known mutations to date.
· *HFE* mutations are present in about 85% of those with hereditary hemochromatosis
· *HFE* related iron overload is an adult onset disorder. Other genes that can
  cause iron overload in children are not included in this chart.
· The risk of iron loading is presently known to be greatest in the C282Y homozygote.
  Heterozygotes, especially compound heterozygotes are also at increased risk of iron
  loading, but likelihood and severity are lower.
· Informed consent: Anyone considering genetic testing should be made aware
  of the consequences such as possible insurance and employer discrimination
  or paternity identification.
· Genetic status provides *NO* information about tissue iron levels. Clinical evaluation
  of serum ferritin and transferrin iron saturation percentage is one way to estimate
  tissue iron status.

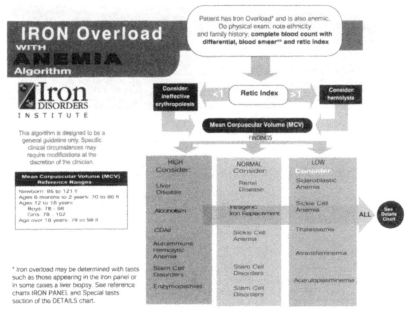

IRON Overload
WITH
ANEMIA
Algorithm

Iron DISORDERS
INSTITUTE

This algorithm is designed to be a general guideline only. Specific clinical circumstances may require modifications at the discretion of the clinician.

Mean Corpuscular Volume (MCV) Reference Ranges

Newborn: 85 to 121 fl
Ages 6 months to 2 years: 70 to 86 fl
Ages 12 to 18 years
 Boys: 78 - 98
 Girls: 78 - 102
Age over 18 years: 78 to 98 fl

* Iron overload may be determined with tests such as those appearing in the iron panel or in some cases a liver biopsy. See reference charts IRON PANEL and Special tests section of the DETAILS chart.

Patient has Iron Overload* and is also anemic. Do physical exam, note ethnicity and family history; **complete blood count with differential, blood smear** and retic index**

Consider: Ineffective erythropoiesis ← <1 — Retic Index — >1 → Consider: hemolysis

Mean Corpuscular Volume (MCV)
FINDINGS

HIGH Consider:	NORMAL Consider:	LOW Consider:
Liver Disease	Renal Disease	Sideroblastic Anemia
Alcoholism	Iatrogenic Iron Replacement	Sickle Cell Anemia
CDAII	Sickle Cell Anemia	Thalassemia
Autoimmune Hemolytic Anemia		Atransferrinemia
Stem Cell Disorders	Stem Cell Disorders	Aceruloplasminemia
Enzymopathies	Stem Cell Disorders	

ALL → See Details Chart

**For excellent images, visit The American Society of Hematology web site. www.hematology.org Click on "education" then on "image bank." For PDF version of copies of chapters from *The Iron Disorders Institute Guide to Anemia*, e-mail your request to. publications@irondisorders.org, or visit the Physician's Section: http://www.irondisorders.org

SELECTED REFERENCE CHARTS AT A GLANCE

DETAILS

Anemias associated with ineffective erythropoiesis are more prone to be associated with de novo iron overload. Conditions with associated iron overload are in the table below.

Condition	Cause/Mechanism	Management of Iron Overload
Sideroblastic Anemia	**Inherited:** Mutations of the X chromosome, autosomes, mitochondrial chromosomes. Iron overload due to ineffective erythropoiesis. **Acquired:** exposure to toxins, medications, nutritional deficiencies, alcoholism, MDS. Iron overload due to chronic hemolysis	EPO with phlebotomy if hemoglobin is sufficient. If not, chelation therapy with Desferal. Beneficial supplements include B6, folic acid and antioxidants.
Thalassemia	**Inherited:** Iron overload due to ineffective hemoglobin production and repeated blood transfusion	Chelation therapy with Desferal. Beneficial supplements include folic acid and antioxidants. Bone marrow transplantation may be useful.
CDA II Congenital dyserythropoietic anemia	**Inherited:** Iron overload due to chronic hemolysis and ineffective erythropoiesis	May require splenectomy to control hemolysis. EPO with phlebotomy if hemoglobin is sufficient. If not, chelation therapy with Desferal. Transfusion support.
Red Cell Enzymopathies such as: Glucose-6 Phosphate Dehydrogenase (G6PD) or Pyruvate kinase deficiency (PKD)	**Inherited: G6PD:** Iron overload is due to chronic hemolysis triggered by specific drugs, especially anti-materials or by foods, especially Fava beans. In **PKD**, iron overload is due to chronic hemolysis or repeated blood transfusion	Avoidance of drugs, foods or conditions that precipitate hemolysis. EPO with phlebotomy if hemoglobin is sufficient. If not, chelation therapy with Desferal.
Sickle Cell Anemia	**Inherited:** Iron Overload due to repeated blood transfusion	Chelation therapy with Desferal. Beneficial supplements include folic acid and antioxidants.
Autoimmune Hemolytic Anemia	**Acquired:** autoimmune response to drugs, systemic autoimmune diseases or idiopathic. Iron overload due to chronic hemolysis	Steroids or other immunosuppressive treatments. EPO with phlebotomy if hemoglobin is sufficient. If not, chelation therapy with Desferal.
Myelodysplastic Syndromes Aplastic Anemia	**Acquired:** stem cell disorder. Iron overload due to repeated blood transfusion	EPO with phlebotomy if hemoglobin is sufficient. If not, chelation therapy with Desferal. Treatment to correct bone marrow dysfunction. Bone marrow transplantation may be necessary in some cases.
Atransferrinemia or hypotransferrinemia Aceruloplasminemia or hypoceruloplasminia	**Inherited:** Iron transport protein deficiencies. Iron overload due to absent or low transferrin. Absent or low ceruloplasmin	Chelation therapy with Desferal. Beneficial supplements include folic acid and antioxidants.

280

Iron Profile in Selected Conditions

Condition	IRON PANEL TESTS						
	Hemoglobin	Serum Iron	Serum Ferritin	Transferrin Iron Saturation Percentage	Total Iron Binding Capacity (TIBC)	Transferrin	Serum Transferrin Receptor
Hemoglobinapathies, Stem cell disorders, Chronic hymolysis Sickle Cell Anemia G6PD Sideroblastic Anemia Thalassemia CDA II Autoimmune Hemolytic Anemia	↓	↑	↑	↑	↓	↓	NORMAL TO HIGH
Aceruloplasminemia	↓	↓	↑ OR NORMAL	↓	↓	↓	NORMAL
Atransferrinemia	NORMAL	↓	↑	↑	↓	↓	NORMAL TO LOW
Hemochromatosis	NORMAL	↑	↑	↑	↓	↓	NORMAL TO LOW
Anemia of Chronic Disease (ACD)	↓	↓	↑ OR NORMAL	↓	↓	↓	NORMAL

NOTE: Many of these conditions occur concomitantly with other illnesses confounding the findings.

Source: Iron Disorders Institute, 2004

symptoms log

Iron Disorders Institute
Providing reliable answers about Iron-Out-of-Balance

Symptoms of an iron imbalance such as iron overload or anemia are not limited to the list provided on this log, which is not intened to prompt self diagnosis. This form is for record-keeping only and its contents should be shared with your physician.

PERSONAL HEALTH PROFILE

ID #

DOB

NAME

DATE Present	Symptom	Comments	DATE Present	Symptom	Comments
	weakness			chronic cough	
	fatigue			sore tongue	
	joint pain			koilonychia	
	lower back pain			bad breath	
	mid back pain			acid reflux	
	abdominal pain			dizziness	
	stomach pain			fainting	
	nausea			weight loss	
	vomiting			weight gain	
	diarrhea			skin color pale	
	constipation			skin color yellow	
	visible blood in stool			skin color bronze	
	stool: pale			skin color:ashen gray/green	
	stool: black			blisters	
	stool: coffee ground			rash	
	urine: pink			frequent bruises	
	urine: dark			frequent nose bleeds	
	urine: foamy			vision problems	
	urination:painful			mental confusion	
	urination: frequent and abundant			lost interest in sex	
	urination: frequent but small amounts			rage/emotional outbursts	
	urination: infrequent			depression	
	thirst:increased			sensitivity to cold	
	headache			sensitivity to heat	
	chest pain			hair loss	
	pain:side of neck			irregular menstruation	
	shortness of breath			difficulty sleeping	
	heartbeat:irregular			blood pressure:high	
	heartbeat:racing			blood pressure:low	
	heartbeat:slow			fever	

LABORATORY	PHONE NUMBER	TREATMENT CENTER	PHONE NUMBER

PHYSICIAN	PHONE NUMBER	PHYSICIAN	PHONE NUMBER

www.irondisorders.org

Iron Disorders Institute
Providing reliable answers about Iron-Out-of-Balance

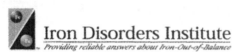

tests

PERSONAL HEALTH PROFILE

NAME ______ DOB ___/___/___ ID # ______

DNA RESULTS

		TEST	TYPICAL REFERENCE RANGES	LAB TEST RESULTS DATE	DATE	DATE	DATE	DATE	DATE
IRON PANEL	OVERLOAD	**Serum Iron**	40-180 mcg/dL						
IRON PANEL	OVERLOAD	**Transferrin Iron Saturation Percentage**	25-35%						
IRON PANEL	OVERLOAD	**Total Iron Binding Capacity**	250-450 mcg/dL						
IRON PANEL	OVERLOAD	**Ferritin** *Refer to* ***Important Reference Ranges*** *Below...*							
IRON PANEL	ANEMIA	**Hemoglobin** (Hgb)	female: 12.0-16.0 g/dL male: 14.0-18.0 g/dL						
IRON PANEL	ANEMIA	**Hematocrit** (Hct)	female: 36.0-48.0% male: 42.0-54.0%						
IRON PANEL	ANEMIA	Serum Transferrin Receptor RAMCO Assay	5.6±0.3 mg/L						
	BLOOD COUNT	Red Blood Count (RBC)	5-10 million/uL						
	BLOOD COUNT	White Blood Cell (WBC)	4-10,000/uL						
	BLOOD COUNT	Red Blood Cell Distribution Width (RDW)	12-16 %						
	BLOOD COUNT	Mean Corpuscular Volume (MCV)	82-98 fL						
	BLOOD COUNT	Mean Corpuscular Hemoglobin (MCH)	27-33 pg						
	BLOOD COUNT	Mean Corpuscular Hemoglobin Concentration (MCHC)	31-36 g/dL						
	BLOOD COUNT	Platelet Count*	140,000-450,000/uL						
	GENERAL	Blood Pressure	<140 over 90						
	GENERAL	Heart Rate (at rest)	<100 bpm						
	GENERAL	Body Mass Index	20-25 ideal 25-27 overweight >27 obese						
	GENERAL	Height*							
	LIPIDS	Cholesterol (Total)	<200 mg/dL						
	LIPIDS	HDL	>35 mg/dL Males >40 mg/dL Females						
	LIPIDS	Triglycerides	<400 mg/dL						
	KIDNEYS	BUN	8-20mg/dL						
	KIDNEYS	Uric Acid	2-6mg/dL						
BIOPSY	LIVER	AST (SGOT)	10-40 IU/L						
BIOPSY	LIVER	ALT (SGPT)	10-40 IU/L						
BIOPSY	LIVER	GGT	0-85 IU/L						
BIOPSY	LIVER	ALP	25-125 IU/L						
ENDOCRINE	PITUITARY & THYROID	Testosterone (total)	Males: 270-1,070 ng/dL Females: 6-86 ng/dL						
ENDOCRINE	PITUITARY & THYROID	TSH	0.5-3.5 mU/L						
ENDOCRINE	PITUITARY & THYROID	T4 (Total)	4.5-12.0 mcg/dL						
ENDOCRINE	PITUITARY & THYROID	T3 (Uptake)	24-39%						
ENDOCRINE	PITUITARY & THYROID	Free Thyroxine Index (T7)	1.2-4.5 ug/dL						
ENDOCRINE	PITUITARY & THYROID	LH*							
ENDOCRINE	PITUITARY & THYROID	FSH*							
ENDOCRINE	PANCREAS	Glucose (fasting)	65-115 mg/dL						
ENDOCRINE	PANCREAS	HGB A1C	4.2-5.9%						
ENDOCRINE	PANCREAS	Amylase (Blood)	25-130 IU/L						

*** Labs vary with respect to ranges. The values listed are only approximate. Normal ranges not provided should be supplied by attending physician.**

Ferritin Important Reference Ranges

Adult Males	up to 300 ng/mL	Male Ages 10-19	23-70 ng/mL	Infants 7-12 Months	60-80 ng/mL
In Treatment	below 100 ng/mL	Female Ages 10-19	6-40 ng/mL	Newborn 1-6 Months	6-410 ng/mL
Ideal Maintenance	25-75 ng/mL	Children Ages 6-9	10-55 ng/mL	Newborn 1-30 Days	6-400 ng/mL
Adult Females	up to 200 ng/mL	Children Ages 1-5	6-24 ng/mL		
In Treatment	below 100 ng/mL				
Ideal Maintenance	25-75 ng/mL				

(**For the definition of "In Treatment", see note on "treatment" page to follow)

This journal is for convenience and record-keeping only and does not represent the limit of diagnostic tests your physician may order on your behalf.

PS2 1/03

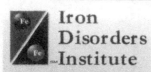

Iron Disorders Institute

Recommendations

Diet

FOR: People with Type I hemochromatosis

Type I hemochromatosis (also called classic hemochromatosis) is an inherited disorder of iron metabolism. People with Type I hemochromatosis absorb more iron from the diet than do people with normal iron metabolism.

Type I hemochromatosis is an adult-onset condition. Though symptoms or abnormal iron tests can be present in teens, usually the first signs occur in 30- to 40-year-old males and in non-menstruating females.

If not treated, iron may continue to build up in the body to toxic levels. Eventually iron-loaded organs such as the heart, liver, pancreas, pituitary and joints cannot function properly. Conditions such as heart failure, cirrhosis, cancer, diabetes, impotence, infertility, depression, arthritis and hypothyroidism can develop.

See recommendations sheets for diagnosing and treatment guidelines and details about inheritance patterns and DNA testing for hemochromatosis.

- **Cut back on consumption of red meat**
  Why: red meat contains the most easily absorbable form of iron called heme iron.

- **Avoid foods high in animal fats**
  Why: fats and iron together can generate free radical activity which is destructive to cells and can damage DNA.

- **Take vitamin C supplements in between meals**
  Why: vitamin C enhances the absorption of iron

- **Cook in ceramic or glassware when possible**
  Why: iron filings from grills or metal skillets can get into the food.

- **Drink alcoholic beverages in moderation**
  Why: Alcohol enhances the absorption of iron.
  Too much alcohol can damage the liver.
  Red wine can be of benefit when consumed in moderation.
  People with cirrhosis should avoid alcohol completely.

- **Avoid sugary foods or beverages.**
  Why: sugar enhances the absorption of iron.

- **Eat lots of fruits and vegetables**
  Why: These foods contain fiber and antioxidants, which inhibit free radical production.
  NOTE: Fruits and vegetables contain non-heme iron which is not easily absorbed. Also, absorption of non-heme iron can be further impaired when consumed with tea, coffee, eggs, fiber or supplemental calcium.

- **Eat nuts, grains, rice and beans**
  Why: These foods are high in fiber and contain non-heme iron.

- **Avoid raw shellfish**
  Why: Shellfish contain a bacterium called *Vibrio vulnificus*, which can be fatal to people with high body iron levels. Also, take care when walking barefoot on beaches where you might step on contaminated shells.

- **Drink tea or coffee with meals when possible (not recommended for people with liver damage).**
  Why: these beverages contain tannins which inhibit the absorption of iron.

Iron Disorders Institute PO BOX 2031 Greenville, SC 29602 864-292-1175 Fax: 864-292-1878 501(c) 3 organization
Mission: reducing pain, suffering and unnecessary death due to disorders of iron through awareness, education and research.

Patient Info Series: HHC Diet May 2004

For updates or a PDF version of this sheet visit our web site: www.irondisorders.org

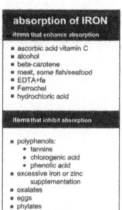

absorption of IRON

items that enhance absorption

- ascorbic acid vitamin C
- alcohol
- beta-carotene
- meat, some fish/seafood
- EDTA+fe
- Ferrochel
- hydrochloric acid

items that inhibit absorption

- polyphenols:
  - tannins
  - chlorogenic acid
  - phenolic acid
- excessive iron or zinc supplementation
- oxalates
- eggs
- phytates
- phosphates in dairy
- calcium

IRON
per 3.2 oz serving MEAT

	total iron MILLIGRAMS	heme iron percentage of total iron	heme iron MILLIGRAMS
VENISON	4.5	51	2.3
LAMB	3.1	55	1.7
BEEF			
RUMP STEAK	2.9	52	1.5
SIRLOIN STEAK	2.5	52	1.3
ROUND STEAK	3.2	50	1.6
TOP ROUND	2.5	48	1.2
GROUND	2.5	40	1.0
BRISKET	2.0	25	0.5
VEAL	1.9	40*	0.7*
PORK	1.3	23	0.3
PROCESSED MEATS			
SAUSAGE (VEAL)	0.7	40*	0.2*
BOILED HAM	0.7	40*	0.2*
LIVER PATE	5.0	16	0.8
CHICKEN	0.6	40*	0.2*
FISH			
COD	0.2	0.0	0.0
MACKEREL	0.7	0.0	0.0
SALMON	0.8	17	0.1
MUSSELS	4.6	48	2.2
LOBSTER	1.6	40*	0.6*
SHRIMP	2.6	40*	1.0*

* resources vary

Meat contains about 40-50% heme iron; the balance is non-heme. The iron in plant-based foods is nearly all non-heme, but some plants do have insignificant traces of heme iron. These plants are not commonly consumed by humans.

Iron Content: Plant-based Foods

Meat substitute:
Tofu, firm 1/4 block....8.5mgs

Nuts, grains, and seeds:
mgs per 1-cup portion
cream of wheat 10
almonds 6.7
cashews 5.3
pistachios 8.7
pumpkin seeds 15.7
sunflower seeds 10.3
rice (white or wild) 6.8
flours & bran:
  rice bran 16.9
  rice flour 6.8
dried fruits: 10 pieces:
  peaches 5.2
  pear 3.7
  prunes 3.0
  raisins 4.0
beans, peas and lentils:
  Split peas 3.4
  Black beans 15.0
  Pintos 12.2

Vegetables:
You need not cut back on vegetables, including spinach. Fruits and vegetables contain a type of iron that is not easily absorbed by the body. In fact, some fruits and vegetables such as raisins and eggplant are high in polyphenols, substances that inhibit the absorption of non-heme iron.

Eggs can also be enjoyed. Though there is about a milligram of iron in a large egg, eggs also contain a protein that inhibits the absorption of iron. This inhibiting action is called the "egg factor."

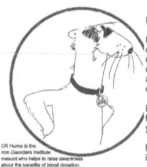

CR Hume is the Iron Disorders Institute mascot who helps to raise awareness about the benefits of blood donation.

Donate blood!

Remember: iron cannot be removed except through blood loss or iron-chelation drugs administered by a health care professional.

Don't believe health food claims that tell you otherwise!

Keep your physician informed!

Iron Disorders Institute PO BOX 2031 Greenville, SC 29602 864-292-1175 Fax: 864-292-1878 501(c) 3 organization
Mission: reducing pain, suffering and unnecessary death due to disorders of iron through awareness, education and research.

Resources

Iron Disorders Institute (IDI)
PO Box 2031
Greenville, SC 29602
Phone: 864-292-1175
Fax: 864-292-1878

*Visit our web site **http://www.irondisorders.org** for*
• books for patients
• updates on our list of genetic labs
• blood centers with an FDA variance to use hemochromatosis blood
  for transfusional purposes
• our national physician registry
• national events for patients and physicians
• our library and PDF versions of physician and patient materials
• a list of IDI's physician and patient services
• Iron Disorders Institute Centers of Excellence, where physicians can
  refer patients or obtain consultation about disorders of iron

Or contact us: 888-565-IRON (4766)

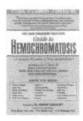 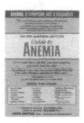 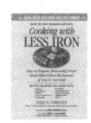

American Academy of Family Physicians
PO Box 11210
Shawnee Mission, KS 66207-1210
800-274-2237
913-906-6000
http://www.aafp.org

American Society of Hematology (ASH)
1900 M Street NW
Suite 200
Washington, DC 20036
Phone: 202-776-0544
Fax: 202-776-0545
http://www.hematology.org/

The American Association for the Study of Liver Diseases
1729 King Street, Suite 200
Alexandria, VA 22314
Phone: 703-299-9766
Fax: 703-299-9622

US Centers for Disease Control and Prevention
To take the healthcare providers online hemochromatosis course, go to www.cdc.gov and search for "hemochromatosis" or visit www.irondisorders.org; go to the healthcare professional portal for the link.

Alcoholism

Al-anon Family Group Headquarters
1600 Corporate Landing Parkway
Virginia Beach, VA 23454
800-356-9996
757-563-1600
http://www.al-anon.alateen.org

Alcoholics Anonymous
PO Box 459
Grand Central Station
New York, NY 10163
212-870-3400
http://www.alcoholics-anony mous.org

National Clearinghouse for Alcohol and Drug Information
PO Box 2345
Rockville, MD 20847
800-729-6686
301-468-2600
http://www.health.org

National Council on Alcoholism and Drug Dependence
20 Exchange Place, Suite 2909
New York, NY 10005
Toll Free: 800-NCA-CALL
Phone: 212-269-7797
Fax: 212-269-7510
http://www.ncadd.org

Arthritis

Arthritis Foundation
1330 West Peachtree Street
Atlanta, GA 30309
800-283-7800
404-872-7100
http://www.arthritis.org

Ankylosing Spondylitis Association
PO Box 5872
Sherman Oaks, CA 91413
800-777-8189
http://www.spondylitis.org

American Juvenile Arthritis Organization
1314 Spring Street NW
Atlanta, GA 30309
800-283-7800
404-872-7100

Blood Disorders

Aplastic Anemia & MDS International Foundation
PO Box 613
Annapolis, MD 21404
800-747-2820
http://www.aplastic.org

Leukemia Society of America
600 Third Street
New York, NY 10016
800-955-4LSA
212-573-8484
http://www.leukemia.org

Cancer

American Cancer Society
1599 Clifton Road NE
Atlanta, GA 30329-4251
800-ACS-2345
404-320-3333
http://www.cancer.org

National Cancer Institute
Cancer Information Service
9000 Rockville Pike
Bethesda, MD 20892
800-4-CANCER
301-496-5583
http://www.cancer.gov

Cardiovascular Disorders

American Heart Association
7272 Greenville Avenue
Dallas, TX 75231
214-373-6300
http://www.amhrt.org

National Heart, Lung, and Blood Institute
Information Center
PO Box 30105
Bethesda, MD 20824-0105
301-251-1222
http://www.nhlbi.nih.org

National Stroke Association
96 Inverness Drive East, Suite 1
Engelwood, CA 80112
800-787-6537
303-649-9299
E-mail: info@stroke.org
http://www.stroke.org

Deafness and Hearing Disorders

American Tinnitus Association
PO Box 5
Portland, OR 97207
503-248-9985
E-mail: tinnitus@ata.org
http://www.ata.org

National Association of the Deaf
814 Thayer Avenue
Silver Spring, MD 20910
301-587-1788
TTY: 301-587-1789
http://www.nad.org

289

Death and Bereavement

The Compassionate Friends, Inc.
PO Box 3696
Oak Brook IL, 60522-3696
Phone: 630-990-0010
Fax: 630-990-0246
http://www.compassionate
friends.org

Hospice Education Institute
PO Box 98
Machiasport, MA 04655
800-331-1620
860-767-1620
E-mail: hospiceall@aol.com
http://www.hospiceworld.org

National Hospice Organization
1901 North Moore Street
Suite 901
Arlington, VA 22209
800-658-8898
703-243-5900
E-mail: drsnho@cais.com
http://www.nho.org

Diabetes

American Diabetes Association
1600 Duke Street
Alexandria, VA 22314
800-232-3472
703-549-1500
http://www.diabetes.org

Juvenile Diabetes Foundation
120 Wall Street, 19th Floor
New York, NY 10005
800-223-1138
http://www.jdfcure.com

National Diabetes Information Clearinghouse
One Information Highway
Bethesda, MD 20892-3560
301-654-3327
http://www.niddk.nih.gov

Digestive Disorders

Crohn's and Colitis Foundation of America
386 Park Avenue South
17th Floor
New York, NY 10016
800-343-3637
http://www.ccfa.org

Digestive Disease National Coalition
507 Capitol Court NE, Suite 200
Washington, DC 20002
202-544-7497
http://www.ddnc.org

National Digestive Diseases Information Clearinghouse
Two Information Highway
Bethesda, MD 20892-3570
301-654-3810

Disabilities and Rehabilitation

Disabled American Veterans
National Headquarters
3725 Alexandria Park
Cold Spring, KY 41076
606-441-7300
http://www.dav.org

290

National Organization on Disability
910 16th Street NW
Suite 600
Washington, DC 20006
202-293-5960
http://www.nod.org

Endocrine Disorders

Pituitary Tumor Network Association
16350 Ventura Blvd., Suite 231
Encino, CA 91436
800-642-9211
805-499-9973
E-mail: ptna@pituitary.com
http://www.pituitary.com

Thyroid Foundation of America
Ruth Sleeper Hall, Room RSL350
40 Parkman Street
Boston, MA 02114
617-726-8500
http://www.tsh.org

Epilepsy

Epilepsy Foundation of America
4351 Garden City Drive
Landover, MD 20785
800-332-1000
301-459-3700
E-mail: postmaster@efa.org
http://www.efa.org

General

The American Medical Association
515 North State Street
Chicago, IL 60610
312-464-5000
http://www.ama-assn.org

The Center for Disease Control and Prevention
1600 Clifton Road NE
Atlanta, GA 30333
404-639-3311
http://www.cdc.gov

National Institutes of Health
9000 Rockville Pike
Bethesda, MD 20892
301-496-4000
http://www.nih.gov

Restless Legs Syndrome Foundation
819 Second Street SW
Rochester, MN 55902-2985
507-287-6465
E-mail: RLSFoundation@rls.org
http://www.rls.org

US Department of Health and Human Services
200 Independence Avenue SW
Washington, DC 20201
202-619-0257
http://www.os.dhhs.gov

US Food and Drug Administration
Office of Consumer Affairs Inquiry
Information Line: 301-827-4420
http://www.fda.gov

291

Genetic Conditions

The Alliance for Genetic Support Groups
800-336-GENE (4363)
http://www.geneticalliance.org

Greenwood Genetic Center
1 Gregor Mendel Circle
Greenwood, SC 29646
888-GGC-GENE (442-4363)
864-941-8100
http://www.ggc.org

National Society of Genetic Counselors
610-872-7608
http://www.nsgc.org

Liver Diseases

American Liver Foundation
75 Maiden Lane, Suite 603
New York, NY 10038
800-GO-Liver (465-4837)
888-4HEP-USA (443-7872)
Phone: 212-668-1000
Fax: 212-483-8179
http://www.liverfoundation.org

American Association for the Study of Liver Diseases
AASLD
1729 King Street, Suite 200
Alexandria, Virginia 22314
Phone: 703-299-9766
Fax: 703-299-9622
Email:aasld@aasld.org
http://www.aasld.org/

National Institute of Diabetes and Digestive and Kidney Diseases (NIDDK)
Center Drive, MSC 2560,
Building 31, room 9A04
Bethesda, MD 20892-2560
www.niddk.nih.gov

Product Information

BMF's Starch-Based Synthetic Iron Chelator
Biomedical Frontiers
1095 Tenth Avenue SE
Minneapolis, MN 55414
Phone: 612-378-0228
Fax: 612-378-3601
Contact: Bo Hedlund, Ph.D.,
president and CEO

Butterfly needle
Becton Dickinson
One Becton Drive
Franklin Lakes, NJ 07417
201-847-6800
http://www.bd.com

CADD micro pump
Sims Deltec, Inc.
1265 Grey Fox Road
St. Paul, MN 55112
Phone: 800-426-2448
Fax: 612-639-2530

Crono pump
Intrapump, Inc.
908 Niagara Falls Blvd., #198
North Tonawanda, NY
14120-2060
Phone: 866-211-7867 x251 or 210
Fax: 800-699-5936
http://www.intrapump.com

Epogen® or Aranesp®
Amgen, Inc. (Headquarters)
Amgen Center
One Amgen Center Drive
Thousand Oaks, CA 91320-1799
Phone: 805-447-1000
Fax: 805-447-1010
http://www.amgen.com

Exjade®: oral iron chelator and Desferal
Customer Interaction Center
Novartis Pharmaceuticals Corp.
One Health Plaza
East Hanover, NJ 07936-1080
Novartis Oncology
888-NOW-NOVA (669-6682)
http://www.novartisoncology.com/home.jsp

Ferriprox: oral iron chelator
Apotex, Inc.
150 Signet Drive
Weston, Ontario M9L 1T9
Phone: 416-749-9300
Fax: 416-401-3835
877-4-APOTEX
General Inquiries: 800-268-4623
http://www.apotex.com/

Grasby pump (sometimes called GRASB)
MarCal Medical, Inc.
1114 Benfield Blvd., Suite H
Millersville, MD 21108
Phone: 800-628-9214
Fax: 410-987-4004
http://www.marcalmedical.com

Hemopurifier™
Aethlon Medical
7825 Fay Avenue, Suite 200
La Jolla, CA 92037
858-456-5777
http://www.aethlonmedical.com

hydroxyurea (Hydrea)
Bristol-Myers Squibb
345 Park Avenue
New York, NY 10154-0037
212-546-4000
http://www.bms.com
Oral Balance
Brotène
Laclede, Inc.
800-922-5856
http://www.laclede.com

Procrit®
Ortho Biotech Products, L.P.
700 U.S. Highway 202
PO Box 670
Raritan, NJ 08869-0670
1-800-325-7504 (prompt #2)
http://www.orthobiotech.com

Topicaine
ESBA Laboratories
800-677-9299
http://www.topicaine.com

For inquiries about clinical trials or updates on product development, visit
www.irondisorders.org
E-mail: info@irondisorders.org

SQUID Technology, Sickle Cell Anemia, or Thalassemia

Children's Hospital & Research Center at Oakland
747 52nd Street
Oakland, CA 94609
510-428-3000
Ellen B. Fung, Ph.D., R.D.
510-428-3885 x4939
efung@mail.cho.org
http://www.childrenshospitaloak
land.org/
or http://www.thalassemia.com

National Cooley's Anemia Foundation
129-09 26th Avenue
Flushing, NY 11354
800-522-7222
718-321-2873
http://www.thalassemia.org

Sickle Cell Information Center, Emory University
PO Box 109
Grady Memorial Hospital
80 Jessie Hill Jr Drive SE
Atlanta, GA 30303
E-mail: aplatt@emory.edu
Phone: 404-616-3572
Fax: 404-616-5998
http://www.scinfo.org

Stroke and Neurological Disorders

Alzheimer's Association
225 North Michigan Avenue
17th Floor
Chicago, IL 60601
800-272-3900
312-335-8700
http://www.alz.org

National Institute of Neurological Disorders and Stroke
Office of Science and Health Reports
PO Box 5801
Bethesda, MD 20824
800-352-9424
301-496-5751
http://www.ninds.nih.gov

Treatment

Visit our web site or call **Iron Disorders Institute** for blood centers with FDA variances to use hemochromatosis blood for transfusional purposes (see page 287).

National Institutes of Health
Warren G. Magnuson
Hemochromatosis Protocol
Bethesda, MD
301-402-3536
Contact: Glorice Mason

294

Glossary

ACD: *See* anemia of chronic disease

aceruloplasminemia: lack of ceruloplasmin, a copper-containing serum protein essential for normal function of transferrin iron transport

acidosis: excessive accumulation of compounds such as carbon dioxide that cause reduction of serum pH values to below 7.4

acquired immune deficiency syndrome (AIDS): caused by a retrovirus that is transmitted congenitally or by contact with infected body fluids; the virus attacks T-lymphocytes, thus markedly increasing risk for opportunistic infections and cancers

adrenals: a pair of endocrine glands that rest above kidneys; the outer layer (cortex) forms an array of steroid hormones; the middle layer (medulla) produces adrenaline (epinephrine)

AIDS: *See* acquired immune deficiency syndrome

alanine transaminase (ALT): liver enzyme (*see also* SGPT); increased serum level indicates liver cell injury

alkaline phosphatase (ALP): liver enzyme that can concentrate in liver and bone; increased serum levels may indicate cirrhosis, hepatoma, or biliary obstruction

alkalosis: elevation of serum pH value due to reduced level of carbon dioxide by prolonged vomiting, too rapid breathing, congestive heart failure

allele: one of the variant forms of a gene at a particular location on a chromosome

alpha-fetoprotein (AFP): oncofetal protein produced by fetal liver during first trimester; increased maternal serum level may indicate neural tube or abdominal wall defect in fetus; increased nonmaternal AFP may indicate hepatoma or other cancers or liver cell necrosis

alveoli: tiny air sacs in the lungs in which exchange of carbon dioxide and oxygen occur

Alzheimer's disease: presenile dementia associated with cortical cerebral sclerosis; a chronic, progressive disorder that accounts for over 50 percent of cases of dementia

amenorrhea: absence of menstruation

amino acids: small molecules that are building blocks of proteins; of twenty essential amino acids, ten must be acquired through diet

aminoglycosides: a class of antibacterial antibiotics that includes amikacin, gentamicin, kanamycin, neomycin, netilomycin, streptomycin, and tobramycin; can combine with iron to cause damage to kidneys and hearing

amosite: a form of asbestos with a high content of iron that is carcinogenic

amylase: an enzyme that digests starch

amyloidosis: disorder in which starch-like glycoproteins (amyloids) accumulate in tissues and impair function

ANA: *See* anti-nuclear antibody

anemia: reduction below normal in number of circulating red blood cells

anemia, aplastic: lack of red blood cell production due to bone marrow failure

anemia, Cooley's: (thalassemia) chronic, hemolytic anemia due to an inherited gene mutation influencing hemoglobin formation

anemia, iron-deficiency: caused by blood loss, lack of iron assimilation, or rapid growth when iron needs exceed intake and stores

anemia of chronic disease (ACD): mild anemia that accompanies the body's inflammatory defense mechanisms during episodes of infection, cancer, and other specific disorders

anemia, pernicious: caused by inadequate absorption of vitamin B_{12} due to the absence of intrinsic factor, a chemical secreted by mucous membranes of stomach

anemia, pyridoxine-responsive: corrected by treatment with pyridoxine (B_6)

anemia, sickle cell (sicklemia): chronic, hemolytic anemia due to an inherited gene mutation influencing hemoglobin formation; during crisis episodes, red blood cells with sickle shape are detected

anemia, sideroblastic: anemia in which iron is deposited prematurely in developing red blood cells which then are impaired in oxygen transport

angiography (arteriography): radiopaque contrast material is injected into the blood vessel during x-ray filming to detect blood flow abnormalities

angiotensin-converting enzyme (ACE) inhibitor: a drug employed to lower blood pressure

anisocytosis: presence of red blood cells with increased variability as measured by red cell distribution width (RDW)

anterior pituitary: the front lobe of the pituitary; its hormone producing cells are very sensitive to iron toxicity

antibody: specific protein(s) formed by B lymphocytes that can combine with and neutralize specific antigen(s)

antigen: a substance that stimulates the formation of a specific antibody and which will combine with that antibody

anti-nuclear antibody (ANA): detected in serum in patients who have systemic lupus erythematosis (SLE), a chronic autoimmune disease

antioxidant: a chemical that can neutralize or destroy oxygen radicals that have been formed by the catalytic action of iron

apheresis: a procedure for treatment of iron overload or sickle cell anemia; the blood is filtered to enable removal of red blood cells or other blood components

apoptosis: programmed cell death, the body's normal method of disposing of damaged, unwanted, or unneeded cells

arrhythmia: lack of normal heartbeat; may be due to iron loading of cardiac cells

arthralgia: pain in a joint

arthropathy: any joint disease

ascites: accumulation of fluid in the abdomen; may be a complication of cirrhosis, congestive heart failure, kidney malfunction, cancer, peritonitis, or various fungal and parasitic diseases

aspartate transaminase (AST): liver enzyme; increased serum level indicates liver cell injury

atherosclerosis: thickening, loss of elasticity, calcification of artery walls

atransferrinemia: congenital disorder in which little or no transferrin is produced

atrophy: loss of mass and function of a tissue or organ

autoimmune disease: a disorder in which the body's immune system attacks itself

autosomal dominant: inheritance in which a gene mutation on a non-sex chromosome carries the defect and is sufficient for expression

autosomal recessive: gene is located on a nonsex chromosome (autosome); inheritance in which two gene mutation copies, one from each parent, are required for expression of the disorder

basal ganglia: collection of nerve cell bodies

benign: noncancerous tumor or growth that does not interfere with normal function

bilirubin: red blood cell waste product in bile; elevated amount in serum and skin causes jaundice

biopsy: removal of a small amount of tissue or fluid, usually by needle, for laboratory examination as an aid in diagnosis

blood urea nitrogen (BUN): a serum test that measures urea nitrogen; used to determine liver and kidney function

bone marrow: soft tissue in sternum and long bones; red portion forms various types of blood cells

bone marrow aspiration: biopsy to determine such conditions as anemias, leukemias, iron deficiency, iron excess, tumors

bone marrow transplant: therapeutic use of bone marrow from healthy, antigen-matched donor in patients who have a variety of neoplastic or metabolic diseases

cachexia: weakness, loss of appetite, emaciation associated with serious infection or cancer

calcification: deposition of blood calcium into tissues in injury, infection or aging; can be part of healing but may lead to impaired organ function

calcium: mineral essential for heartbeat regulation, muscle contraction, nerve impulse transmission, formation of bones and teeth

Candida: a genus of yeast (fungi) that normally occurs in the mouth, intestine, and vagina; abnormal growth of Candida results in infection called candidiasis

carcinogen: a chemical or radioactive agent that induces normal cells to become malignant

cardiomyopathy: condition in which heart muscle cells are damaged

cardiotoxicity: damage to heart muscle cells as by certain anti-cancer drugs (e.g., adriamycin) that combine with iron; an iron-trapping agent (dexrazoxane) may be employed with the anti-cancer drug

case-control study: comparison of cases with healthy controls matched for such factors as age and gender

celiac disease: congenital (present at birth) disorder caused by an allergic intolerance to gluten, a protein constituent of most grains

cerebellum: the portion of the brain lying below the cerebrum and above the pons and medulla

cerebrospinal fluid (CSF): a clear, normally colorless, and blood-free fluid that cushions and nourishes the brain and spinal cord

ceruloplasmin (Cp): a copper-containing serum protein essential for the normal transport of iron by transferrin

chelator: a chemical that can tightly bind one or more transition series metals such as iron, manganese, zinc, or copper

cholelithiasis: gallstones

cholesterol: principal animal sterol; normally present in all body tissues, especially brain, spinal cord, and all animal fats

chondrosarcoma: a cancer arising in cartilage cells

chromosome: nuclear structure that contains the genes

chrysotile: form of asbestos that is comprised mainly of magnesium (rather than iron) silicate and which is much less carcinogenic than forms that contain high iron

cirrhosis: a chronic, progressive, inflammatory disease of liver; degeneration and death of parenchymal (functional) liver cells; distortion of normal architectural pattern of liver

colitis: inflammatory condition of large intestine

collagen: albuminoid substance of the white fibers of connective tissue, cartilage, and bone

colony-stimulating factors: cytokines (hormones) that stimulate the formation of various kinds of blood cells

colostrum: the first milk secreted after the birth of the child; has an unusually high content of lactoferrin, which is instrumental in suppressing potential pathogenic bacteria in the infant intestine

compound heterozygote: in hereditary hemochromatosis, a patient who has inherited a single CY mutation and a single HD mutation

congenital: existing at birth

connective tissue disease (collagen disease): various autoimmune conditions characterized by inflammatory changes in small blood vessels and connective tissue

coronary: encircling, for example, the blood vessels that supply the heart muscle; a "coronary" indicates blockage of blood supply to the heart

coronary thrombosis: blood clot obstructing flow in a coronary artery

cortisol: steroid hormone produced in cells of adrenal cortex

creatinine: waste product of protein metabolism; increased level in serum indicates kidney insufficiency

crocidolite: form of asbestos with very high content of iron silicate; thus, highly carcinogenic

Crohn's disease: chronic autoimmune inflammatory condition of various sites in gastrointestinal tract

cytokine: hormone-like peptides produced by various cells that act on other cells to stimulate or inhibit their function

cytopenia: a deficiency of cells in the blood

cytotoxic: destructive to cells

DCT1: divalent cation transporter #1; enables enterocytes to accumulate various essential metal ions from diet

Delaney amendment: passed by US Congress in the 1970s to prevent adulteration of US foods by carcinogens; unfortunately, iron (a well-known carcinogen) was exempted because its addition to foods in the United States had begun in earlier decades

Deferiprone: oral iron chelating drug used by thalassemic patients in India and Europe; not yet available in the United States

deoxyribonucleic acid (DNA): the chemical in the cell nucleus that carries the genetic instructions for producing new cells

Desferal: injectable iron chelating drug used by thalassemic patients worldwide

diabetes (mellitus): inability to metabolize glucose due to lack of insulin production (type 1) or lack of insulin efficacy or availability (type 2)

dialysis: filtration of waste products from body fluids of patients with kidney insufficiency

dilated cardiomyopathy: heart muscle disease causing enlargement of chambers and impairment of pumping efficiency

Down syndrome: congenital neurological disorder; iron loading and neuropathology similar to that of Alzheimer's disease

doxorubicin: an antibiotic used to treat several forms of cancer; an example is adriamycin

dyserythropoiesis: abnormal red blood cell synthesis; abnormal chromatin pattern, bizarre shapes, nuclear fragmentation

echocardiography: a test that bounces sound waves off the heart to produce pictures of its internal structures

electrocardiogram: measurement of electrical activity during heart-beats

electrophoresis: separation of molecules by size and electrical charge; by electric current the molecules can be forced through a gel with pores of a size that will separate specific molecules

endocarditis: serious bacterial infection of the membrane lining the heart and of the valves or heart muscle

endocrine glands: organs such as pituitary, pancreas, adrenals, thyroid, parathyroid that secrete hormones that regulate other body systems

endothelium: cells that form the inner lining of the heart, blood vessels, lymph channels, and various body cavities

enterocytes: cells in lining of small intestine that function in absorption of specific nutrients from diet

enzymes: proteins formed by living cells that catalyze specific chemical changes

enzymopathy: disease that results from inability by the patient's cells to form a specific enzyme

erythrocyte: red blood cell

erythropoietin (EPO): a hormone produced by the kidneys that stimulates the formation of red blood cells in the bone marrow

esophageal varices: enlarged veins in lining of esophagus subject to severe bleeding; often appear in patients who have liver disease

estrogen: female sex hormone produced by ovaries

erythrocyte sedimentation rate (ESR): test for evidence of inflammatory activity

ferritin: a large protein formed by nearly all living cells to store excess iron; synthesis is increased during infectious and neoplastic cell invasions as well as in response to iron loading

ferroportin: an iron export protein; a mutation in the ferroportin gene may lead to high macrophage iron and is associated with African siderosis

fibrosis: abnormal formation of connective or scar tissue

folic acid: part of the B-complex of vitamins; needed for normal synthesis and function of red and white blood cells

frataxin: a mitochondrial protein; deficiency results in mitochondrial iron accumulation, deficits in mitochondrial enzymes, and cell death

gamma globulin: fraction of serum proteins that contain anti-body molecules

gamma glutamyl transpeptidase (GGT): an enzyme predominantly in liver; increased levels in serum indicate liver disease such as hepatitis, cirrhosis

gastrointestinal tract: esophagus, stomach, liver, pancreas, gall bladder

gene amplification: an increase in the copies of any particular piece of DNA

gene expression: the process by which proteins are made from the instruction coded by DNA

genetic code: adenine (A), thymine (T), guanine (G), and cytosine (C) are the letters of the DNA code; each gene's code combines the four bases in various ways to spell 3-letter words that specify the sequence of amino acids that will comprise the proteins

genetic marker: a segment of DNA with an identifiable physical location on a chromosome and whose inheritance can be followed

genetic mutation: a substitution of one of the DNA bases to result in an altered amino acid insertion in the gene product

gene transfer: insertion of unre-lated DNA into the cells of an organism

germ line: inherited material that is passed on to the offspring

globulins: class of proteins soluble in dilute saline and differentiated from albumens by molecular size and charge

glucose-6-phosphate dehydroge-nase (G6PD): an enzyme; inability to form the enzyme is inherited; the deficiency can result in red blood cell hemolysis if sulfonamide or specific antimalarial drugs are used; repeated hemolysis can lead to iron loading

glycogen: carbohydrate polymer formed from glucose, stored mainly in liver

gonadotroph: gonad-stimulating hormone produced by anterior pituitary

granulocyte: circulating white blood cell; at site of invasion, cell releases its granules which contain anti-infective agents including lactoferrin, a powerful iron-binding protein

granuloma: a focalized nodule of inflammatory tissue at an invasion site

growth hormone (GH): a hormone produced by the anterior pituitary that stimulates cell growth

HA-A: *See* hepatitis-associated antigen

haptoglobin: a liver protein secreted into serum to combine with hemoglobin released from lysed red blood cells; persons who inherit inability to make efficient types of haptoglobin have elevated serum iron

HbA1c: a monitor of blood sugar variation over time; elevation indicates periods of blood sugar elevation

HBV: hepatitis B virus

HCV: hepatitis C virus

Helicobacter pylori: gram negative bacterium that grows in stomach mucosa and which derives nutritional iron from human lactoferrin; associated in some, but not all, persons with gastritis, ulcers, and stomach cancer

hematocrit: the percentage of the whole blood volume that is occupied by the formed elements (red cells, white cells, platelets)

hematuria: blood in urine

heme: the iron containing porphyrin within the hemoglobin molecule

hemochromatosis: genetic metabolic disorder, mainly in Caucasians, in which excessive absorption of iron may accumulate in liver, pancreas, heart, anterior pituitary, skin, joints, etc. to result in decay of functions of the involved organs

hemoglobin: the respiratory protein of erythrocytes using the porphyrin iron to take up oxygen or to release it

hemoglobin electrophoresis: a test that identifies abnormal forms of the protein as in hemoglobin C and H disease, sickle cell disease, and various forms of thalassemia

hemoglobinopathy: a disease in which abnormal hemoglobin molecules are formed

hemolysis: lysis (rupture) of cell membrane of red blood cells to release hemoglobin into the environment

hemolytic jaundice: severe hemolytic anemia that results in a high level of free bilirubin and which leads to a jaundiced appearance

hemorrhage: escape of blood from circulatory system

hemosiderin: insoluble complex of ferric hydroxide and protein debris derived from excessive ferritin in iron-loaded cells

hemosiderosis: excessive iron in tissues; associated with a great variety of inherited metabolic disorders or from environmental exposure to iron-containing substances

hepatitis A: viral infection of liver contracted by ingestion of contaminated food or water; a vaccine is available

hepatitis-associated antigen (HA-A): a protein used to detect hepatitis A

hepatitis B: viral infection of liver contracted by exposure to contaminated blood and other body fluids, contaminated needles, etc.; a vaccine is available

hepatitis C: viral infection of liver contracted by exposure to contaminated blood and other body fluids, contaminated needles, etc.; a vaccine is not yet available

hepatitis, chronic: inflammation of the liver persisting for more than six months; can be due to hepatitis B or C, alcohol, drugs, toxic chemicals, or autoimmune processes

hepatocellular injury: damage to liver cells

hepatoma: malignant tumor whose primary site is the liver

hepatotoxicity: destructive effect on the liver caused by alcohol or other chemicals

hepcidin: liver hormone that inhibits intestinal absorption of excessive iron and, during inflammatory episodes, suppresses macrophage release of iron

heterozygote: an individual who has two dissimilar mutations of a gene; a carrier of a gene mutation

HFE: protein that combines with transferrin receptor to suppress cellular uptake of excessive iron; specific mutations in the *HFE* gene can result in hemochromatosis

histology: the microscopic study of cells and tissues

HIV: human immunodeficiency virus; *see also* acquired immune deficiency syndrome

HLA: human leukocyte antigen; used in determining compatibility of tissue transplants for host recipients

homozygote: an individual who has two identical members of a mutated gene

hormone: chemical produced by cells in one tissue or gland that acts on cells in other tissues; *see also* cytokine

Huntington's disease: chronic, progressive hereditary chorea (irregular movements, speech disturbance, increasing dementia)

hypercalcemia: elevated level of serum calcium; often associated with cancers

hypersplenism: proliferation of splenic cells associated with hemolytic conditions

hypertrophic cardiomyopathy: thickening of heart muscle walls, interfering with normal heart function

hypochromic erythrocytes: subnormal content of hemoglobin in cells

hypoferremia: subnormal content of serum iron

hypothyroidism: underactive thyroid gland; may occur in hemochromatosis if anterior pituitary (which normally stimulates thyroid) is injured by iron

hypoxia: lowered availability of oxygen

hysterectomy: total or partial removal of uterus; may be followed by onset of iron loading

ichthyosis: dry harsh skin with adherent scales

idiopathic: condition for which no cause is yet known

immunoglobulins (IgA, IgG, IgM): antibodies

infarction: a portion of tissue that undergoes necrosis (cell death) due to loss of blood supply

infection: condition caused by invasion of bacterial, fungal, protozoan, or viral pathogens

inflammation: the reaction of tissues to injury

insulin: the anti-diabetic hormone produced by pancreatic beta cells

interferons: specific cytokines that participate in inflammatory defense

interstitial: occupies space between tissues

intravenous: into a vein

intrinsic factor: hormone produced in stomach mucosa essential for assimilation of vitamin B_{12} from diet

iron dextran: polysaccharide complex of iron employed for intramuscular or intravenous injection of the metal

iron doping: consumption or injection of excessive amounts of iron with the hope of improving athletic performance

iron panel: series of tests that measure levels of iron in serum and other tissues

iron overload: a potentially fatal condition in which iron accumulates in various tissues as in some hemolytic anemias, hemochromatosis, and excessive number of blood transfusions

ischemia: decreased blood supply to a body organ or part

jaundice: elevated bilirubin in blood due to liver disease, resulting in yellow whites of eyes and skin, dark urine

juvenile hemochromatosis: onset of iron loading prior to age thirty

ketoacidosis: a complication of inadequately treated diabetes mellitus; may also occur in starvation

knockout: inactivation of specific genes in yeast or mice to determine identity of specific function coded by the gene

koilonychia: atrophic deformity of the nails

Kupffer cells: fixed macrophages that line liver sinusoids

lactoferrin: a protein that strongly combines with iron in body fluids and tissues to deprive invading pathogens of the metal

lamina: a thin flat layer or membrane

Langerhans islets: collection of cells in the pancreas that produce insulin

LDL: *See* low density lipoprotein

Legionnaire's disease: a severe, often fatal, noncontagious pneumonia due to inhalation of the pathogen, often from water-borne aerosols

leukemia: white blood cell neoplasm resulting in high concentration of the malignant cells in the blood

leukocyte: circulating white blood cells (neutrophils or granulocytes, eosinophils, basophils)

lipase: fat splitting enzyme in blood and pancreatic secretion

liver function tests: serum assay of levels of such liver enzymes as ALT (SGPT), AST (SGOT), GGT, and ALP; elevation is modest in iron loading, much higher in viral hepatitis

locus: the place on a chromosome where a specific gene is located

lymph: fluid in lymphatic vessels

low density lipoprotein (LDL): combines with cholesterol in plaque formation

lymphocyte: circulating white blood cell required for antibody synthesis (B cell) or for inducing cell mediated immunity (T cell)

lymphoma: cancer of a lymphocyte node

lysozyme: enzyme in body fluids that digests bacterial cell walls

macrophage: large white blood cell in spleen, lymph nodes, and many tissue locations; scavenge debris, recycle aged erythrocyte membranes and hemoglobin, phagocytose and kill microbial invaders

malabsorption: inadequate assimilation of nutrients from the small intestine

malignant: dangerous to life; cancerous

melanoma: a cancer derived from cells that contain melanin pigment

Mendelian inheritance: manner in which genes are passed to offspring; examples include autosomal dominant, autosomal recessive, and sex-linked genes

metabolism: chemical processes that consist of building cell constituents (anabolism) and digesting cell constituents (catabolism)

metacarpals: bones of the hand to which finger bones are attached

metastasis: spread of cancer cells or infectious microbes from their original location to other tissues of the body

microcytosis: abnormally small erythrocytes

microbes: bacteria, fungi, protozoa; some are pathogenic

mitochondria: self-replicating portion of the cell; metabolic function provides energy to the host cell

monocyte: circulating macrophage

multiple myeloma: malignancy beginning in plasma cells of bone marrow

myocardial infarction (MI): heart attack

myoglobin: small globular protein with a heme porphyrin in muscle; stores oxygen needed for muscle function

NASH: *See* non-alcoholic steatohepatitis

neoplasia: a new and abnormal formation of tissue as a tumor

necrotizing enterocolitis: severe infectious bacterial invasion of intestinal lining in non–breast-fed infants who lack maternal lactoferrin

nephrotoxicity: damage to kidneys

neuropathy: damage to nerve tissue

neutropenia: white blood cell count below normal

neutrophil: *see* granulocyte

non-alcoholic steatohepatitis (NASH): fatty liver not caused by alcohol consumption; can be associated with C282Y mutation; patients have elevated serum ferritin, insulin resistance

oncogene: a gene that can cause transformation of normal cells into cancer cells

oncology: study of cancer

307

osteoarthritis: degenerate joint disease; can be an early sign of iron loading

osteoporosis: loss of bony substance, producing brittleness and bone softness; in some cases, associated with iron loading

pancreas: a large gland in upper portion of abdomen with an exocrine and endocrine function; in former, digestive enzymes are secreted into intestine; in latter, insulin is secreted into blood

parathyroid: four small endocrine glands in neck behind thyroid gland; hormone secreted controls calcium and phosphate metabolism

parenchyma: cells in an organ that are responsible for specific function(s) of the organ; for example, the hepatocytes in the liver

parenteral: subcutaneous, intramuscular, or intravenous injection of drugs or nutrients to bypass the intestinal route

Parkinson's disease: a neuropathy involving a rhythmic tremor and rigidity of muscle action; associated with accumulation of iron in substantia nigra portion of brain

pericardial: pertaining to membranes surrounding the heart

pernicious anemia: chronic anemia that occurs with Vitamin B$_{12}$ deficiency due to lack of intrinsic factor

phagocyte: *see* macrophage

petechiae: dot-size hemorrhages into the skin or mucous membranes

phenotype: an observed trait or characteristic; for example, the increased intestinal absorption of iron in hemochromatosis

phlebotomy: therapeutic withdrawal of blood

phytates: natural compounds in grains that suppress intestinal absorption of excessive nonheme iron

plasma: the liquid portion of the blood and lymph

platelets: small, colorless disks in blood that are essential for clotting

platonychia: thickened spots in center of fingernails

polycythemia: above-normal level of red blood cells

porphyria: pathologic levels of porphyrins in body fluids, feces, urine

porphyria cutanea tarda (PCT): photosensitivity, increased skin porphyrins; hepatic dysfunction; associated with iron loading and often with hepatitis C

porphyrins: small molecules that contain heme; present in hemoglobin, myoglobin, cytochromes

308

preeclampsia: toxic complication of pregnancy; increased blood pressure and serum iron; kidney damage; edema

prostate specific antigen (PSA): level may rise in some cases of prostate cancer

proteins: large molecules comprised of chains of amino acids; include enzymes, antibodies, and many structural components of cells and tissues

pruritus: itching

pulmonary edema: fluid accumulation in lungs

pyelonephritis: bacterial infection of one or both kidneys

pyridoxine: vitamin B_6

Q-T wave: an electrocardiogram measure; in iron-loaded heart (and also in congestive heart failure) the Q-T wave is lengthened

quantitative phlebotomy: calculation of total body iron by means of the number of pints of blood phlebotomized

recessive trait: for phenotypic expression, both parents had to have contributed the genetic mutation

red cell indices: tests for size, concentration of hemoglobin in red cells

Reed-Sternberg cell: indicates presence of Hodgkin's disease

renal: pertaining to kidney

restless legs syndrome: increased need to move extremities; decreased level of iron in substantia nigra; possible defect in transferrin receptor synthesis

reticulocytes: young, immature red blood cells

reticuloendothelial system (RES): monocyte/macrophage system; cells primarily involved in defense against microbial and neoplastic cell invaders and in disposal of breakdown products of aged body cells

retina: the light-receptive layer and terminal expansion of the optic nerve in the eye

retinopathy of prematurity: damage to retina in premature infants by exposure of child to excessive iron and oxygen

rheumatoid arthritis: chronic, autoimmune, inflammatory disease of joints; symptoms can be intensified by parenteral iron

sarcoidosis: chronic inflammatory disease of unknown origin that causes small lumps (nodules) in various tissues

septicemia: bacterial infection in which the pathogens have invaded and are multiplying in the blood serum: blood plasma minus fibrinogen

serum glutamic-oxaloacetic transaminase (SGOT): a test used in cases of suspected coronary occlusion or liver diseases such as hepatitis or cirrhosis

serum glutamic-pyruvate transaminase (SGPT): an enzyme released into the blood by injury or disease affecting the liver

sickle cell anemia: See anemia, sickle cell

sideroblastic anemia: See anemia, sideroblastic

sideroblasts: immature red blood cells that contain excess iron

siderosis: a general term for iron loading

Sjogren's syndrome: an autoimmune disorder characterized by dryness of the mouth and eyes and recurrent salivary gland enlargement

splenectomy: surgical removal of spleen

splenomegaly: enlarged spleen

substantia nigra: a broad, thick plate of large, pigmented nerve cells in the brain; iron loading is associated with development of Parkinson's disease; iron deficit with restless legs syndrome

sudden infant death syndrome (SIDS): unexpected death of normal child under six months of age; no known cause; condition is associated with postnatal iron loading

synovial membrane: thin lining membrane of a joint

systemic lupus erythematosis (SLE): a chronic autoimmune disease; in some cases, may be a long-term complication of measles

T cell: See lymphocyte

thalassemia (Cooley's anemia): inherited disorder in which abnormal hemoglobin is formed; required repeated blood transfusions result in iron loading with especial impairment of functions of pituitary, heart, and pancreas; prevalent in countries bordering the Mediterranean, in the Middle East, and in India and Southeast Asia

thyroid stimulating hormone (TSH): compound secreted by the anterior pituitary gland to control the release of thyroid hormone from the thyroid gland

total iron binding capacity (TIBC): measurement of the quantity of iron needed to saturate the binding activity of serum transferrin

toxemia of pregnancy: sequel to untreated preeclampsia

transaminases: enzymes that transfer an amino group from various amino acids to alpha-ketoglutaric acid to form glutamic acid

transferrin (siderophilin): protein that transports iron through serum, lymph and cerebrospinal fluid; functions also to remove free (nonprotein bound) iron from these fluids

tremolite: form of asbestos consisting entirely of iron silicate; highly carcinogenic, especially when used as a whitewash covering in homes

triglyceride: ester of glycerol in which the three hydroxyl groups are combined with a fatty acid

TSH: *See* thyroid stimulating hormone

unbound iron binding capacity (UIBC): the difference between the TIBC and the serum iron; high in iron-deficiency anemia and low in iron overload

urea: the end product of protein catabolism

vascular: pertaining to blood vessels

ventricular fibrillation: rapid, irregular quivering of heart's ventricles with no effective heartbeat; can be associated with iron loading of heart muscle

Vibrio vulnificus: a species of gram-negative bacteria in coastal seawater and in shellfish; requires highly saturated transferrin iron to grow in body; wounds in coastal waterways and ingestion of raw shellfish can be fatal to iron-loaded patients

villi: minute, elongated projections from membrane surfaces

Wilson's disease: inherited disorder of copper metabolism; accumulation of the metal in liver, erythrocytes, central nervous system; anemia, tremors, liver dysfunction, dementia

Yersinia: genus of gram-negative bacteria; some species grow in iron-loaded body fluids, others require iron-loaded macrophages

zinc: an essential metal required for protein synthesis, insulin stability, vision, reproductive functions, wound healing; iron supplements can interfere with normal acquisition of dietary zinc

Index

life expectancy and, 193, 218
liver biopsy and, 200
mice with, 56
misdiagnoses of, 9
mortality and, 25, 61, 265
MRI imaging in, 79
neonatal, 18, 53, 204, 211
online study course for, xvi, 288
organization, xv,
osteoporosis in, 120
patients with, 8, 9, 11, 54, 68, 124, 127, 222, 262,
patients, untreated, 70
PCT may accompany, 126
spleens in, 60
subgroup of, 17,
therapy for, 215–16, 218
types of, 29–30, 47
under-diagnosis of, 32
untreated, 143
viral hepatitis in, 58
hemodialysis, 14, 180, 234
hemoglobin synthesis, 14, 59, 92
hemoglobin values
  stillbirths and, 253
  low birthweight and, 252
  preterm birth and, 252
hemojuvelin gene, 19, 203
hemolysis, 5, 13, 17, 53, 60, 148, 211, 302–3
Hemopurifier, 234
hemosiderin, 47, 49, 53, 103, 110, 117, 124–25, 163, 214, 303
hemosiderosis, 18, 110–11, 303
heparin flush, 221
hepatic iron index, 36
hepatic stellate cells, 53, 58

hepatocytes, 12, 18, 35–36, 48, 53, 55–56, 163, 166, 308
hepatoma, 138, 295, 304
hepatomegaly, 19, 197, 201
hepcidin, 25, 36–37, 46–48, 55–56, 63–65, 166, 226, 232, 304
hephaestin, 45–46
heterozygote, 12, 18, 27–30, 35–36, 48, 56, 92, 299, 304
HFE, 7–8, 12–13, 16, 19, 26–32, 35–36, 45–46, 48, 53, 55–56, 59, 63–64, 92, 94, 112, 116, 125, 137, 203, 215, 304
  knockout mice, 56
high density lipoprotein (HDL), 95
hippocampus, 80
Hispanics, 171
histidine, 27
HLA, 25–26, 304
HLA-A, 26
HLA-B, 26
HLA-C, 26
HLA-D, 26
homologs, 27–28
homozygote, 7, 13, 16, 27–28, 29, 30–33, 35–36, 55, 63, 69, 92, 137, 201, 203, 304
hormones, 7, 9, 47, 67, 125, 295, 299, 301
human immunodeficiency virus (HIV), 146, 304
human leukocyte antigen, 25, 304
Hunt, Janet, 244
hydroxyurea, 232–33, 294
hyperchlolesteremia, 33
hyperferritinemia, 17, 63

reticuloendothelial system (RES), 13, 18, 55, 309
retinal degeneration, 16, 129
retinopathy, 178, 309
rheumatoid arthritis (RA), 109, 116–18
RHuEPO, 222
ringed sideroblasts, 15, 59
Rush, Benjamin, 262
salmonellosis, 145–46, 152, 155, 177, 258
sarcomas, 124, 139
Schade, Arthur, 161–62, 166
schizophrenia, 82
screening, 116, 204
Scripps Research, 31, 172
selenium, 218, 234
septicemias, 142, 144
serum ferritin
    acute-phase reactant, 210
    apheresis, 220
    chelation therapy, 227
    cirrhosis index, 201
    elevated, 16, 31–33, 35, 54, 59, 69, 71, 117, 193, 197, 200, 204, 215
    elevated, naturally, 211
    examined, 75
    fasting, not affected by, 196
    forced-sustained anemia and, 214
    haptoglobin, values and 148
    increased in, 12, 18, 69
    inflammatory response, elevated in, 97, 174, 216
    levels in patients, 32
    lowered, 58, 69, 166
    measuring, 193, 226
    meat-eaters, of, 69–70

phlebotomy, 216–17, 262
red cell indices, improved, 222
restless legs syndrome and, 213
rising rapidly, 14
routine metabolic panel, as part of, x
values, 55, 94
vegetarians, of, 69–70
women, in, 148
serum glutamic oxaloacetic transaminase, 198
serum insulin, 69
serum transaminases, 54, 58
SGOT, 198, 306, 310
Shakespeare, William, 161
sickle cell anemia, 5, 60, 203, 210, 223, 232–33, 292, 297, 310
sicklemia, 146, 264, 296
    mortality, 14
sideroblastic anemia (SA), 5, 14–15, 59, 203, 223, 296, 310
siderophilins, 163–64, 167
siderophore receptors, 142
silica, 103, 106
Simon, Marcel, 7
skin color changes, 11
skin hyperpigmentation, 123–24
skin pigmentation, 77, 192, 262
slit-lamp examination, 225
Smith, James, 218
smoking, 93, 106, 108–10, 117, 128–29, 146, 152, 156, 212, 263–64
smooth endoplasmic reticulum, 53
soy protein, 244